Equine Pathology and Laboratory Diagnostics

Editors

BRUCE K. WOBESER
COLLEEN DUNCAN

VETERINARY CLINICS OF NORTH AMERICA: EQUINE PRACTICE

www.vetequine.theclinics.com

Consulting Editor
THOMAS J. DIVERS

August 2015 • Volume 31 • Number 2

ELSEVIER

1600 John F. Kennedy Boulevard • Suite 1800 • Philadelphia, Pennsylvania, 19103-2899

http://www.vetequine.theclinics.com

VETERINARY CLINICS OF NORTH AMERICA: EQUINE PRACTICE Volume 31, Number 2
August 2015 ISSN 0749-0739, ISBN-13: 978-0-323-39362-1

Editor: Patrick Manley
Developmental Editor: Donald Mumford

Veterinary Clinics of North America: Equine Practice (ISSN 0749-0739) is published in April, August, and December by Elsevier Inc., 360 Park Avenue South, New York, NY 10010-1710. Business and Editorial Offices: 1600 John F. Kennedy Blvd., Suite 1800, Philadelphia, PA 19103-2899. Subscription prices are $270.00 per year (domestic individuals), $431.00 per year (domestic institutions), $130.00 per year (domestic students/residents), $315.00 per year (Canadian individuals), $543.00 per year (Canadian institutions), $365.00 per year (international individuals), $543.00 per year (international institutions), and $180.00 per year (international and Canadian students/residents). To receive student/resident rate, orders must be accompanied by name of affiliated institution, date of term, and the signature of program/residency coordinator on institution letterhead. Orders will be billed at individual rate until proof of status is received. Foreign air speed delivery is included in all *Clinics* subscription prices. All prices are subject to change without notice. **POSTMASTER:** Send address changes to *Veterinary Clinics of North America: Equine Practice*, 3251 Riverport Lane, Maryland Heights, MO 63043. Customer Service (orders, claims, online, change of address): Elsevier Health Sciences Division, Subscription **Customer Service, 3251 Riverport Lane, Maryland Heights, MO 63043. Tel: 1-800-654-2452 (U.S. and Canada); 314-447-8871 (outside U.S. and Canada). Fax: 314-447-8029. E-mail: journalscustomerservice-usa@elsevier.com (for print support);** E-mail: **journalsonlinesupport-usa@elsevier.com (for online support).**

Reprints. For copies of 100 or more of articles in this publication, please contact the Commercial Reprints Department, Elsevier Inc., 360 Park Avenue South, New York, NY 10010-1710. Tel.: 212-633-3874; Fax: 212-633-3820; E-mail: reprints@elsevier.com.

Veterinary Clinics of North America: Equine Practice is covered in *MEDLINE/PubMed (Index Medicus), Excerpta Medica, Current Contents/Agriculture, Biology and Environmental Sciences,* and ISI.

Contributors

CONSULTING EDITOR

THOMAS J. DIVERS, DVM
Diplomate, American College of Veterinary Internal Medicine; Diplomate, American College of Veterinary Emergency and Critical Care; Steffen Professor of Veterinary Medicine, Section Chief, Section of Large Animal Medicine, College of Veterinary Medicine, Cornell University, Ithaca, New York

EDITORS

BRUCE K. WOBESER, DVM, MVetSc, PhD
Diplomate, American College of Veterinary Pathologists; Assistant Professor of Anatomic Pathology; Department of Veterinary Pathology, Western College of Veterinary Medicine, University of Saskatchewan, Saskatoon, Saskatchewan, Canada

COLLEEN DUNCAN, DVM, MSc, PhD
Diplomate, American College of Veterinary Pathology; Diplomate, American College of Veterinary Preventative Medicine; Associate Professor, Departments of Microbiology, Immunology and Pathology, Veterinary Diagnostic Laboratory, College of Veterinary Medicine and Biomedical Sciences, Colorado State University, Fort Collins, Colorado

AUTHORS

AHMAD AL-DISSI, BVetSc, MSc, PhD
Diplomate, American College of Veterinary Pathologists; Department of Veterinary Pathology, Western College of Veterinary Medicine, University of Saskatchewan, Saskatoon, Saskatchewan, Canada

LUIS G. ARROYO, DVM, DVSc, PhD
Diplomate, American College of Veterinary Internal Medicine (Large Animal); Associate Professor, Department of Clinical Studies, Ontario Veterinary College, University of Guelph, Guelph, Ontario, Canada

CLAUDIO BARROS, DVM, PhD
Laboratory of Anatomic Pathology, College of Veterinary Medicine and Animal Husbandry, Federal University of Mato Grosso do Sul, Campo Grande, Mato Grosso do Sul, Brazil

BIANCA S. BAUER, DVM, MSc
Diplomate, American College of Veterinary Ophthalmologists; Associate Professor, Small Animal Clinical Sciences, Western College of Veterinary Medicine, University of Saskatchewan, Saskatoon, Saskatchewan, Canada

JAMES E. BRYANT, DVM
Diplomate, American College of Veterinary Surgeons; Pilchuck Veterinary Hospital and Equine Referral Center, Snohomish, Washington

SANTIAGO S. DIAB, DVM
Diplomate, American College of Veterinary Pathology; Assistant Professor of Clinical Pathology, California Animal Health and Food Safety Laboratory, School of Veterinary Medicine, University of California, Davis, Davis, California

COLLEEN DUNCAN, DVM, MSc, PhD
Diplomate, American College of Veterinary Pathology; Diplomate, American College of Veterinary Preventative Medicine; Associate Professor, Departments of Microbiology, Immunology and Pathology, Veterinary Diagnostic Laboratory, College of Veterinary Medicine and Biomedical Sciences, Colorado State University, Fort Collins, Colorado

CHAD FRANK, DVM, MSc
Diplomate, American College of Veterinary Pathology; Assistant Professor, Departments of Microbiology, Immunology and Pathology, Veterinary Diagnostic Laboratory, Colorado State University, Fort Collins, Colorado

JOANNE HEWSON, DVM, PhD
Diplomate, American College of Veterinary Internal Medicine (Large Animal); Associate Professor, Department of Clinical Studies, Ontario Veterinary College, University of Guelph, Guelph, Ontario, Canada

CHRISTOPHER E. KAWCAK, DVM, PhD
Diplomate, American College of Veterinary Surgeons; Diplomate, American College of Veterinary Sports Medicine and Rehabilitation; Professor, Equine Orthopaedic Research Center, College of Veterinary Medicine and Biomedical Sciences, Colorado State University, Fort Collins, Colorado

SALLY J. LESTER, DVM, MVSc
Diplomate, American College of Veterinary Pathology; Clinical and Anatomic, Pilchuck Veterinary Hospital and Equine Referral Center, Snohomish, Washington

DENNIS J. MADDEN, BS
Veterinary Diagnostic Laboratory, Colorado State University, Fort Collins, Colorado

SHANNON McLELAND, DVM
Diplomate, American College of Veterinary Pathologists; Postdoctoral Fellow, Departments of Microbiology, Immunology and Pathology, College of Veterinary Medicine and Biomedical Sciences, Colorado State University, Fort Collins, Colorado

WENDY H. MOLLAT, DVM
Diplomate, American College of Veterinary Internal Medicine; Pilchuck Veterinary Hospital and Equine Referral Center, Snohomish, Washington

FRANCES J. PEAT, BVSc, PGCertSc
Resident, Equine Sports Medicine, Equine Orthopaedic Research Center, College of Veterinary Medicine and Biomedical Sciences, Colorado State University, Fort Collins, Colorado

RAQUEL RECH, DVM, MSc, PhD
Diplomate, American College of Veterinary Pathologists; Department of Veterinary Pathobiology, College of Veterinary Medicine and Biomedical Sciences, Texas A&M University, College Station, Texas

TIMOTHY A. SNIDER, DVM, PhD
Diplomate, American College of Veterinary Pathologists; Department of Pathobiology, Oklahoma State University, Stillwater, Oklahoma

FRANCISCO A. UZAL, DVM, MSc, PhD
Diplomate, American College of Veterinary Pathology; Professor of Diagnostic Pathology, California Animal Health and Food Safety Laboratory, San Bernardino, California

BRUCE K. WOBESER, DVM, MVetSc, PhD
Diplomate, American College of Veterinary Pathologists; Assistant Professor of Anatomic Pathology; Department of Veterinary Pathology, Western College of Veterinary Medicine, University of Saskatchewan, Saskatoon, Saskatchewan, Canada

Contents

Evaluation of the upper and lower respiratory tract of horses requires strategic selection of possible diagnostic tests based on location of suspected pathologic lesions and purpose of testing and must also include consideration of patient status. This article discusses the various diagnostic modalities that may be applied to the respiratory system of horses under field conditions, indications for use, and aspects of sample collection, handling, and laboratory processing that can impact test results and ultimately a successful diagnosis in cases of respiratory disease.

The gastrointestinal system of horses is affected by a large variety of inflammatory infectious and noninfectious conditions. The most prevalent form of gastritis is associated with ulceration of the pars esophagea. Although the diagnostic techniques for alimentary diseases of horses have improved significantly over the past few years, difficulties still exist in establishing the causes of a significant number of enteric diseases in this species. This problem is compounded by several agents of enteric disease also being found in the intestine of clinically normal horses, which questions the validity of the mere detection of these agents in the intestine.

Skin disease in horses is a common and potentially challenging clinical problem. Information pertaining to skin disease is lacking in horses when compared with that in other companion animal species. Certainly, both horse-specific and location-specific patterns are present, but these can often be confounded by other factors. There are many possible ways in which to organize skin disease; in this article, they are organized based loosely on their most common clinical feature. Space limits the number of conditions that can be described here, and those chosen were seen relatively frequently in a multiinstitutional study of equine biopsies.

Uncommon diseases of the equine urinary system span a variety of etiologies and frequently have nonspecific clinical presentations. Because of the infrequency of equine urinary disease and inconsistencies in clinical symptoms, diagnosis and subsequent treatment of urinary disease in this species may be challenging. This article reviews various diseases of the equine urinary system, morphologies, and potential discriminating clinical and clinicopathologic presentations to aid the clinician in determining a definitive diagnosis in practice.

Timothy A. Snider

Reproductive disease is relatively common in the horse, resulting in a variable, yet significant, economic impact on individual horsemen as well as the entire industry. Diverse expertise from the veterinary community ensures and improves individual and population health of the horse. From a pathology and diagnostics perspective, this review provides a comprehensive overview of pathology of the male and female equine reproductive tract. Recognition by clinical and gross features is emphasized, although some essential histologic parameters are included, as appropriate. Where relevant, discussion of ancillary diagnostic tests and approaches are included for some diseases and lesions.

Frances J. Peat and Christopher E. Kawcak

The current understanding of pathology as it relates to common diseases of the equine musculoskeletal system is reviewed. Conditions are organized under the fundamental categories of developmental, exercise-induced, infectious, and miscellaneous pathology. The overview of developmental pathology incorporates the new classification system of juvenile osteochondral conditions. Discussion of exercise-induced pathology emphasizes increased understanding of the contribution of cumulative microdamage caused by repetitive cyclic loading. Miscellaneous musculoskeletal pathology focuses on laminitis, which current knowledge indicates should be regarded as a clinical syndrome with a variety of possible distinct mechanisms of structural failure that are outlined in this overview.

Bianca S. Bauer

Although not comprehensive of all ocular conditions in the equine species, this article concentrates on various ophthalmic conditions observed in the horse where laboratory diagnostics are recommended. The importance of laboratory diagnostic testing cannot be underestimated with equine ophthalmic disease. In many cases, laboratory diagnostics can aid in obtaining an early diagnosis and determining appropriate therapy, which in turn, can provide a better prognosis. In unfortunate cases where ocular disease results in a blind, painful eye necessitating enucleation, light microscopic evaluation is *imperative* to determine or confirm the cause of the blindness and provide a prognosis for the contralateral eye.

VETERINARY CLINICS OF
NORTH AMERICA: EQUINE PRACTICE

THE CLINICS ARE NOW AVAILABLE ONLINE!
Access your subscription at:
www.theclinics.com

Preface

Equine Pathology and Diagnostics for the Practicing Veterinarian

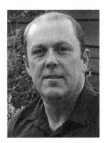 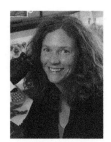

Bruce K. Wobeser, DVM, MVetSc, PhD, DACVP

Colleen Duncan, DVM, MSc, PhD, DACVP, DACVPM

Editors

This is the first issue of *Veterinary Clinics of North America: Equine Practice* that has been entirely devoted to pathology and diagnostics. The need for such an issue highlights both the continuous stream of new information in the field of diagnostics and the emergence and evolution of equine diseases that can provide a diagnostic challenge for veterinarians. While some equine pathology subjects have been covered in individual issues, a single issue devoted to the broad category of diagnostic pathology will hopefully be a useful single resource for practitioners.

This issue begins with articles describing a generalized approach to both the necropsy of the horse and clinical pathology and a broad review of equine toxicology. A wide variety of diseases can affect horses; there is no single approach that will work in all cases, but this generalized approach is suitable for the vast majority of cases and provides a template for use in specialized cases. Following these introductory articles, the majority of this issue was created by experts in various specific organ systems from across North America who selected those diseases that they believe are the most important for equine practitioners in North America. These include both classic diseases and those just newly emerging. In addition to these, there is advice for the selection and treatment of samples for the diagnosis of disease for which the cause is unknown to the practitioner.

As editors, we would sincerely like to thank all of the contributors for their efforts in producing this issue. It was a great pleasure to work with such a wide group of experts,

Vet Clin Equine 31 (2015) xi–xii
http://dx.doi.org/10.1016/j.cveq.2015.05.001
0749-0739/15/$ – see front matter © 2015 Elsevier Inc. All rights reserved.

who were so giving of their time and knowledge to produce an issue that it is hoped will be useful to all equine practitioners.

Bruce K. Wobeser, DVM, MVetSc, PhD, DACVP
Department of Veterinary Pathology
Western College of Veterinary Medicine
University of Saskatchewan
52 Campus Drive
Saskatoon, Saskatchewan S7N 5B4, Canada

Colleen Duncan, DVM, MSc, PhD, DACVP, DACVPM
Department of Microbiology, Immunology
and Pathology
College of Veterinary Medicine and Biomedical Sciences
Colorado State University
300 West Drake Avenue
Fort Collins, CO 80524, USA

E-mail addresses:
Bruce.wobeser@usask.ca (B.K. Wobeser)
Colleen.duncan@colostate.edu (C. Duncan)

Field Necropsy of the Horse

Chad Frank, DVM, MSc*, Dennis J. Madden, BS,
Colleen Duncan, DVM, MSc, PhD

KEYWORDS

- Equine • Necropsy • Postmortem examination • Mortality • Investigation

KEY POINTS

- Prior to initiating a necropsy, consideration should be given to equipment, location, sampling, disposal and clean up.
- Use of a standardized approach will enable the practitioner to be better prepared to identify true pathologic lesions versus changes of minimal significance.
- On completion of the necropsy, observations should be recorded and assessed in the context of any clinical questions.
- If necessary, formalin-fixed and/or fresh tissues may be submitted to a diagnostic laboratory for further evaluation.
- In addition to the biologic samples, the laboratory-specific submission form should be completed including a brief history and necropsy findings along with specific diagnostic test requests or questions.

INTRODUCTION

This article provides an overview of the equine necropsy that can be used by veterinarians in the field. Use of a systematic process enables the practitioner to develop a familiarity with normal anatomic positioning and tissue appearance such that abnormalities are quickly identified. Although an exhaustive review of equine pathology is beyond the scope of this article, there are several excellent resources on equine pathology[1,2] that may be used to aid in the interpretation of changes identified. Additionally, several articles elsewhere in this issue focus on disease processes in specific body systems.

Field Versus Laboratory Examination

Logistical factors often influence the decision to perform the postmortem examination in the field or have the carcass transported to a diagnostic laboratory with necropsy

Veterinary Diagnostic Laboratory, Colorado State University, 300 West Drake Avenue, Fort Collins, CO 80524, USA
* Corresponding author.
E-mail address: chad.frank@colostate.edu

facilities. For animals dying on farm, transport requires not only a trailer of appropriate size, but also the ability to winch the carcass onto the trailer. Given that many horses are housed on small acreages such equipment may not be readily available on farm; however, commercial services are often available to facilitate postmortem animal transport. It is helpful for veterinary clinics to have this information readily available to inform clients of disposal options regardless of whether or not necropsy is desired. In the case of elective euthanasia, where the animal can be safely and humanely transported, it may be possible to euthanize the animal at the laboratory or have a staff veterinarian perform the euthanasia at the laboratory. Because the policy regarding euthanasia at laboratories varies significantly between facilities it is important to contact the laboratory to ascertain that this is an option before transporting the horse. There are often additional costs incurred by having the work done at a laboratory that preclude a client from selecting that option.

There are some benefits to having the examination be conducted in a laboratory situation. Many horses are insured for mortality and the insurance company may require a complete postmortem examination be conducted. Requirements for the level of detail (ie, gross or histologic examination) vary widely by company and policy type; in the case of highly valued horses it may be necessary that examination be done by a certified veterinary pathologist. The responsibility of communicating with the insurance company, and therefore the decision, is ultimately borne by the owner; however, the benefits and weaknesses of a field or laboratory postmortem examination may not be completely understood by the client and it is therefore important for the veterinarian to understand the expectations of the owner and insurance agency before making a decision. Similarly, in cases where foul play or other illegal actions may have been involved, it is beneficial to have the necropsy performed by specialists who are familiar with such case investigations. Finally, in cases where it is challenging to dispose of an equine carcass safely on site or in the local area, transport of the animal to the laboratory may be necessary.

Safety Considerations

Before conducting a necropsy, consideration must be given to safety of all parties involved. Although it is possible for a single veterinarian to perform a complete postmortem examination, the assistance of another person minimizes physical exertion and the duration of the procedure. It is advisable, however, to keep the number of people actually assisting in the procedure to a minimum to prevent accidents or lesions being missed by the veterinarian. Proper equipment is required for safety because dull knives are more likely to slip and cause accidental harm. Although zoonotic diseases are relatively uncommon in horses in North America, before initiating a postmortem examination consideration must be given to any potential public health risks associated with the necropsy.

It is important to pick a site for the necropsy that is practical and minimizes any biosecurity risks associated with the procedure. In general, it is easiest to perform the necropsy in a location that can be easily accessed by the equipment needed to collect or dispose of the remains and where access to scavengers can be restricted. A surface that can be cleaned and disinfected, such as a concrete pad, is preferable to grass or dirt.

Equipment

Having the appropriate equipment prepared and readily accessible makes it physically and logistically easier to perform necropsies in the field. Basic necropsy equipment is listed in **Box 1** and is outlined with ordering information by Mason and Madden.[3]

Box 1
Minimal equipment for equine field necropsy kit

- Sharp knife
- Sharpening steel
- Rib cutters (garden shears)
- Formalin
- Whirl-paks or other sterile containers
- Scissors
- Forceps
- Rubber gloves
- Cold sterile kit
- Cleaver or saw for brain removal

A digital camera is extremely helpful for documenting lesions to include in a final report and also to solicit feedback from other veterinarians or diagnosticians.

Disposal of Carcasses

Determining the method of disposal before initiating the necropsy is important because it may influence protocols, such as handling of viscera. Timely and appropriate removal of a carcass is also important for biosecurity and environmental protection. In many locations there are commercial services available that pick up and dispose of the carcass, other times they transport it to a location for disposal identified by the client. Some transport companies are unwilling to transport an animal after necropsy, or may require the carcass be sewn up before transport. In the case of the latter, it is usually impossible to include all of the abdominal viscera with the carcass so this must be collected, and sometimes disposed of, separately. In other cases, transport companies may be willing to transport a carcass that has been opened, but nothing removed. In these cases it may be possible to perform a quick and targeted postmortem examination without removal of the viscera.

In general, burial is the most common method of carcass disposal. Specific requirements for burial are variable, but in general include regulations regarding the distance away from any well or open water, depth of burial as it relates to both groundwater and surface, and location of the burial ground in the context of water runoff and erosion. Because chemical euthanasia can result in secondary toxicity to scavengers with access to the carcass, arranging for complete burial immediately after performing the necropsy is important. Some landfills allow disposal of dead animals, but others do not. Even those accepting carcasses may have specific transport requirements, such as covered cargo rules. Animal composting is available in some areas, but these typically do not accept carcasses from animals chemically euthanized.

NECROPSY PROCEDURE

One of the most important procedural considerations of any species necropsy is that the procedure be performed systematically in the same manner each time. Routine positioning and protocol enable the prosector to rapidly identify abnormalities necessitating more detailed or modified prosection techniques. The protocol presented here (**Box 2**) is based on the authors' experiences with some modifications for a field

---

Box 2
Stepwise approach to the equine field necropsy

1. Incise skin along midline
2. Reflect limbs dorsally
3. Open abdominal cavity
4. Open thoracic cavity
5. All system examination ± sample collection
6. Examine thoracic viscera
7. Examine gastrointestinal tract
8. Examine other abdominal viscera
9. Remove brain
10. Other systems as necessary

---

situation. In some cases where only a specific organ system is of interest, it may be decided to not conduct a complete examination; regardless, it is important that the approach to the system in question be consistent.

Sample collection is performed throughout the necropsy procedure. In general, it is best to collect a full set of tissues on all animals such that diagnostics can be optimized. A section of all organs should be collected for histopathology (**Box 3**). These sections should be a maximum of 1 cm thick and should be representative of any changes seen on necropsy. Where the tissue is variable in appearance, multiple representative sections should be included. Tissue should be fixed in 10% neutral buffered formalin with a tissue to formalin ratio of 1:10. Additional samples for microbiology, toxicology, or other tests should be collected in sterile containers or whirl-paks and kept refrigerated (**Box 4**).

Box 3
Routine formalin-fixed tissues for collection:

- Lung
- Heart (left ventricular papillary muscle, interventricular septum, right ventricular free wall)
- Liver
- Spleen
- Kidney
- Thyroid gland
- Adrenal gland
- Pancreas
- Stomach
- Small intestine (multiple)
- Large intestine (multiple)
- Brain (whole)

> **Box 4**
> **Additional samples for consideration**
>
> - Microbiology
>   - Affected organ or tissue in question
>   - Lung/liver/kidney for systemic disease
> - Toxicology: liver, kidney, stomach contents, fat
> - Parasitology: feces
> - Specialty diagnostics (discussed elsewhere in this issue)

Positioning and Opening of the Carcass

The horse should be positioned in right lateral recumbency. Puncture the skin in the left axilla and extend the incision cranially toward the ramus of the mandible with the knife blade parallel to the body, cutting from the subcutaneous tissue outward. Similarly, extend the incision caudally to the perineum, taking care to not puncture a taut abdomen. In male horses, deviate the incision from midline to above (left of) the penis and prepuce. Abduct the left fore and hind limbs by incising the soft tissue beneath the scapula and disarticulating the coxofemoral joint (**Fig. 1**A).

To open the abdominal cavity, incise the musculature along the caudal border of the rib cage with the knife blade parallel to the body to minimize inadvertent puncture of the intestinal tract. After an opening is made in the abdominal cavity, insert your hand and the handle of the knife into the abdomen with the back of the blade resting

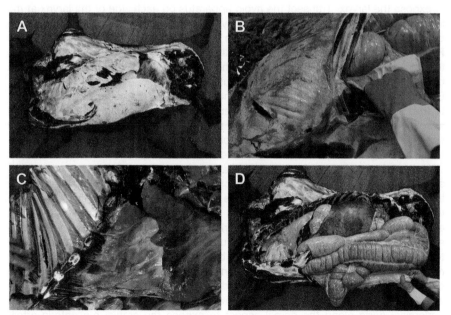

Fig. 1. (*A*) Equine in right lateral recumbency with limbs and skin reflected. (*B*) Opening the abdominal cavity is best achieved by cutting the body wall from the inside outward to avoid puncturing the intestinal tract. (*C*) The ribs can be reflected ventrally by scoring them at the costochondral junction. (*D*) Equine in right lateral recumbency with both thorax and abdomen open and ready for examination.

between your thumb and forefinger (see **Fig. 1**B). Extend the cut along the caudal border of the ribs, and then along the dorsal body wall, adjacent to the transverse processes of the lumbar vertebrae, to the pelvis and finally down to ventral midline, reflecting the body wall ventrally. Leave the abdominal wall flap attached, because it may be needed to close the abdomen following completion of the necropsy.

To open the thoracic cavity, the diaphragm must first be punctured to check for negative pressure, and cut away from the ribs. Cut each rib just below the angle of the rib and reflect them ventrally. After a few ribs are cut, make a handhold by incising the intercostal muscles near the center of the rib cage. This allows an assistant to apply ventral tension on the rib cage to help with removal. The rib cage can be completely reflected by scoring the costochondral junction with the ribs under tension (see **Fig. 1**C). Alternatively, the ventral aspect of all ribs can be completely transected with the rib cutters. If warranted, bone marrow may be collected from the rib at this time.

When the abdominal and thoracic cavities are opened, and before removal of any viscera, it is appropriate to do a complete assessment of the carcass and, if indicated, collect tissues for ancillary laboratory tests before contamination (see **Fig. 1**D). Equine colic is commonly associated with intestinal displacements or torsions that are readily identified in situ; common locations for displacements and entrapments are presented in **Fig. 2**.

Thoracic viscera can be removed en bloc with the trachea, esophagus, larynx, and tongue (the pluck) or left within the thoracic cavity, depending on the desired method of disposal (**Fig. 3**A). Remove the tongue ventrally between the mandibles after incising the soft tissues along the medial aspect of the bone to the mandibular symphysis. Keep tension on the tongue and incise the soft palate and connective tissue to expose the larynx. Transect the hyoid apparatus on each side of the larynx at the joint between the stylohyoid and keratohyoid bones; this joint is easily identifiable by palpating the larynx for the less than 90° angle between the two bones (see **Fig. 3**B). Continue to cut the dorsal soft tissue, extracting the larynx and reflecting the trachea and esophagus through the thoracic inlet. The guttural pouches should be examined after reflecting the larynx, pharynx, and tongue caudally (see **Fig. 3**C). Extend the cut through the mediastinum and along the ventral aspect of the vertebrae to the diaphragm. To remove the pluck en bloc, the aorta, cranial vena cava, and esophagus are transected at the level of the diaphragm; then, free the pericardial sac from the sternum and the pluck can be removed from the body cavity. Alternatively, the lungs and heart can be left in the thoracic cavity for examination.

Abdominal viscera are best removed in a stepwise process and examined systematically as described later (**Fig. 4**A). The spleen should be reflected cranial by cutting the suspensory ligament. Avoid cutting the splenic artery and vein in the hilus. Incise the dorsal perirenal fat and bluntly dissect the left kidney ventrally to expose the left adrenal. Pull the left kidney toward the urinary bladder while cutting the renal vein and artery from the anterior extremity. The ureter should remain intact from the kidney to the bladder. The small colon is removed by transecting it at the aboral and oral end, respectively. Tying off the transverse colon and aboral duodenum at the level of the duodenal-colic ligament is recommended (see **Fig. 4**B). Trim the small intestine away from the mesentery all the way down to the ileum (see **Fig. 4**C). Open the abdominal aorta along the dorsal aspect to expose the cranial mesenteric artery and examine for evidence of *Stronglus vulgaris* larval migration (see **Fig. 4**D). The large colon, cecum, and pancreas can be removed en bloc by cutting across the cranial mesenteric artery just below the aorta. The right adrenal and kidney can now be examined in a similar fashion as the left side. Open the stomach along the greater curvature.

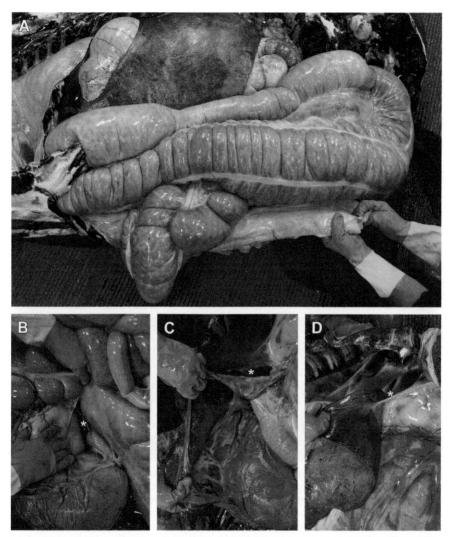

Fig. 2. (A) Equine in right lateral recumbency with the abdominal wall reflected ventrally. On opening the abdominal cavity the apex of the cecum, left ventral colon, pelvic flexure, left dorsal colon, spleen, and body of the stomach are visualized. Note the prominent bands and sacculations of the left ventral colon. (B–D) Anatomic locations of sites of intestinal entrapment include (B) epiploic foramen (*asterisk*), (C) gastrosplenic ligament (*asterisk*), and (D) nephrosplenic ligament (*asterisk*).

SYSTEM-SPECIFIC EXAMINATION
The Pluck (Cardiopulmonary and Thyroids)

The thyroid glands should be examined and sampled for histopathology if abnormal. Incise the dorsal aspect of the larynx and open the trachea to the level of the tracheal bifurcation and the proximal aspect of the mainstem bronchi and examine. To examine the lungs in situ, grasp the caudodorsal aspect of the left caudal lung lobe and reflect it cranially to the thoracic inlet by cutting mediastinal tissues and transecting the left main stem bronchus. Open and examine the pulmonary artery and vein (see

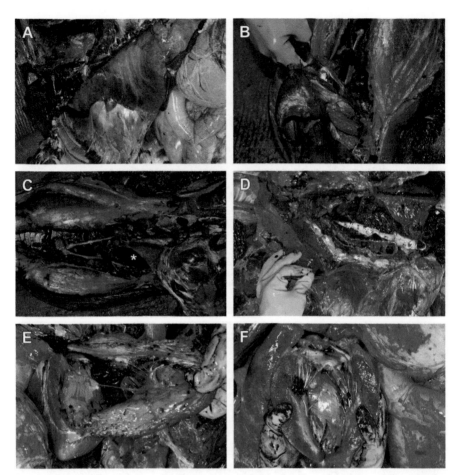

Fig. 3. (*A*) Overview of the equine thoracic cavity with the ribs reflected ventrally. (*B*) After the tongue is reflected caudally and the soft palate transected, the hyoid apparatus is identified by palpating the 90° angle between the stylohyoid and keratohyoid bones. Transect the hyoid bones at the site of articulation. (*C*) Caudoventral reflection of the tongue, larynx, and pharynx allows visualization of the guttural pouches (*asterisk*). (*D*) Examination of the mainstem bronchus and pulmonary artery and vein. Note the smooth intimal surface of the vein and artery, which are located dorsally and ventrally to the bronchus, respectively. (*E*) Opening the right atrium and ventricle. The cut should follow the normal blood flow through the right atrium into the right ventricle along the interventricular septum and out the pulmonary outflow tract. (*F*) Opening the left atrium and ventricle. After an opening is made in the left atrium, the remainder of the left atrium and left ventricle are opened by making a single cut through the left ventricular free wall. The aortic outflow tract is located beneath the mitral valve leaflet.

Fig. 3D). After examining the vessels, the bronchi should be opened and examined. The right lung lobes can be exposed and examined by reflecting the tongue, trachea, and esophagus caudally. The lungs should be serial sectioned, approximately 1 inch thick (breadloafed), and palpated throughout with sections collected from multiple locations (cranial and caudal) for histopathology.

After opening and examining the pericardial sac, the heart can be removed from or remain attached to the pulmonary system for examination. Open the heart by following

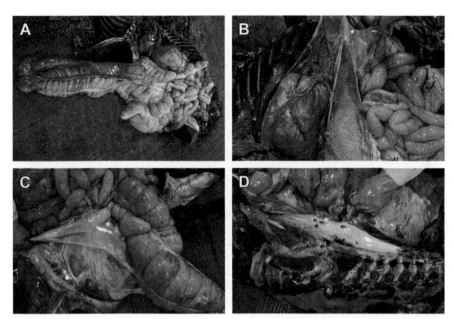

Fig. 4. (*A*) Overview of the equine gastrointestinal tract. The large colon and cecum have been reflected ventrally to allow visualization of the entire gastrointestinal tract. (*B*) The small intestine is extracted from the abdominal cavity by transecting the duodenum adjacent to the duodenal-colic ligament (*asterisk*), cutting along the mesenteric attachments, and then transecting the ileum adjacent to the ileocecal ligament. The right dorsal colon has been opened to examine for evidence of nonsteroidal anti-inflammatory drug–induced right dorsal colitis. (*C*) Identification of the ileocecal ligament (*asterisk*). (*D*) Examination of the cranial mesenteric artery for evidence of *Strongylus vulgaris* larval migration. The cranial mesenteric and renal arteries form a triangular structure with the cranial mesenteric artery located most rostrally (*asterisk*). Open the cranial mesenteric artery with scissors and examine for evidence of thrombosis or intimal roughening.

the blood flow from the right atrium along the interventricular septum to the pulmonary outflow tract (see **Fig. 3**E). Open the left side of the heart by making an opening in the left atrium and then the left ventricle with a single incision through the left ventricular free wall (see **Fig. 3**F). Open the aortic outflow track by incising through the left AV valve and extending the incision along the aorta. Each of the heart valves, the cardiac musculature, and the intimal surface of the great vessels should be examined systematically. The relative thicknesses of the ventricular walls should be compared and at least one full-thickness (left papillary muscle) section of tissue should be collected for histopathology.

Gastrointestinal

The gastrointestinal system should undergo a cursory, survey examination after opening the abdominal and thoracic cavities. After the thoracic viscera has been removed, and before removal of the gastrointestinal tract, a more detailed examination of the placement of the intestine may be conducted. It is not uncommon for the equine intestine to shift post mortem when the carcass is manipulated before necropsy. As such, any displaced viscera must be examined for corroborative evidence that the change occurred antemortem (ie, vascular compromise).

Each component of the gastrointestinal tract should be examined systematically. Representative sections, if not the entirety, of the small and large intestine should be opened and examined with appropriate histologic and microbiologic samples collected. Because the mucosal surface is easily damaged and undergoes rapid autolysis, care must be taken to minimally handle samples. Special attention should be paid to areas prone to particular lesions (ie, nonsteroidal anti-inflammatory drug–associated ulcers of the right dorsal colon). Where intestinal microbiology is warranted, an entire loop of intestine and contents can be collected and tied off at each end for submission to the diagnostic laboratory. If intestinal disease appears restricted to the aboral intestine fecal samples may suffice.

Urogenital

Kidneys and adjacent adrenal glands (**Fig. 5**A) should be sectioned longitudinally on midline, facilitating the examination of the renal cortex, medulla, and pelvis (see **Fig. 5**B). Close examination of the pelvis should be conducted on horses receiving nonsteroidal anti-inflammatory drugs. Histologic sections should include cortex and medulla including the papillary crest. The bladder should be incised and the mucosal surface examined and tissues collected for histopathology if necessary. The reproductive system should be examined grossly, and if there is a history of reproductive failure, collection of all segments of the reproductive tract may be warranted.

Hepatic

The liver should be serially sectioned (see **Fig. 5**C) then palpated and examined for uniform appearance and consistency (see **Fig. 5**D). If ancillary testing is desired, sterile samples of liver should be collected, because this is an ideal organ for toxicologic testing and cultures when systemic infection is suspected.

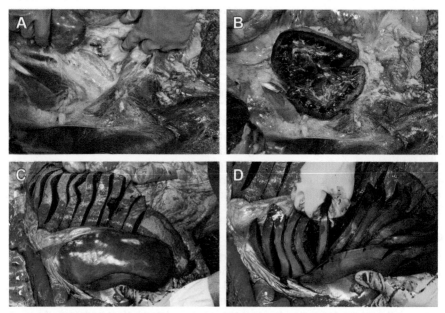

Fig. 5. (*A*) The left adrenal gland is located adjacent to the left kidney. (*B*) Kidney transected for examination. (*C*) Spleen "breadloafed" for examination, liver adjacent. (*D*) Liver "breadloafed" for examination and palpated for consistency.

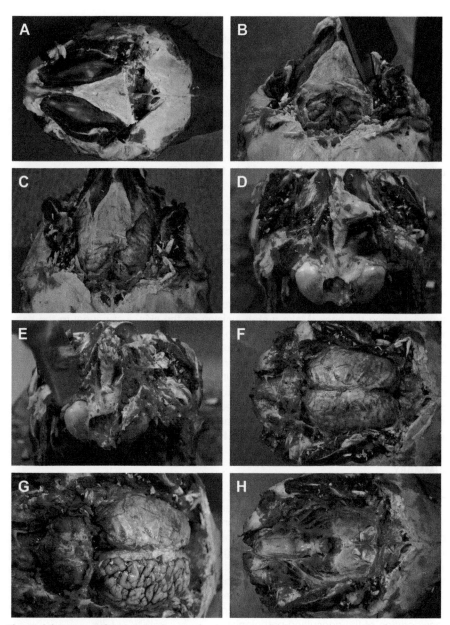

Fig. 6. (*A*) Remove the temporalis muscles to expose the bone and open the frontal sinus. (*B*) Open the cranial vault behind the frontal sinus and continue caudally by striking downward (*tangentially*) and chiseling away bone. (*C*) This technique exposes the brain without damage. (*D*) Remove the nuchal crest. (*E*) Continue cutting tangentially toward the foramen magnum. (*F*) Remove the calvarium to expose the brain. (*G*) Cut away the dura matter to free the brain. (*H*) The pituitary gland must be collected after the brain has been removed.

Musculoskeletal System

Complete examination of the equine musculoskeletal system can be challenging to do in the field and is therefore not commonly performed. However, when medical history includes lameness in a particular location, it may be desirable to perform a focused dissection in that location to confirm the clinical diagnosis. Where bone lesions in that location are expected or have been identified radiographically, it may be indicated to isolate the effected bone and section it using a hand or power saw. In foals or other animals where sepsis is suspected, gross examination of multiple joints may aid in the confirmation of this diagnosis. While the horse is in right lateral recumbence, opening the stifle by incising along the lateral aspect of the joint and reflecting the patella medially facilitates examination of the joint fluid for fibrin. The joint fluid should be viscous and clear to light yellow in color.

Brain Removal

Examination of the brain is critical in cases of unexpected death or neurologic disease. If the latter is suspected it may be most appropriate to ship the entire skull intact to a diagnostic laboratory that can extract the brain using appropriate biosecurity that minimizes exposure to rabies or other zoonotic diseases. In cases where zoonotic diseases are unlikely, the brain can be removed in the field using either a handsaw or a cleaver. To remove the head from the carcass, the head should be pulled dorsally, hyperextending the neck. Make a stab incision on the skin, just caudal to the base of the ears, and extend the incision through the skin along the ramus of the mandible. Transect the cervical hypaxial muscles to expose the atlanto-occipital joint. Incise the ventral atlanto-occipital membrane and dura mater to expose the spinal cord. At this point a needle and syringe is used for collection of cerebral spinal fluid, if desired. Insert the tip of the blade into the atlanto-occipital joint to transect the spinal cord, joint capsule, and lateral atlanto-occipital ligaments. Reflect the head dorsally and transect the nuchal ligament, muscles, and dorsal skin to remove the head. A stepwise approach to brain removal is presented in **Fig. 6**.

SUMMARY

On completion of the necropsy, observations should be recorded and assessed in the context of any clinical questions. If necessary, formalin-fixed and/or fresh tissues may be submitted to a diagnostic laboratory for further evaluation. In addition to the biologic samples, the laboratory-specific submission form should be completed including a brief history and necropsy findings along with specific diagnostic test requests or questions. Because only small sections of tissue are provided to the laboratory, accurate and complete descriptions of all changes identified at necropsy are important. Descriptive features of lesions to be included are summarized in **Box 5**. Digital photographs may also be emailed (or photographs sent) to the diagnostic laboratory for consideration of the consulting pathologist.

Box 5
Lesion description should include the following information

- Tissue and specific location within tissue
- Shape, color, consistency, size of lesions
- Percent of involved tissue/organ

Fresh tissues should be chilled and sent with coolant packs as soon as possible. Shipping of formalin-fixed tissues requires a sealable container with additional plastic to prevent leakage during transport. Because proper fixation of tissues requires a 1:10 tissue to formalin ratio, it may be desirable to allow tissues to fully fix (∼4 days) before shipping them. At this time, tissues can be shipped in a container with sufficient formalin to keep them damp, but the complete volume need not be sent.

Necropsy is an invaluable diagnostic tool that can be used not only to determine cause of death, but also answer a range of clinical questions, provide legal documentation, and serve as a source of education to the client and practitioner. By following the systematic steps outlined in this article the practitioner can confidently perform a thorough field necropsy to enhance the chances of achieving a diagnosis and to gain a better understanding of the case.

REFERENCES

1. Buergelt CD, Del Piero F. Color atlas of equine pathology. Hoboken, (NJ): Wiley-Blackwell; 2014.
2. Knottenbelt DC, Pascoe RR. Color atlas of diseases and disorders of the horse. Maryland Heights (MO): Mosby; 1994.
3. Mason GL, Madden DJ. Performing the field necropsy examination. Vet Clin North Am Food Anim Pract 2007;23(3):503–26.

Overview of Clinical Pathology and the Horse

Sally J. Lester, DVM, MVSc*, Wendy H. Mollat, DVM, James E. Bryant, DVM

KEYWORDS

- Quality assurance • Hematology • Chemistry • Cytology

KEY POINTS

- Quality assurance is an essential aspect of laboratory diagnostics.
- Leukocyte morphology helps in assessing inflammatory and infectious conditions.
- Serum/plasma iron, lactate levels, and cardiac troponin levels are important parameters that can be measured routinely in horses.
- The assessment of total nucleated cell counts and protein levels is essential for the diagnosis of effusions in horses.
- Endocrine testing procedures for the diagnosis of metabolic abnormalities in horses, along with a brief overview of these conditions, provides a basis for diagnosis.

QUALITY ASSURANCE

In order to have confidence in the accuracy of laboratory results and their interpretation, a quality assurance (QA) system must be in place, whether this is in a clinic laboratory or a reference laboratory. The basic tenets of QA (**Table 1**) include the preanalytical phase (sample quality), analytical phase (instrumentation), and postanalytical phase (reporting of results).

In summary, standard preanalytical procedures relate to submission of specimens, types of blood tubes, and how they are handled (ie, how long can they sit on the counter[1,2]) as well as training checklists for personnel submitting the samples or running the tests. The analytical phase incorporates standard operating procedures (SOPs) for each test, personnel training, evaluation of control materials including the appropriate analyte levels in the controls, numbers of controls run daily (they must be run daily), and what to do if the controls are not within established parameters. The postanalytical phase encompasses establishment of reference intervals for your practice region, including age and breed-related differences, and result interpretation, including the effects of sample quality (hemolysis, lipemia, and icterus) on the

Pilchuck Veterinary Hospital and Equine Referral Center, 11308 92nd Street Southeast, Snohomish, WA 98290, USA
* Corresponding author.
E-mail address: slpathd@aol.com

Vet Clin Equine 31 (2015) 247–268
http://dx.doi.org/10.1016/j.cveq.2015.04.004
0749-0739/15/$ – see front matter Published by Elsevier Inc.

Table 1				
Tenets of a QA program				
Preanalytic	Samples required for tests	Documentation of the tests that are ordered	Handling of the samples, including refrigeration, separation of clotted samples	Centrifuge maintenance and calibration. Refrigeration temperature charts
Analytic	Methodology protocols	Quality control materials and details Maintenance of machines	Reference interval establishment	Interferograms documenting the effects of hemolysis, lipemia, and icterus on test results
Postanalytic	Accurate reporting of results	Timely reporting of results	Verification that results are released or checked	Tabulation of abnormal results

interpretation. There must be designated personnel that run the tests, devise SOPs, and have adequate training in laboratory QA. A doctor within the practice should be designated to oversee the laboratory and the technical staff and should also receive training in QA and laboratory testing.[3–6]

There are numerous machines now available for in-clinic complete blood counts (CBCs) and chemistry tests, both point-of-care (POC) and bench-top models; however, all have drawbacks; it is prudent that the cost of these machines, supplies, support, and reliability as well as accuracy and precision are evaluated. The major advantage to in-clinic testing is a rapid turnaround time for results, whereas the disadvantages include acceptance of the printed results as accurate, the cost of running these tests, and the lack of expertise in maintaining the machines and establishing QA. Continuing education programs dealing with QA at conferences and on networks, such as the Veterinary Information Network, are becoming more common. It is beyond the scope of this article to assess these machines, but a list of references is given that may be helpful for determining their utility.[7–12]

Reference intervals should be established for your practice population, as these will vary in different areas of the country and also with the breeds that are present within a practice area. If you are using a reference laboratory, then it is important to understand how their reference intervals were established and whether they fit with your practice.[13–18]

HEMATOLOGY

The basic assessment of hematology parameters includes a CBC with manual differential and fibrinogen levels and may also include a spun packed cell volume (PCV) and plasma protein (PP) level (total solids).[19,20] The parameters, PP (total solids) plus PCV and evaluation of a stained smear can provide the basic information needed to determine if there is an inflammatory condition present and an anemia or protein decrease and can also be used to monitor the animal and determine if there is progression of the disease.

The microhematocrit centrifuge needs routine maintenance including checking the speed with a tachometer and changing brushes on a regular basis. The color of the plasma should be recorded in the patient file, as lipemia may be a clue to metabolic diseases; icterus will increase with liver disease/anorexia; and hemolysis may indicate either trouble with collection or breakdown of red cells.

The Erythron

Erythrocytosis in horses is associated with splenic contraction or with dehydration. Often with splenic contraction there will be an increase in mature small lymphocytes; whereas with dehydration increases in serum total protein, albumin, and sodium may occur. Primary polycythemias are rare in horses but have been reported as paraneoplastic syndromes in association with hepatocellular carcinoma and metastatic carcinoma.[21]

Anemia is not uncommon and can result from loss of red cells (hemolysis or blood loss) or the failure to produce these cells (**Fig. 1**). In adult horses the peripheral blood smear provides little indication of a response to anemia. It is possible to follow mean corpuscular volume levels as these will increase with a regenerative response, but CBCs would need to be monitored every 3 to 4 days to discern this trend.[22] In general a clinical history, level of total protein (TP) and albumin to rule out hemorrhage, and bilirubin levels will be more helpful than the peripheral smear in determining the cause of the anemia (hemorrhage/hemolysis).

Evaluation of the smear is important in the identification of *Theileria equi, Babesia* spp, *Anaplasma phagocytophilum*, or *Mycoplasma* spp; serologic tests are also available for these organisms.[23–25]

Anemia that is the result of an inadequate marrow response is more consistently diagnosed by evaluation of chemistry, ultrasound, and physical examination findings, which may identify the underlying cause, such as liver disease. A nonregenerative anemia results from an insufficient bone marrow response that can be the result of

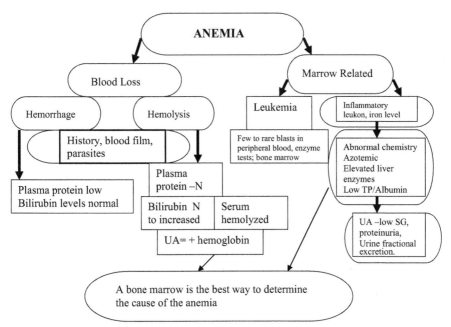

Fig. 1. Potential causes and diagnostic investigation of equine anemia. N, normal; SG, specific gravity; TP, total protein; UA, urinalysis.

a primary marrow problem (myelodysplasia or neoplasia) or a reflection of other disease processes and the influences of cytokines on the marrow. Inflammatory diseases result in increases in the acute phase protein hepcidin; this protein blocks ferroportin, which then causes cells to retain iron.[23] Anemia develops when there is insufficient iron for red cell production. Chronic liver disease is also associated with increased hepcidin levels, whereas chronic kidney disease results in a combination of increased hepcidin levels (this protein is excreted by the kidney) and lack of the erythropoietin stimulus to the marrow.[26–28] The best procedure to determine if an anemia is regenerative or nonregenerative is to perform a bone marrow aspirate or core biopsy.

In foals in the 0- to 3-day age range, regenerative responses may be detected with increased reticulocytosis in the peripheral blood; this can be helpful in detecting the presence of neonatal isoerythrolysis.[29]

The Leukon

Neutrophil responses

The inflammatory process may be evaluated by the leukogram with special attention to the neutrophils and fibrinogen levels (**Table 2**). The horse has only a moderate storage pool of mature neutrophils; thus, with significant inflammation a drain on the numbers of neutrophils will occur. If the demand for these cells is marked, the numbers will drop rapidly; this is accompanied by release of cells that are less than mature and exhibit toxic change. Toxic change in horses includes Döhle bodies in the cytoplasm, increased cytoplasmic basophilia that may be accompanied by cytoplasmic vacuolation, and granules that become more prominent.[30] These changes are the result of the increased stimulus to neutropoiesis with early release of these cells from the marrow; the changes are not occurring within the peripheral circulation. The increased basophilia reflects persistence of cytoplasmic RNA; the vacuoles reflect dispersion of the granules or breakdown of these granules, whereas Döhle bodies are a reflection of retained endoplasmic reticulum (**Fig. 2**).

The nuclear chromatin will appear lacey; segmentation of the nucleus will be decreased, which will lead to the presence of bands in the peripheral circulation.[31,32] Endotoxemia and conditions such as *Salmonella sp* infections and acute pleuropneumonia are common causes of neutropenia in the horse. Ulceration of the dorsal colon,

| | | | Chronic | Chronic Localized |
Analyte	Early Sepsis/ Endotoxemia	Established Endotoxemia	Chronic Inflammatory Disease	Chronic Localized Inflammatory Disease
TNCC	↓	↓	Slight ↑	Often normal ↑
Neutrophils	↓	↓	↑	Normal ↑
PCV	↑	↓↑	↓	Normal
Fibrinogen	Normal	After 36–48 h ↑	↑	↑
Morphology of neutrophils	Slight toxic change	Moderate to marked toxic change	Normal to slight toxic change	Normal
Band	+/−	↑	Unlikely	Unlikely
Serum iron	↓	↓	Slightly decreased	Often normal

Table 2
Responses to inflammation

Abbreviation: TNCC, total nucleated cell counts.

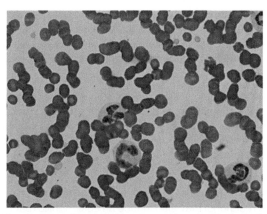

Fig. 2. Peripheral blood neutrophils, lymphocyte, and band with toxic change. Note band is larger than the neutrophil; granules are more prominent; and the chromatin is less clumped (wright-giemsa, original magnification ×50).

whether the result of nonsteroidal antiinflammatory drugs, circulatory changes, or impaction, can lead to a leucopenia. Less common causes include marrow-related disorders, such as neoplasia with altered maturation (myeloproliferative disease) and toxic injury to the marrow; both conditions usually result in decreases in more than one cell line.

Fibrinogen levels will increase after inflammation has been present for at least 36 hours; often the increase is not noted until 48 hours as the heat precipitation method, although a reasonable evaluation of elevated levels is a semiquantitative test rather than a precise estimate of the fibrinogen levels. Iron levels are a better indicator of acute inflammation as they start to decrease within 4 hours of a systemic inflammatory response, and persistently low levels warrants a guarded prognosis. Serum amyloid A is another indicator of the acute phase reaction in horses.[19,20,33]

Following a decrease in neutrophil levels with acute inflammation, the neutrophil counts will increase as the marrow responds (4–5 days); but this increase also depends on a reduction in neutrophil loss to tissues and the ability of the marrow production to exceed demand.[31,32] The increase in neutrophils may be accompanied by a monocytosis; the persistence of a monocytosis indicates that the inflammatory process has become chronic. Neutrophilia may also be accompanied by an increase in lymphocytes as the adaptive immune response develops.

Lymphoid responses
Lymphocytosis is common as a fear response, which is especially prominent in young animals and reflects splenic and lymphatic contraction. When associated with established inflammation and a persistence of cytokines and foreign antigen, the increased lymphoid population may be linked to a corresponding increase in levels of globulins. (Protein electrophoresis may be required to detect this increase in immunoglobulins.) Lymphocytosis can be seen with chronic pleuritis/pneumonia. Reactive lymphocytes are not uncommon and can be detected on the blood smear as large round cells with marked cytoplasmic basophilia. It should also be noted that EDTA is a mitogen, and prolonged exposure (hours) will result in increased numbers of reactive lymphocytes in the blood smears.

Lymphopenia is usually the result of increased cortisol levels, which alter lymphocyte kinetics and cause a decrease in their efflux from lymphoid tissues as well as redistribution within hematopoietic tissues. The effects of steroids will persist as long as cortisol levels are increased and over time will also result in lympholysis. In a sick animal, the return of lymphocytes to within reference intervals is considered a good prognostic indicator, whereas persistent lymphopenia is considered a poor prognostic indicator.

Monocyte responses

Monocytopenia is not identified, as the reference interval includes *zero*. Monocytosis is the result of cytokine stimulation and often coexists with a neutrophilia. Monocytes are the precursors for tissue macrophages and are involved both in the innate and adaptive immune responses. They are actively involved in phagocytosis of debris and may indicate tissue necrosis.

Eosinophil responses

Eosinophilia can occur with parasitic migration through tissues. Hypersensitivity reactions (diffuse insect reactions) may also induce an eosinophilic reaction. Hypereosinophilic syndromes are not uncommon in horses and involve the intestinal tract, skin, respiratory system, or all of these organs; but less than 20% of the literature reported cases exhibited eosinophilia.[34–36]

Basophil responses

Changes in basophils are difficult to interpret; little is known about the cell kinetics as so few are normally present within the peripheral blood. The increases may parallel those associated with eosinophils and include parasitism, hypersensitivity reactions, or neoplasia.

Platelets

Platelets may be increased with chronic inflammation or with low-grade blood loss. Increases can also occur along with epinephrine contraction of the spleen or in association with iron deficiency, production of interleukin 6 by neoplastic cells, and exercise.

Thrombocytopenia may result from immune-mediated destruction of these cells, sequestration or altered distribution with endotoxemia, marrow injury (toxins/anoxia), and with organisms such as *Anaplasma phagocytophilum*.[25] Spurious thrombocytopenia and neutropenia can occur with EDTA artifact.[37]

FLUID EVALUATION

Abdominocentesis, thoracocentesis, and arthrocentesis are important procedures in equine practice. Total nucleated cell counts (TNCC) provide a great deal of information when combined with an evaluation of a sediment smear and with the total solids (plasma protein) of the fluid. The appearance of the neutrophils, including the presence or absence of microorganisms, will allow for a rapid assessment of the prognosis (**Table 3**).

White cell counts and red cell counts can be evaluated with most automated impedance counters, but it is essential that fluid be collected in EDTA and the sample be well mixed. Any particulate debris will cause problems/obstruction of the apertures and damage to the instrument. Evaluation of the sediment smear along with the protein levels and PCV can characterize the disease process.[38–46]

The PP (total solids) should be used to determine the pathogenesis of the fluid development. Fluids with low protein levels (less than 1.5 g/dL) are considered pure transudates; this implies that water has leaked from vessels as a result of altered fluid forces, including hydrostatic and oncotic pressures. Transudates occur when total

Table 3
Fluid cytology

Analyte	Normal Body Cavity Fluid	Colic with Intact Intestine	Colic with Developing Peritonitis (Exudate)	Pleuritis; Milky Fluid Occurs with Lymphatic Leakage	Joint Fluid Normals May Vary with Site
WBC (TNCC) 10.3/µl	<5000[a]	1000–8000	>5000[b]	>5000	<1000
RBC 10.6/µl	0	Scant	>20,000	Variable	0 But can increase because of tap
TP (total solids) g/dl	0–1.5	1.0–3.0	2.5–4.0	2.0–4.0	<2.0
Cytology	Mononuclear cells	70% Or greater mononuclear cells present with nontoxic neutrophils	Shift to neutrophils with toxic change; organisms present if the GI breeched	Mixed cells, with neutrophils predominant; organisms difficult to find	Mononuclear cells only; viscosity is high in normal joint fluids

Abbreviations: GI, gastrointestinal; RBC, red blood cell; WBC, white blood cell.
[a] Various references define total counts as 1500 to 10,000 cells; 5000 is more consistently used.
[b] Foals younger than 1 month should have TNCC counts less than 1500/µ; TNCC greater than 2000 suggests exudation in foals.

serum protein/albumin levels are low (<3.0 TP; <1.5 serum albumin), with increased capillary pressures before damage to endothelium, or with leakage from low protein lymphatic fluid. Low protein transudates in the pleural cavity are uncommon as altered hydrostatic pressures result in pulmonary edema rather than pleural effusion.

Increased protein levels in fluids, whether or not accompanied by increased cellularity, imply a disruption of the vasculature such that protein within the intravascular compartment is able to enter the interstitial tissues or body cavities. These fluids may be accompanied by an influx of cells if there is an inflammatory component (cytokine production) that results in cellular egress through the endothelium. The transudates with elevated protein levels are referred to as high protein transudates, and these can occur with conditions such as portal hypertension or obstruction of circulation (masses). The cellularity of these fluids is usually less than expected with an exudate, but there may be overlap between these conditions. Evaluation of thoracic fluid may also identify neoplastic conditions, such as metastatic melanoma; these fluids are usually high protein transudates with low or moderate cellularity (**Fig. 3**).

Exudates are considered to have a TP greater than 3.6 g/dL and an increased cellularity with increased numbers of neutrophils. The actual nucleated cell count for a fluid to be considered an exudate is variable throughout the literature; the interpretation should also be based on the distribution of the cells, the integrity of the cell population, and the presence or absence of organisms.

BIOCHEMICAL CHANGES

Most diagnostic chemistry tests are based on a panel approach rather than single analytes. This approach allows for a comprehensive overview of multiple systems,

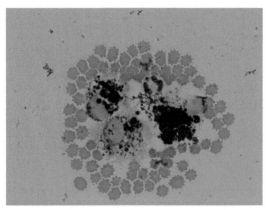

Fig. 3. Cytospin preparation; melanoma in chest fluid; neutrophil and red cells (wright-giemsa, original magnification ×100).

with liver disease and renal disease detected by specific tests, whereas other disease processes are inferred by combinations of altered parameters. Biochemical parameters that can be evaluated include liver enzymes (aspartic aminotransferase [AST], gamma glutamyltransferase [GGT], sorbital dehydrogenase [SDH]); blood urea nitrogen (BUN); creatinine, TP and albumin; acute phase responders, such as iron and serum amyloid A; and specific cardiac markers, such as cardiac troponin I. Electrolytes are important parameters in the horse with enteric disease, especially when coupled with lactate levels.

Cardiac troponin I levels are helpful with enteric disease and also with cardiac dysfunction. Cardiac troponin I methodologies are variable; unfortunately not all methods will accurately assess this analyte, and some may cross-react with skeletal muscle troponin leading to confusion and distrust over the results.[47,48] Cardiac troponin I levels in serum are very low, with values ranging from 0.0 to 0.1 ng/mL, which may also be the limit of detection of most assays, so modest or early increases in these levels may be difficult to determine and depend on the specific assay. The troponins are a complex of 2 subunits; troponin C (CTNC) binds calcium, troponin I (CTNI) is an inhibitor, and troponin T (CTNT) bonds tropomysin. The subunits do exist as several isoforms, which are present in cardiac muscle and slow and fast twitch skeletal muscle. Cardiac troponin is present in circulation as 3 forms: bound to a complex with CTNC, bound with both CTNC and CTNT, or free. There are also low levels of free troponin within the myofibrils, which are responsible for the initial increase in these levels in serum; then as the myofibril injury continues and the membrane is destroyed, a more sustained elevation develops. Most methodologies are immunologic with antibody developed to the specific troponin and to unique regions of the protein. The levels increase rapidly after myocardial injury; in humans the levels peak in 8 hours, and levels diminish quickly, although still detectable 4 to 5 days after injury.[49,50] In horses one study of injected troponin I indicated a rapid clearance with a half-life ($t_{1/2}$) of 0.47 hours, which would indicate a similar clearance as reported in humans.[51] Troponin levels and their behavior in association with anesthesia, racing, training, and endurance exercise has also been studied.[52–56] Increased CTNI levels in horses with colic support a less favorable prognosis and are associated with increased ventricular arrhythmias postoperatively. In one study, the combination of high CTNI levels postoperatively and high lactate levels preoperatively were significantly associated with nonsurvival.[57,58]

Enteric Diseases

Altered electrolytes occur with enteric disease with decreases in sodium and chloride levels, which may be accompanied by increased total carbon dioxide (TCO_2). The increases in TCO_2 are more prominent with ileus or obstructive conditions, whereas the decreases in sodium/chloride occur with effusion of fluid into the intestinal tract. Serum TP levels may drop if this effusion reflects loss of mucosal integrity. The levels of TP and albumin are often low or at the low end of the reference interval with chronic malabsorption syndromes, including intestinal lymphoma.[59,60] A fecal examination for parasites should be routine for any enteric disease.

Conditions generally referred to as colic require a clinical evaluation including rectal palpation as well as evaluation of clinical pathology panels. In general when there are significant changes in the laboratory parameters, time is of the essence. Such parameters are listed in **Table 4**.

Abdominal pain evaluation

The level of glucose in the serum is a predictor of outcome, as significant increases occur with stress, catecholamine release, and high levels greater than 200 mg/dL occur as a preterminal event. Lactate levels are helpful in determining prognosis, and ratios of serum to peritoneal lactate and or serial measurement of plasma lactate may be better at predicting ongoing disease and prognosis than a single measurement. Lactate levels in plasma increase over time because of anaerobic glycolysis; so samples should be collected in either sodium fluoride or heparin-containing tubes and processed rapidly. Whole-blood measurement of lactate can also be done with blood gas machines and some POC instruments; but correlation of POC instruments to blood gas machines indicates a bias, and higher values for pH are more common with POC instruments. Reference intervals specific to the instrument are required for accurate determination.[61] Elevation of PP (total solids) coupled with PCV will aid in determining fluid shifts and the extent of dehydration. However, these parameters should be interpreted cautiously once the animal is receiving parenteral fluid therapy. Measurement of lactate, pH, and glucose in the abdominal fluid may also be helpful as glucose declines along with pH with increased bacterial activity, whereas lactate increases. Cytologic evaluation of abdominal fluid is necessary for all colic cases. The color and quantity of abdominal fluid along with the refractometer protein levels should be recorded. Evaluation of direct and concentrated smears (centrifuge the fluid at 2500 rpm for a minimum of 5 minutes and make a smear of the button of cells that forms in the bottom of the tube) allows for identification of cell types. A shift from mononuclear cells to neutrophils indicates the severity of the inflammation, whereas organisms within neutrophils indicate rupture of the gastrointestinal tract; increased red cells with macrophages exhibiting erythrophagy indicate a predominantly hemorrhagic event; more modest increased red cells in the fluid may reflect serosal leakage and/or intestinal necrosis. It is important that organisms be identified within cells rather than in the background as debris on slides and accidental puncture of a distended intestinal segment can result in bacteria in the background rather than within cells (**Fig. 4**)

The fluid should also be interpreted in light of the clinical history and duration of signs. Fluid obtained when there has been a very recent intestinal rupture is often consistent with a low cell transudate as there has not been enough time for cells to increase or for sufficient protein to leak into the fluid to increase the protein levels. Other chemistry tests that can be run on abdominal fluid include creatinine and potassium levels, which when compared with serum levels and interpreted along with altered serum electrolytes will aid in the diagnosis of bladder rupture. A ratio

Table 4
Colic interpretation

	Medical Colic	Surgical Colic Without Strangulation	Colic with Strangulation	Ruptured Viscous
TP/albumin	Normal to increased	Normal to increased	Levels often decreased but may increase with dehydration	Decreased levels caused by fluid shifts, hemorrhage, shock
Serum lactate	Levels less than 2 × reference	Levels in plasma greater than 2 × reference; increased levels in abdominal fluid as compared with peripheral blood	Ratio of peripheral blood lactate to abdominal fluid should be one or less in normal animals; lactate levels more than 3 × reference, poor prognosis	Serial measurement of lactate with increasing levels from baseline is poor prognostic indicator and may predict loss of intestinal integrity
Serum glucose	Within reference	Modest increased glucose	Glucose elevated 1.5 × reference	Glucose 2 × reference or higher
Serum iron	Within reference	Normal to slight decrease	Decreased levels suggest sepsis	Decreased levels
CBC	WBCs within reference, slight neutrophilia, lymphopenia	WBCs within reference, bands may be present and toxic change apparent	WBCs often low with bands, toxic change moderate	Severe leucopenia, neutropenia, and left shift; marked toxic change
Abdominal fluid	Transudate with nucleated cells counts less than 5000	Protein levels that exceed 1.5 should be correlated to lactate level TNCC <10,000	Cell counts often higher than 10,000, protein levels consistent with high protein transudate	Cell counts may be low if rupture very acute, bacteria present within neutrophils; TNCC increase with time from rupture and cells exhibit more disintegration

Abbreviations: CBC, complete blood count; WBCs, white blood cells.

of 2:1 abdominal fluid creatinine to serum creatinine is predictive of a bladder rupture. Amylase and lipase levels may be run on abdominal fluid and elevated levels (values are close to zero in normal abdominal fluid) support pancreatic disease. Serum biochemistry parameters, such as lactate, are expected to return to reference intervals if the disease process is corrected; persistence of high levels (over 24 hours) is a poor prognostic indicator.[62,63]

After anesthesia, creatinine levels should be monitored as anoxia/circulatory shifts associated with shock and with anesthesia will result in tubular necrosis and can give

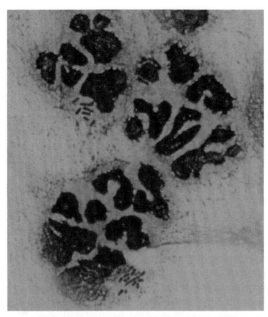

Fig. 4. Disintegrating neutrophils, with mixed bacteria; peritoneal fluid after gastrointestinal rupture (wright-giemsa, original magnification ×100).

rise to significant renal injury, which interferes with renal function. Sequential CTNI levels are a sensitive indictor of myocardial damage, which occurs with systemic inflammatory responses as well as in association with sepsis, anoxia, and fluid shifts.

Infectious enteric disease
Infectious causes related to enteric disease in horses can occur in adults and foals as well as complicating hospital confinement or stressful conditions. The common infectious causes include *Salmonella* sp, *Lawsonia* sp (mainly young horses), neorickettsiosis, and altered intestinal flora with increased toxigenic *Escherichia coli* and *Clostridium difficile* or *Clostridium perfringens* toxins. The hallmark of these conditions is often a sustained decline in neutrophil count with significant toxic changes observed in the neutrophils; this is often coupled to a loss of mucosal integrity and declines in serum TP and albumin levels. An enzyme-linked immunosorbent assay test for *C difficile* toxin A and B in feces is an aid in diagnosis; but a definitive diagnosis would also include anaerobic fecal culture followed by polymerase chain reaction (PCR) on the isolated organisms to establish that these organisms can produce toxins. Evaluation of histologic specimens of intestinal lesions may be necessary to substantiate the cause of the enteritis. PCR evaluation of diarrheic fecal samples is rewarding for establishing an infectious cause.[64–68]

Malabsorptive enteric disease
Malabsorption occurs in the horse when there is damage to the intestinal mucosa/submucosa, which can result from inflammation that develops as the result of antigen/antibody reactions, food intolerance, and true hypersensitivity lesions. The role of the cyathostomes must also be considered as they encyst and then can emerge in large numbers with disruption in the mucosa/submucosa that triggers fibrosis, which impedes absorption.[59,68] Inflammatory bowel disease characterized by lymphocytic/eosinophilic infiltrates, although nonspecific as to cause, is a relatively newly

recognized cause of malabsorption.[35] Enteric lymphoma is also recognized as a cause for malabsorption.[60] Hypereosinophilic syndromes, whether as a specific disease entity with multiple organ system involvement or when limited to the gastrointestinal tract, are increasingly common in horses and result in significant malabsorption accompanied by decreasing levels of serum albumin and recurrent syndromes that include diarrhea, colic, and weight loss. These lesions tend to be progressive and ultimately will lead to fibrosis within the intestinal tract mediated by cytokines responsive to the eosinophilic infiltrates, such as transforming growth factor α.[34–36] Ultrasound and laparoscopic evaluation may be helpful, but biopsy is the mainstay of diagnosis.[68]

Glucose tolerance tests may be used to document decreased intestinal absorption; values should increase after the administration of glucose if mucosal absorption is present (**Box 1**).

Post operative enteric considerations

Postoperative ileus is a serious complication of abdominal/intestinal surgery in horses and may also be caused by or predispose to endotoxemia and sepsis. Excessive reflux is a hallmark of this condition; although criteria vary, it is generally agreed that the presence of nasogastric reflux that exceeds 4 L at any intubation or greater than 2 L of fluid per hour would fit the criteria of postoperative reflux. Decreases in sodium and chloride in serum along with a significant decline in neutrophils and toxic changes may occur as the condition progresses. Lactate levels remain elevated rather than declining as expected with correction of the original pathology.[69]

Liver Disease

Although acute disorders occur in horses, the presentation of most horses with liver disease will be of a chronic progressive condition. In adult horses, liver disease often results from food-related plant toxins, such as pyrrolizidine alkaloids, alsike clover, and ryegrass, whereas toxins such as arsenic and phenols are uncommon but reported causes. Liver enzymes along with bile acids and biopsies are important for determining prognosis and also disease progression.[70,71]

AST and SDH are enzymes that directly reflect hepatocellular disease and leak from these cells, whereas alkaline phosphatase (ALP) and GGT are considered biliary related or cholestatic indicators and are induced by disease processes rather than leakage enzymes (**Table 5**). GGT may also elevate with dorsal colon displacement and as a nonspecific finding with induction from medications or supplements; nonspecific increases in GGT tend to be less than 2 times the reference intervals. Bilirubin levels may also indicate cholestatic disease; but total bilirubin can increase with anorexia up to 5 times the reference interval, which makes the test a less specific indictor of hepatic function. Bile acids are an assessment of hepatic function as these are produced within the liver excreted through the biliary system and then reabsorbed in the ileum and recirculated and then removed from circulation by the hepatocytes. This transport requires active and functional hepatocytes as well as an intact excretory system and normal circulation.

Bile acid levels to some extent reflect the degree of hepatic compromise; however, as fibrosis in the liver develops, circulatory interference will decrease uptake and loss of hepatocytes will decrease production. As liver failure develops, bile acid levels may not reflect the extent of dysfunction.

The prognostic significance of liver enzymes is related to their decrease in accordance with their $t_{1/2}$. Declining levels may indicate that the injury to the liver is not ongoing; however, these must be interpreted in light of the changes in TP and albumin as well as the clinical assessment of the animal. When viable hepatocytes are lost with

Box 1
Diagnostic tests for metabolic diseases in horses

Glucose tolerance test

- Collect a baseline serum/plasma sample (process quickly as glucose levels decline). A 12-hour fast is preferred or only feed grass hay.

- Administer glucose 1 g/kg as a 20% solution given by nasogastric tube.

- Collect serum/plasma samples at 1, 2, and 4 hours after administration.

Glucose levels should increase at least 80% more than baseline by 2 hours (peak response) and then gradually decrease.

Dexamethasone suppression test

- Take the baseline cortisol at 0 hours at 5 to 7 pm.

- Inject dexamethasone at 40 μg/kg (0.04 mg/kg); an average horse is 20 mg.

- Collect the next sample at 15 hours after injection and the next at 19 hours after injection.

The normal horse will have undetectable cortisol levels at 15 and 19 hours, whereas the horse with PPID dysfunction will have levels greater than the lower limit of detection of the test (27–30 nmol/L) at 15 or 19 hours; horses with developing PPID may suppress at 15 hours but not at 19 hours.

TRH response test

- Take a baseline sample (EDTA should be spun immediately, and place plasma in plastic vials).

- Inject 1 mg TRH IV (0.5 mg for ponies).

- Collect a second EDTA sample at 10 minutes and at 30 minutes. Separate and handle plasma appropriately as previously discussed.

- If testing for hypothyroidism, collect serum samples at 2 and 4 hours after administration. Measure T4 and T3.

A normal horse will have a doubling of the T4 values by 4 hours and a doubling of T3 values at 2 hours.

A horse with PPID may have modestly increased ACTH levels at 0 hours but will have markedly elevated levels at 10 or 30 minutes after TRH injection (interpret in light of your laboratory reference intervals).

Test for insulin resistance (oral)

Feed 1 flake of grass hay at 10 PM, and start the test the following morning at 8 AM.

Oral glucose challenge

- Collect a 0-hour baseline serum sample for glucose and insulin determination.

- Administer light Karo syrup (ACH Food Companies, Inc, Cordova, TN) (15 mL/100 kg by mouth).

- Collect a second serum sample at 60 and 90 minutes and measure glucose and insulin.

A normal horse will increase insulin levels to maintain normoglycemia, but insulin levels will seldom exceed the reference intervals at 60 and 90 minutes. Glucose levels will return to baseline within 45 to 60 minutes in normal horses. Horses with insulin resistance will maintain insulin levels greater than 4 times the baseline, and glucose levels will remain greater than the reference at 60 or 90 minutes.

Abbreviations: ACTH, corticotropin; IV, intravenous; PPID, pituitary pars intermedia dysfunction; TRH, thyrotropin-releasing hormone.

Table 5
Biochemical changes associated with liver disease in the horse

Analyte	$T_{1/2}$	Peak	Acute	Chronic	Information
SDH	12 h	12–24 h	Increases detected 12 h after injury and continue as long as injury is ongoing.	There are often normal levels.	SDH should return to reference levels rapidly; if there is a slow decline, fibrosis or ongoing injury is present.
AST	12–36 h	24–36 h	Increased levels develop after 3 d and then will continue to increase.	Elevated levels persist longer than SDH.	Progressive decline in AST levels when monitored on a weekly to monthly basis can indicate a good prognosis if clinical signs and appetite are improving.
GGT	3 d	7 d	It is induced but takes days to be detected.	Declining values may indicate resolution or hepatic failure.	Induction can occur with medication supplements and intestinal disease. Decline in values with resolution may take months.
ALP	3–5 d	5–6 d	Once induced, levels are maintained longer than GGT levels.	Declining values may indicate resolution or hepatic failure.	Decline in values is prolonged and may take months.
Bile acids	1–2 d	Variable	There is an increase within 12 h.	Values may decline as the lesion becomes chronic.	They are recirculated 10 times in 24 h.
Iron	Unknown	Marked increase within 12 h of acute hepatocellular injury	Variable levels depend on the degree of hepatocellular necrosis.	Elevated levels decline within hours of resolution. Levels remain low if inflammation persists.	Levels decrease to 10%–20% of the reference within 12 h when sepsis develops.
Albumin	20 d	May be high with dehydration	It is normal.	Levels decline with chronicity, at the low end of the reference or less.	Stability of albumin levels over months indicates a better prognosis.

a chronic injury, the liver enzymes will decrease, so caution should be used in interpreting declines in AST or SDH. GGT and ALP have a longer $t_{1/2}$ than the hepatocellular enzymes, so there will be a more gradual decline in these enzymes. Albumin is produced solely by the liver; if the disease becomes chronic, a gradual decline in albumin levels will occur. Albumin in the horse has a $t_{1/2}$ of 20 days; thus, declines are of prognostic significance but take considerable time to develop. BUN levels may be low with liver disease, but this is considered an insensitive indicator of disease. Serum iron levels are elevated when there is significant hepatocellular necrosis but will decline as the liver disease becomes chronic and when there is significant inflammatory/infectious components.[70,72–74]

Triglycerides should be measured to determine if hepatic lipidosis is present.[75] Triglycerides may also be measured in chylous effusions, which can develop with lipidosis and with intestinal lymphatic obstructions.

Changes in the complete blood count (CBC) do occur with liver disease, especially when these are the result of bacterial infections (ascending from the gastrointestinal tract) or primary infectious disease, such as Tyzzer disease (foals), and with choleliths as these are often associated with necrosis of liver tissue. Neutrophilia may occur and be accompanied by a monocytosis and lymphopenia. Anemia will develop with chronicity. Biopsy of the liver is a relatively simple procedure and is necessary to determine specific causes for the liver disease.

Musculoskeletal Disease

Evaluation of skeletal muscle injury includes the assessment of the muscle enzymes, creatinine kinase (CK) and AST. These enzymes have different half-lives and when used in concert can predict the resolution of muscle injuries as well as the initiation. The $t_{1/2}$ of CK is 2 hours, whereas the $t_{1/2}$ of AST is variable but has been considered to range from 12 hours to 7 days. The CK levels peak at 6 to 12 hours after an insult, whereas the AST peaks at 24 to 36 hours after an insult. CK is a cytosolic enzyme that is released rapidly from injured muscle, whereas more sustained release will occur with AST as this is both cytosolic and nuclear. Because the $t_{1/2}$ of CK is short, declines occur more rapidly than declines in AST; this difference can be used to monitor resolution of the injury.[76]

Diseases of the Urinary System

The evaluation of urine is a critical part of the evaluation of renal function and should be part of the evaluation in all clinically ill horses. Routine examination of sediment as well as urine specific gravity (SG) and dipstick levels should be part of the urinalysis.

The urine SG in horses is normally more than 1.020, with ranges given of 1.020 to 1.050; the pH ranges from 7.5 to 8.5. In foals 0 to 3 days old, the values are significantly lower, with an SG of 1.001 to 1.012; the pH is 6 to 7. The isothenuric range in adult horses is considered to be 1.008 to 1.014. Evaluation of electrolyte fractional excretion is of value for determining tubular injury. Fractional excretions also vary between foals and adults, with normal foals having a fractional excretion of sodium 0.3%, potassium 11.6 ± 8.7, and phosphorus of 1.19 ± 1.47, whereas an adult horse has a fractional excretion of sodium less than 1%, potassium excretion of 20% to 75%, and phosphorus excretion of 0% to 1.0%. Calcium excretion is also double in adult horses as opposed to foals.[77–81]

Both BUN and creatinine can be used as markers of renal insufficiency; but neither test is as sensitive as SG, which is less than 1.020 when there has been loss of 50% of the renal function, while neither BUN nor creatinine increase until 70% of the renal function is lost. The increase in BUN and creatinine is an indication of a decrease in glomerular filtration rate. Creatinine levels vary with the breed; horses with a large muscle mass, such as quarter horses, will have creatinine values that may exceed the reference interval. Creatinine values may be 4 to 5 times higher in foals in the first 12 to 24 hours if there was placental insufficiency. These values will rapidly decline to reference intervals within 3 days. Calcium levels are commonly increased over the reference interval with renal disease in horses in part because of the high calcium intake associated with feeds and the active excretion of calcium by the kidney in horses. Phosphorus levels in serum are elevated with decreased glomerular filtration in most mammalian species; but in horses these levels are often normal or decreased, which may reflect anorexia, high serum calcium levels, and also the polyuria that decreases phosphorus reabsorption in the distal tubules.

Neurologic Disease

Evaluation of cerebrospinal fluid (CSF) is important in determining the cause of neurologic disease in the horse. Elevations in protein levels as well as the cellular composition of this fluid are important. Most procedures now involve cytospin concentration of cells, which essentially will secure any cells present in the fluid. A shift in the cell population from macrophages and lymphocytes to neutrophils indicates bacterial/fungal infections, whereas a predominance and increase in mononuclear cells can be seen with protozoal and viral diseases. Evaluation of CSF fluid for the presence of equine protozoal myeloencephalitis–specific antibodies is considered the most accurate method of determining the disease presence.[82]

Respiratory Disease

Chronic respiratory conditions as well as acute pneumonia are not uncommon processes in horses. Transtracheal wash (TTW) and bronchioalveolar lavage (BAL) are important diagnostic tools. Fluid obtained should always be cultured; cytologic evaluation should include a description of the quantity of fluid, color, clarity, cell counts, and both direct and sediment cytologic evaluation. Cytologic evaluation including the percentage of various cell types is the most sensitive method of determining the underlying pathology within the lung. A standard counting procedure, such as 500 cell counts, or total counts within cytospin preparations that are specific volumes of fluids helps to define the significance of the different cell populations. Increased numbers of neutrophils are associated with inflammatory conditions, including those related to chronic lower airway disease; hemorrhage as indicated by macrophages containing both red cells and hemosideron and increased numbers of mast cells may also occur with chronic lower respiratory conditions. The definition of normal BAL is variable as there are many factors that need to be considered, including the timing of the collection (before/after exercise), the environment of the horse, and the volume of fluid that was given and retrieved.[83–86] Normal BAL fluid is of low cellularity, with a predominance of round cells (macrophages/lymphoid) with neutrophils not exceeding 4% of the nucleated cells (**Figs. 5** and **6**).

Pleuropneumonia can develop from many infectious causes in the horse and may be concurrent with pneumonia or develop after more acute pneumonic symptoms have diminished. There are many predisposing causes, including stress/transport and nutrition. Diagnosis of this condition includes thoracocentesis and TTW. Pleural fluid in this condition is an exudate with protein values exceeding 3.5 g/dL and high TNCC with a predominance of neutrophils, many of which may be degenerate. As this condition becomes chronic and fibrosis develops, it may be difficult to retrieve substantial fluid with a thoracocentesis. Culture, both aerobic and anaerobic, is essential for the diagnosis and to determine the appropriate antibiotic therapy. CBC changes common

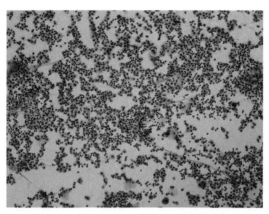

Fig. 5. BAL from horse with chronic lower airway disease; note giant cells (wright-giemsa, original magnification ×10).

to this condition include elevated mature neutrophils count with monocytosis, elevated serum protein, and globulin levels with a polyclonal gammopathy.[87,88]

Metabolic Diseases

Various metabolic syndromes have been identified in the horse, the 2 most common of which are excessive production of corticotropin (ACTH) and insulin resistance whether as a consequence of excessive ACTH or as a primary diagnosis of insulin dysregulation. ACTH levels should always be interpreted according to the laboratory-established reference intervals. These levels will depend on the population of horses in the region as well as the photoperiods; in most regions, levels tend to be higher in the fall and lower in the spring and summer.

Most horses with pituitary pars intermedia dysfunction will be diagnosed from the plasma ACTH level; there is a subset for which other testing maybe necessary to confirm the diagnosis. These tests include the dexamethasone suppression test and the thyroid-releasing hormone (TRH) stimulation test (see **Box 1**).

Insulin measurements will also vary with the methodology and are specific to the laboratory and to your population of horses. A single fasting insulin level that is 2 times

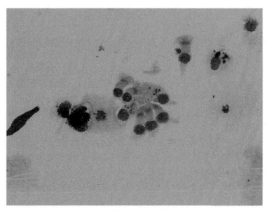

Fig. 6. TTW from horse with prior hemorrhage; note ciliated epithelium and hemosideron in macrophages (wright-giemsa, original magnification ×40).

more than the reference interval is adequate to diagnosis insulin resistance, but dynamic testing using oral sugar tests with measurement of serum glucose and insulin levels can be necessary to accurately assess insulin dysregulation.[88–91]

Hypothyroidism is a rare condition in horses, although low thyroxine levels may occur with other disease processes, medications such as phenylbutazone, and exercise. To determine if hypothyroidism is truly present, a thyrotropin-releasing hormone stimulation test would be needed.[91–93]

REFERENCES

1. Rendle DJ, Heller J, Hughes KJ, et al. Stability of common biochemical analytes in equine blood stored at room temperature. Equine Vet J 2009;41(5):428–32.
2. Clark P, Mogg TD, Tvedten HW, et al. Artifactual changes in equine blood following storage, detected using the Advia 120 hematology analyzer. Vet Clin Pathol 2002;31(2):90–4.
3. Bell R, Harr K, Rishniw M, et al. Survey of point of care instrumentation, analysis and quality assurance in veterinary practice. Vet Clin Pathol 2014;43:185–92.
4. Cian F, Villiers E, Archer J, et al. Use of six sigma work sheets for assessment of interval and external failure costs associated with candidate quality control rules for the ADVIA 120 hematology analyzer. Vet Clin Pathol 2014;43:164–71.
5. Lester SJ, Harr K, Rishniw M, et al. Current quality assurance concepts and considerations for quality control of in-clinic biochemistry testing. J Am Vet Med Assoc 2013;241:182–92.
6. Farr AJ, Freeman KP. Quality control validation, application of sigma metrics and performance comparison between two biochemistry analyzers in a commercial veterinary laboratory. J Vet Diagn Invest 2008;20(5):536–44.
7. Bauer N, Nakagawa J, Dunker C, et al. Evaluation of the automated hematology analyzer Sysmex XT-2000iV compared to the Advia 2120 for its use in dogs, cats and horses: part 1–precision, linearity and accuracy of complete blood cell count. J Vet Diagn Invest 2011;23(6):1168–80.
8. Bauer N, Nakagawa J, Dunker C, et al. Evaluation of the automated hematology analyzer Sysmex XT2000iV compared to the ADVIA 2120 for its use in dogs, cats and horses. Part 11: accuracy of leukocyte differential and reticulocyte count, impact of anticoagulant and sample aging. J Vet Diagn Invest 2012;24(1):74–89.
9. Bienzle D, Stanton JB, Embry JM, et al. Evaluation of an in-house centrifugal hematology analyzer for use in veterinary practice. J Am Vet Med Assoc 2000; 217(8):1195–200.
10. Rodoff S, Arndt G, Botterina B, et al. Clinical evaluation of the CA530-Vet hematology analyzer for use in veterinary practice. Vet Clin Pathol 2007;36(2):155–66.
11. Flatland B, Breickner LC, Fry MM. Analytical performance of a dry chemistry analyzer designed for in clinic use. Vet Clin Pathol 2014;43(2):206–17.
12. Vassmuth AK, Riond B, Hofmann-Lehmann R, et al. Evaluation of the mythic 18 hematology analyzer for use with canine, feline and equine samples. J Vet Diagn Invest 2011;23(3):436–53.
13. Adamu L, Noraniza M, Rasedee A, et al. Effect of age and performance on physical, hematological and biochemical parameters in endurance horses. J Equine Vet Sci 2013;33:415–20.
14. Harvey RW, Aquith RL, McNulty PK, et al. Hematology of foals up to one year old. Equine Vet J 1994;16(4):347–53.
15. Jarvey JW, Pate MG, Kivipleto J, et al. Clinical biochemistry of pregnant and nursing mares. Vet Clin Pathol 2005;34(3):248–54.

16. Snow DH, Riddle C, Salmon PW. Haematology response to racing and training exercise in thoroughbred horses with particular reference to the leukocyte response. Equine Vet J 1983;15(2):141–4.
17. Zobba R, Ardu M, Niccolini S, et al. Physical, hematological and biochemical response to acute intense exercise in polo horses. J Equine Vet Sci 2011;31(9):542–8.
18. Poso AR, Soveri T, Oksanen HE. The effect of exercise on blood parameters in Standardbred and Finnish-bred horses. Acta Vet Scand 1983;24(2):170–84.
19. Corradini I, Armengou L, Viu J, et al. Parallel testing of plasma iron and fibrinogen concentrations to detect systemic inflammation in hospitalized horses. J Vet Emerg Crit Care (San Antonio) 2014;24(4):414–20.
20. Borges AS, Divers TJ, Stokol T, et al. Serum iron and plasma fibrinogen concentrations as indicators of systemic inflammatory diseases in horses. J Vet Intern Med 2007;21(3):489–94.
21. Lording PM. Erythrocyte. Vet Clin North Am Equine Pract 2008;24:225–37.
22. Cooper C, Sears W, Bienzle D. Reticulocyte changes after experimental anemia and erythropoietin treatment in horses. J Appl Physiol (1985) 2005;99:915–21.
23. Rubino G, Lacinio R, Bramante G, et al. Hematology and some blood chemical parameters as a function of tick-borne disease (TBD) signs in horses. J Equine Vet Sci 2006;26(10):475–80.
24. Dieckmann SM, Winkler M, Groebel K, et al. Haemotrophic mycoplasma infection in horses. Vet Microbiol 2010;145:351–3.
25. Dziegiel B, Adaszek L, Kalinowki M, et al. Equine granulocytic anaplasmosis. Res Vet Sci 2013;95(2):316–20.
26. Oliveira-filho JP, Badial PR, Cunha PH, et al. Lipopolysaccharide infusion upregulated hepcidin mRNA expression in equine liver. Innate Immun 2011;18(3):438–46.
27. Ganz T, Nemeth E. Regulation of iron acquisition and iron distribution in mammals. Biochim Biophys Acta 2006;1763:690–9.
28. Gisbert JP, Gomollon F. An update on iron physiology. World J Gastroenterol 2009;15(37):4617–26.
29. O'Neill E, Horney B, Burton S. What is your diagnosis? Blood loss in a foal. Vet Clin Pathol 2014;43(2):287–8.
30. Weiss DJ, Evanson OA. Evaluation of activated neutrophils in the blood of horses with colic. Am J Vet Res 2003;64(11):1364–8.
31. Carrick JB, Begg AP. Peripheral blood leukocytes. Vet Clin North Am Equine Pract 2008;24:239–59.
32. Hurley DJ, Parks RJ, Reber AJ, et al. Dynamic changes in circulating leukocytes during induction of equine laminitis with black walnut extract. Vet Immunol Immunopathol 2006;110:195–206.
33. Belgrave RL, Dickey MM, Arheart KL, et al. Assessment of serum amyloid A testing in horses and its clinical application in a specialized equine practice. J Am Vet Med Assoc 2013;243(1):113–9.
34. Edwards GB, Kelly DF, Proudman CJ. Segmental eosinophilic colitis: a review of 22 cases. Equine Vet J Suppl 2000;32:86–93.
35. Makinen PE, Archer DC, Baptise KE, et al. Characterization of the inflammatory reaction in equine idiopathic focal eosinophilic enteritis and diffuse eosinophilic enteritis. Equine Vet J 2008;40(4):386–92.
36. Booster L, Verryken K, Bauwens C, et al. Equine multisystemic eosinophilic epitheliotropic disease: a case report and review of the literature. N Z Vet J 2013;61(3):177–82.
37. Hinchcliff KW, Kociba GJ, Mitten LA. Diagnosis of EDTA-dependent pseudo-thrombocytopenia in a horse. J Am Vet Med Assoc 1993;203(12):1715–6.

38. Duesterdieck-Zellmer KF, Riehl JH, Firshman AM, et al. Effects of abdominocentesis technique on peritoneal fluid and clinical variables in horses. Equine Vet Educ 2014;26(5):262–8.

39. Ekmann A, Rigdal M, Gondahl G. Automated counting of nucleated cells in equine synovial fluid without and with hyaluronidase pretreatment. Vet Clin Pathol 2010;39(1):83–9.

40. Garma-Acila A. Cytology of 100 samples of abdominal fluid from 100 horses with abdominal disease. Equine Vet J 1998;30:435–44.

41. Koreneck NL, Andrews FM, Maddux JM, et al. Determination of total protein concentration and viscosity of synovial fluid from the tibiotarsal joints of horses. Am J Vet Res 1992;53(5):781–4.

42. Krista KM, White NA, Barrett JK, et al. Evaluation of neutrophils apoptosis in horses with acute abdominal disease. Am J Vet Res 2013;74(7):999–1004.

43. Nelson AW. Analysis of equine peritoneal fluid. Vet Clin North Am Large Anim Pract 1979;1:267–74.

44. Roquet I, Hendrick S, Carmalt JL. The effect of blood contamination on equine synovial fluid analysis. Vet Comp Orthop Traumatol 2012;25(6):460–5.

45. Seabaugh KA, Goodrich LR, Morley PS, et al. Comparisons of peritoneal fluid values after laparoscopic cryptorchidectomy using a vessel-sealing device (Ligasure) versus a ligating loop and removal of the descended testis. Vet Surg 2013;42:600–6.

46. Tulamo RM, Bramladge LR, Gabel AA. Sequential clinical and synovial fluid changes associated with acute infectious arthritis in the horse. Equine Vet J 1989;21(5):325–31.

47. Apple FS, Collinson PO. Analytical characteristics of high-sensitivity cardiac troponin assays. Clin Chem 2012;58(1):54–61.

48. Rishniw M, Simpson KW. Cloning and sequencing of equine cardiac troponin I and confirmation of its usefulness as a target analyte for commercial troponin I analyzers. J Vet Diagn Invest 2005;17(6):582–4.

49. Rossi TM, Pyel WG, Maxie MG, et al. Troponin assays in the assessment of the equine myocardium. Equine Vet J 2014;46:270–5.

50. Nath LC, Anderson GA, Hinchcliff KW, et al. Serum cardiac troponin I concentrations in horses with cardiac disease. Aust Vet J 2012;90(9):351–7.

51. Kraus MS, Kaufer BB, Damiani A, et al. Elimination half-life of intravenously administered equine cardiac troponin I in healthy ponies. Equine Vet J 2013; 45(1):56–9.

52. Holbrook TC, Birks EK, Sleeper NN, et al. Endurance exercise is associated with increased plasma cardiac troponin I in horses. Equine Vet J Suppl 2006;36:27–31.

53. Nostell K, Haagstrom J. Resting concentrations of cardiac troponin I in fit horses and effect of racing. J Vet Cardiol 2008;10(2):105–9.

54. Phillips W, Giguere S, Franklin RP, et al. Cardiac troponin I in pastured and race training thoroughbred horses. J Vet Intern Med 2003;17:597–9.

55. Slack J, Boston R, Driessen B, et al. Effect of general anesthesia on plasma cardiac troponin I concentrations in healthy horses. J Vet Cardiol 2011;13(30):163–9.

56. Slack J, Boston RC, Soma L, et al. Cardiac troponin I in racing standardbreds. J Vet Intern Med 2012;27(5):1202–8.

57. SecoDias OM, Durando MM, Birks EK, et al. Cardiac troponin I concentrations in horses with colic. J Am Vet Med Assoc 2014;245:118–25.

58. Radcliffe RM, Divers TJ, Fletcher DJ, et al. Evaluation of L-lactate and cardiac troponin I in horses undergoing emergency abdominal surgery. J Vet Emerg Crit Care (San Antonio) 2012;22(3):313–9.

59. Mair TS, Pearson GR, Divers TJ. Malabsorption syndromes in the horse. Equine Vet Educ 2006;18:299–306.
60. Meyer J, Delay J, Bienzle D. Clinical, laboratory and histopathological features of equine lymphoma. Vet Pathol 2006;43:914–24.
61. Saulez MN, Cebra CK. Comparative biochemical analyses of venous blood and peritoneal fluid from horses with colic using a portable analyser and an in-house analyser. Vet Rec 2005;157(8):217–23.
62. Van Den Biim R, Butler CM, Sloet van Oldruitenborgh-Oosterbaan MM. The usability of peritoneal lactate concentration as a prognostic marker in horses with severe colic admitted to a veterinary teaching hospital. Equine Vet Educ 2010;22(8):420–5.
63. Johnston K, Holcombe SJ, Haputman JG. Plasma lactate as a predictor of colonic viability and survival after 360 degrees volvulus of the ascending colon in horses. Vet Surg 2007;36(6):563–7.
64. Pusteria N, Mapes S, Johnson C, et al. Comparison of feces versus rectal swabs for the molecular detection of Lawsonia intracellularis in foals with equine proliferative enteropathy. J Vet Diagn Invest 2010;24(3):622–7.
65. Bertin FR, Reising A, Slovis NM, et al. Clinical and clinicopathological factors associated with survival in 44 horses with equine neorickettsiosis (Potomac horse fever). J Vet Intern Med 2013;27:1528–34.
66. Diab SS, Rodriguez-Bartos A, Uzal FA. Pathology and diagnostic criteria of clostridium difficile enteric infection in horses. Vet Pathol 2013;50(6):1028–36.
67. Vannucci FA, Gebhart CJ. Recent advances in understanding the pathogenesis of Lawsonia intracellularis infections. Vet Pathol 2014;51(2):465–77.
68. Schumacher J, Edwards JF, Cohen ND. Chronic idiopathic inflammatory bowel disease of the horse. J Vet Intern Med 2000;14:258–65.
69. Lefebvre D, Pirie RS, Handel IG, et al. Clinical features and management of postoperative ileus (POI): survey of diplomates of the European Colleges of Equine Internal Medicine (ECEIM) and Veterinary Surgeons (ECVS). Equine Vet J 2014;9:545–53.
70. Durham AE, Newton JR, Smith KC, et al. Retrospective analysis of historical, clinical, ultrasonographic, serum biochemical and haematological data in prognostic evaluation of equine liver disease. Equine Vet J 2003;35(6):542–7.
71. Durham AE, Smith KC, Newton JR, et al. Development and application of a scoring system for prognostic evaluation of equine liver biopsies. Equine Vet J 2003;35(6):534–40.
72. Peek SF, Divers TJ. Medical treatment of cholangiohepatitic and cholelithiasis in mature horses: 9 cases (1991–1998). Equine Vet J 2000;32(4):301–6.
73. Peek SF. Cholangiohepatitis in the mature horse. Equine Vet Educ 2004;16:94–9.
74. Smith MR, Stevens KB, Durham AE, et al. Equine hepatic disease: the effect of patient and case specific variable on risk and prognosis. Equine Vet J 2003;35(6):549–52.
75. Dunkel B, McKenzie HC. Severe triglyceridemia in clinically ill horses: diagnosis, treatment and outcome. Equine Vet J 2003;35(6):590–5.
76. Snow DH, Harris P. Enzymes as markers of physical fitness and training of racing horses. Adv Clin Enzymolo 1988;6:251–8.
77. Bayly WM, Brobst DF, Elfers RS, et al. Serum and urinary biochemistry and enzyme changes in ponies with acute renal failure. Cornell Vet 1986;76(3):306–16.
78. Cohen ND, Peck KE, Smith SA, et al. Values of urine specific gravity for thoroughbred horses treated with furosemide prior to racing compared to untreated horses 2000. J Vet Diagn Invest 2002;14(3):231–5.

79. Divers TJ, Whitlock RH, Byars TD, et al. Acute renal failure in six horses resulting from hemodynamic causes. Equine Vet J 1987;19(1):178–84.
80. Edwards DH, Brownlee MA, Hutchins DR. Indices of renal function values in eight normal foals from birth to 56 days. Aust Vet J 1990;67(7):251–4.
81. Lefebvre HP, Dossin O, Trumel C, et al. Fractional excretion tests: a critical review of methods and applications in domestic animals. Vet Clin Pathol 2008;37(1):4–20.
82. Reed SM, Howe DK, Morrow JK, et al. Accurate antemortem diagnosis of equine protozoal myeloencephalitis (EPM) based on detection of intrathecal antibodies against sarcocystic neurona using the SNSAG2 and SnSAG4/3 Elisas. J Vet Intern Med 2013;27(12):1193–200.
83. Evans DL, Kiddell I, Smith SL. Pulmonary function measurements immediately after exercise are correlated with neutrophils percentage in tracheal aspirates in horses with poor racing performance. Res Vet Sci 2011;90(3):510–5.
84. Ivester KM, Couetil LL, Moore GE, et al. Environmental exposures and airway inflammation in young thoroughbred horses. J Vet Intern Med 2014;28:918–24.
85. Nolen-Watson RD, Harris M, Agnew ME, et al. Clinical and diagnostic features of inflammatory airway disease subtypes in horses examined because of poor performance: 98 cases (2004–2010). J Am Vet Med Assoc 2013;242(8):1138–45.
86. Fernandez NJ, Hecker KG, Gilroy CV, et al. Reliability of 400 cell and 5-field leukocyte differential counts for equine bronchioalveolar lavage fluid. Vet Clin Pathol 2013;42(1):92–8.
87. Copas V. Diagnosis and treatment of equine pleuropneumonia. Pract 2011;33(4):155–62.
88. Collins MB, Hodgson DR, Hutchins DR. Pleural effusion associated with acute and chronic pleuropneumonia and pleuritis secondary to thoracic wounds in horses: 43 cases (1982–1992). J Am Vet Med Assoc 1994;205(12):1753–8.
89. Beech J, Boston R, Lindborg S. Comparison of cortisol and ACTH responses after administration of thyrotropin releasing hormone in normal horses and those with pituitary pars intermedia dysfunction. J Vet Intern Med 2011;25:1431–8.
90. Durham AE, McGowan CM, Fey K, et al. Pituitary pars intermedia dysfunction: diagnosis and treatment. Equine Vet Educ 2014;26(4):216–23.
91. Frank N, Tadros EM. Insulin dysregulation. Equine Vet J 2014;46:102–22.
92. Morris DD, Garcia MC. Effects of phenylbutazone and anabolic steroids on adrenal and thyroid function tests in healthy horses. Am J Vet Res 1985;46(2):359–64.
93. Hilderbran AC, Breuhause BA, Refsal KR. Nonthyroidal illness syndrome in adult horses. J Vet Intern Med 2014;28:609–17.

Toxicology for the Equine Practitioner

Ahmad Al-Dissi, BVetSc, MSc, PhD

KEYWORDS

- Toxicology • Pathology • Equine • Gross lesions • Diagnosis

KEY POINTS

- The identification of gross lesions produced by toxins by equine practitioners is often the first step in formulating a diagnostic plan.
- Two structural toxicoses of the nervous system in horse which produce gross lesions are equine nigropallidal encephalomalacia (ENPE) and equine leukoencephalomalacia (ELM).
- The most common toxin responsible for liver failure in horses is pyrrolizidine alkaloid (PA).
- Red maple toxicosis and chronic sorghum poisoning produce detectable gross lesions within the kidney and urinary bladder, respectively.
- Toxicoses producing gross myocardial lesions in horses include a few plants, such as white snake root, and ionophore antimicrobials.
- Common gastrointestinal toxicosis producing gross lesions within the GI tract include Bister Beetle (Cantharidin) Toxicosis and Nonsteroidal Anti-inflammatory Drugs.

INTRODUCTION

A wide variety of toxins cause diseases in the horse and are investigated routinely by veterinarians and veterinary pathologists trying to identify the cause of illness and death. A complete investigation always involves performing a thorough necropsy and requires macroscopic and microscopic examination of lesions and a variety of laboratory testing to obtain an accurate diagnosis. The identification of gross lesions by equine practitioners is often the first step in formulating a diagnostic plan. Therefore, the accurate identification of such lesions is invaluable for making a correct diagnosis.

A comprehensive discussion of equine toxicoses is beyond the scope of this article, which provides a brief description of selected common toxins producing detectable gross lesions in horses in North America. Thus, this article should be useful to equine practitioners and veterinary pathologists investigating a toxicology-related death. An organ system approach has been adopted.

Department of Veterinary Pathology, Western College of Veterinary Medicine, University of Saskatchewan, 52 Campus Drive, Saskatoon, Saskatchewan S7N 5B4, Canada
E-mail address: ahmad.aldissi@usask.ca

Vet Clin Equine 31 (2015) 269–279
http://dx.doi.org/10.1016/j.cveq.2015.04.009   vetequine.theclinics.com

TOXINS AFFECTING THE NERVOUS SYSTEM

Toxins affecting the nervous system can be categorized into two main groups based on mechanism of toxicoses: structural toxicoses and functional toxicoses. Toxins affecting the structure of the nervous system may harm one or more of three components (neurons, axons, or myelin) resulting in a neuropathy, axonopathy, or myelinopathy, respectively. Structural toxicoses commonly result in detectable lesions at the gross and/or microscopic level, which facilitate their diagnosis. However, functional toxicoses do not result in detectable lesions and exert their effects by interfering with neurotransmitter synthesis, storage, release, binding, reuptake, or degradation. Alteration of action potential mediated by effects on sodium, potassium, chloride, or calcium channels can also result in functional toxicoses.[1] The diagnosis of functional toxicoses can be difficult and often requires laboratory testing. This section focuses on two structural toxicoses of the horse: equine nigropallidal encephalomalacia (ENPE) and equine leukoencephalomalacia (ELM).

Equine Nigropallidal Encephalomalacia

ENPE is a disease of horses with resemblance to Parkinson disease. Two plants in the Asteraceae family are known to cause ENPE: yellow star-thistle (*Centaurea solstitialis*) and Russian knapweed (*Acroptilon repens*). Repin, a constituent within the two toxic plants, is thought to be the toxic principle responsible for the development of this disease.[2] The exact mechanism by which repin causes ENPE is uncertain. However, a limited body of experimental evidence points to a role for the glutathione redox system.[3,4] Other compounds, such as cynaropicrin and solstitialin, have been found to be cytotoxic in primary cultures of rat substantia nigra cells and may also be involved.[5]

Clinical signs often appear suddenly after the prolonged ingestion of the toxic plants for 4 to 11 weeks and include paralysis of the lip and tongue with inability to eat and drink resulting in emaciation and death.[6,7] Complete blood count and serum chemistry are often normal, and there seems to be no way to predict the onset of this disease.

Grossly and histologically, ENPE results in bilateral, symmetric, focal necrosis and malacia of the globus pallidus and/or substantia nigra. Such lesions may bear resemblance to Parkinson disease in which the substania nigra compacta displays loss of dopaminergic neurons and Lewy body formation.[8] However, a recent report examining brain lesions in 10 horses affected by ENPE showed that ENPE lesions are actually present within the substanitia nigra reticulata, with sparing of cell bodies of dopaminergic neurons in substania nigra compacta. It was suggested that ENPE may serve as a large animal model of environmentally acquired toxic parkinsonism, with clinical phenotype directly attributable to lesions in globus pallidus and substantia nigra pars reticulata rather than to the destruction of dopaminergic neurons.[9] Diagnosis of ENPE is often confirmed by postmortem examination of the brain; however, MRI can be used to detect lesions in affected areas of the brain antemortem.

Equine Leukoencephalomalacia

ELM is caused by ingestion of corn contaminated with the fungus *Fusarium moniliforme*, which grows in warm and moist conditions and produces a group of mycotoxins known as fumonisins.[10] Fumonisins are natural contaminants of corn and corn-based rations and also occur infrequently in sorghum, asparagus, rice, beer, and mung beans.[11]

The exact mechanism by which fumonisins cause ELM is unknown; however, fumonisin B1 is thought to be the primary mycotoxin responsible for the development of the disease. Fumonisin B1 is known to interfere with sphingolipid biosynthesis by inhibiting the enzyme ceramide synthase, which results in the accumulation of bioactive intermediates of sphingolipid metabolism leading to cell death.[12,13]

Horses are very susceptible to fumonisin B1 toxicity, which mainly targets the central nervous system; however, lesions within the liver and less commonly the heart may also be found.[10] Neurotoxicity occurs after 3 to 4 weeks of daily ingestion of contaminated feed. Clinical signs appear suddenly and include tongue paralysis, aimless circling, incoordination, head pressing, and blindness. The clinical course of the disease can be short with death occurring shortly after the sudden onset of clinical signs. The disorder may occur as an outbreak with morbidity reaching 100% and older horses being more susceptible. Grossly, the surface of the brain may be unaltered, although gyri overlying areas of leukoencephalomalacia may appear slightly flattened.

Diagnosis requires sectioning the brain to examine the white matter, which often has random malacic foci of variable sizes that appear as a soft, pulpy, gray depression within the white matter. More severe cases display white matter cavitation and marked hemorrhage. Histologically, the areas of malacia are mainly in the white matter but a few small loci may be seen in the cortex. The irregular cavitations may follow or surround blood vessels, with edema and separation of the white matter at the periphery of cavitated areas. Infiltrations with eosinophils and plasma cells are often present. Lesions can also be found within the brainstem and the spinal cord; however, the gray matter is often more affected than the white matter particularly within the spinal cord. Liver lesions are similar to those found in aflatoxicosis.[10] Diagnosis is often made at necropsy by detecting appropriate lesions with associated history and clinical signs.

TOXINS AFFECTING THE LIVER AND BILIARY SYSTEM

The liver is highly susceptible to toxins because of its role in excretion of xenobiotics. Toxins taken orally reach the liver through the portal system and are metabolized by a group of enzymes known as mixed-function oxidases. These enzymes usually increase the water solubility of metabolized compounds but occasionally produce more toxic metabolites. Depending on the dose and the duration of exposure the toxic injury results in hepatic necrosis, fibrosis, bile duct proliferation, regeneration, and variable degrees of inflammation. Toxins affecting the liver include natural toxins produced by plants and fungi and industrial toxins, such as chemicals, drugs, and heavy metals. The most common toxin responsible for liver failure in horses is pyrrolizidine alkaloid (PA). Less common causes include mycotoxicosis and alsike clover poisoning. This section only focuses on PA toxicosis.

Pyrrolizidine Alkaloid Toxicosis

PAs are a group of different compounds found in more than 6000 plants. Most of the toxic plant species contain more than one PA, of which approximately 600 have been chemically identified to date. In North America, PA toxicity is caused by the prolonged ingestion of four plant genera: (1) Senecio, (2) Crotalaria, (3) Cynoglossum, and (4) Amsinckia. Senecio species are the most common source of PA poisoning worldwide.[14,15] Three species of Senecio are responsible for most PA poisoning in the western United States: (1) tansy ragwort (S jacobaea), (2) threadleaf or wooly groundsel (S douglasii var. longilobus),[16] and (3) Riddell's groundsel (S riddellii).[17,18] The PA content of Senecio plants generally increases with maturation and reaches a maximum just before the opening of the flower buds.[19] The greatest amount of PAs is found within flowers, whereas seeds of Crotalaria and Amsinckia concentrate high levels of PA.[20,21]

PA poisoning in horses occurs after chronic exposure, with exposure times ranging from 2 weeks to several months. Poisoning can occur at any time of the year after pasture grazing or ingestion of contaminated hay or grain, because fresh and dried plants are considered toxic.[22] Toxicity is mediated by PA metabolites, which are dehydropyrrolizidine derivatives (pyrrolic esters) that bind and disrupt DNA, RNA, and other cellular proteins.[23] Therefore, most PAs are primarily hepatotoxic and inhibit DNA synthesis and mitosis.[24] A few hepatocytes are able to replicate their DNA without undergoing mitosis resulting in the formation of large hepatocytes or "megalocytes," which are seen histologically. Megalocyte formation is not pathognomonic for PA toxicity because it is also seen in aflatoxicosis. Rarely the lung and the kidney are also affected in PA toxicoses. A wide range of tissues are affected when *Crotalaria* is the cause of PA toxicity; notably, monocrotaline causes diffuse lung injury, leading to pulmonary edema and fibrosis.[22]

Clinically, horses display signs of hepatic encephalopathy with head-pressing and compulsive walking. Photosensitization may be seen in surviving animals.[22] On gross examination, the liver can become firm secondary to fibrosis and atrophic because hepatocytes are lost faster than they can be replaced. Multiple regenerative nodules can also be seen except when the toxicosis is caused by *Heliotropium* ingestion. Histologically, there is diffuse fibrosis, bile ductule proliferation hepatocellular necrosis, and megalocytosis.[25]

PA plants can be readily identified through examination of the total diet including grain, hay, silage, haylage, and pasture. A few laboratories also offer pyrrole analysis of blood and liver tissue, although this is not routinely performed on suspect cases.[22] Differential diagnosis for toxins affecting the equine liver include alsike clover and aflatoxicosis, both of which are uncommon in horses.

TOXINS AFFECTING THE URINARY SYSTEM

The kidney is a primary target for toxicity because of its high perfusion. Toxins affecting the kidney can be categorized into two groups: exogenous toxins and endogenous toxins. Exogenous toxins include a long list of chemicals, drugs, plants, and metals, whereas endogenous toxins include hemoglobin myoglobin and bilirubin. Both endogenous and exogenous toxins cause tubular necrosis with proximal convoluted tubules being most susceptible. With the exception of hemoglobinuric nephrosis, acute renal toxicity is difficult to detect grossly, but often results in pale and swollen cortex, which bulges on cut section. Regeneration can occur if tubular basement membrane remained intact. Chronic toxicoses result in renal fibrosis causing the kidney to be pale and shrunken with irregular surface. Unlike the kidney, lesions within the urinary bladder are easily detected grossly. Two toxins can cause gross lesions within the equine urinary bladder and include cantharidin toxicoses and chronic cyanide poisoning. This section discusses two toxicoses producing detectable gross lesions within the renal system: red maple and sorghum toxicoses. Cantharidin toxicosis is discussed later with the gastrointestinal (GI) system.

Red Maple Toxicosis

Although red maple is not considered a primary renal toxicosis, gross changes within the kidney provide an important clue for the diagnosis. Red maple (*Acer rubrum*), which is also called soft maple or swamp, is a tree native to the eastern part of North America. The ingestion of red maple leaves is known to cause oxidative damage to red blood cells causing severe hemolytic anemia in multiple species.[26] Gallic acid and tannic acid are believed to be the primary oxidants within red maple; however, pyrogallol, a metabolite of gallic acid, may also contribute to oxidant-induced damage. In vitro studies have shown that pyrogallol has a higher capacity to induce methemoglobin in equine erythrocytes than tannic acid and gallic acid.[27] Toxicity can occur during the spring and the fall because fresh and dry leaves are toxic. However, toxicity is more often associated with ingestion of wilted or dried leaves during the fall, which may remain toxic for weeks or more. Ingestion of 1.5 to 3 g of leaves per kilogram body-weight in horses results in a hemolytic crisis resulting in death within 18 to 24 hours in severe cases.

Clinical signs may develop within 2 to 6 days and include depression, lethargy, tachycardia, tachypnea with icteric mucous membranes, and hemoglobinuria (dark brown urine). Pregnant mares may abort without showing any clinical signs.[28,29] Hematologic abnormalities include anemia, methemoglobinemia, increased mean corpuscular hemoglobin concentration (MCHC) and mean corpuscular hemoglobin (MCH), free plasma hemoglobin, anisocytosis, poikilocytosis, eccentrocytes, lysed erythrocytes that produce fragments or membrane ghosts, agglutination, and Heinz bodies.[29]

Grossly dark brown to black kidneys from hemoglobinuric nephrosis, generalized icterus, and splenomegaly are seen. Histologic lesions include renal tubular epithelial degeneration and necrosis with intratubular hemoglobin casts and hepatocyte degeneration in centrilobular areas.[25] Diagnosis is based on history of ingestion of plant material with appropriate clinical signs and hematologic and pathologic findings. Differential diagnoses include copper and nitrate toxicosis, equine infectious anemia, and babesiosis.

Sorghum Toxicosis

Chronic sorghum consumption in horses, and less commonly cattle, results in cystitis and posterior ataxia (sorghum cystitis and ataxia syndrome). Although sorghum toxicity is not a primary toxicosis of the urinary system, gross lesions are often found within the urinary bladder. Sorghum species are drought-tolerant plants found primarily in the southwestern United States. The syndrome develops in horses after grazing hybrid Sudan pastures for weeks to months and produces axonal degeneration and myelomalacia in the spinal cord and cauda equina.[30,31]

Clinically, horses present with posterior ataxia, progressing to irreversible flaccid paralysis, and urinary incontinence caused by overflow from a distended, atonic bladder and resulting in alopecia on the hind legs. The loss of urinary bladder function is related to axonal degeneration, and demyelination within the spinal cord and the cauda equina predisposes horses to cystitis. Perineal muscle relaxation, protrusion of the penis, and tail paresis can also be seen. Fatal poisoning is infrequent, although affected horses may die from cystitis and pyelonephritis. Treatment with antibiotics can be helpful, but a full recovery is rare if ataxia develops. Lathyrogenic nitriles, such as β-cyanoalanine, cyanogenic glycosides, and nitrates, have been suggested as causative agents.[32,33]

Gross alopecia of the hind limbs is often present. The bladder mucosa can be thick and hemorrhagic and the urine may be red or contain pus. Similar lesions can be found within the renal pelvis caused by an ascending infection. Histologically, there is axonal degeneration and demyelination at all levels of the cord but most prominent caudally in ventral and lateral funiculi. Lesions within the urinary bladder and the kidney include neutrophilic to lymphoplasmacytic inflammation with necrosis and hemorrhage.[25] Diagnosis depends on the history of sorghum consumption and the clinical signs of posterior ataxia and urinary incontinence and gross and histologic lesions.[1]

TOXINS AFFECTING THE CARDIOVASCULAR SYSTEM

Drugs, chemicals, and plants can produce toxic effects on the heart. Common equine myocardial toxicoses in North America include ionophore antimicrobials (eg, monensin, lasalocid), blister beetles (discussed later), many plants, and rarely mycotoxins.

Most plant toxicoses affecting the equine myocardium result in sudden onset of clinical signs and fall into the alkaloid and glycoside groups. An alkaloid is a nitrogen base containing organic compound that has a pharmacologic effect in animals and humans. Plant-derived toxic alkaloids generally affect the passage of ions across membranes leading to various disturbances causing cardiac arrhythmia. A glycoside is a molecule containing a sugar group that is bound to another functional group via a glycosidic bond. Cardiac glycosides inhibit the transmembrane sodium-potassium ATPase pump causing a rise in intracellular sodium and calcium, which in turn results in increased force of myocardial contraction. Toxicoses resulting from the accidental ingestion of plants containing toxic alkaloids and cardiac glycosides usually produce minimal or no gross lesions in horses and can be difficult to diagnose. Toxicoses producing gross myocardial lesions in horses include a few plants, such as white snake root, and ionophore antimicrobials, which are discussed briefly.

Ionophore Toxicosis

Ionophores are added to bovine and poultry rations to increase feed efficiency and weight gain of beef and dairy cattle and control coccidiosis, respectively. Examples include monensin, lasalocid, salinomycin, narasin, and maduramicin.[34] Ionophores affect cellular transmembrane transport of electrolytes and, when present in excess, ionophores damage skeletal and cardiac muscles. Ionophores form complexes with cations, such as Na^+ and Ca^+, to facilitate their transport across cell membranes in exchange for H^+ and K^+ ions. The increase in intracellular Ca^+ and Na^+ is thought to result in cell membrane injury and dysfunction causing mitochondrial swelling and decreased ATP production.[35]

Horses are very susceptible to ionophore toxicity even at extremely low concentrations. Toxicity occurs through the consumption of ruminant feed containing ionophores; horse feed accidentally contaminated in a mill producing horse, poultry, and cattle feeds; and horse feed accidentally mixed with ionophores.[1] Clinical findings include anorexia, stiffness, and weakness especially in hind quarters progressing to ataxia. Polyurea and myoglobin urea may also be present. Subsequent congestive heart failure may be seen in surviving animals.[36]

Ionophores cause acute cardiac rhabdomyocyte degeneration and necrosis. Postmortem lesions of ionophore toxicity may be difficult to detect in acute cases dying within 24 hours. Unlike sheep and swine, in which skeletal muscles are the main site of damage, gross lesions in horses are mainly present within the heart where ill-defined pale streaks may be visible in the myocardium.[25] Microscopic lesions of ionophore toxicity typically are monophasic (ie, of the same duration) and indicate a single insult. Lesions of severe acute myocardial loss and necrosis are often found in acute toxicity, whereas myocardial fibrosis and loss is seen in chronic sublethal doses.[25]

Diagnosis of poisoning depends on history of ingestion of ionophore-contaminated feed; clinical signs of excessive intolerance, heart failure, and myoglobinurea; and elevated serum muscle enzymes. Confirmation can be made by analyzing feed and stomach content for ionophores.[1]

White Snake Root (Eupatorium rugosum)

White snakeroot is found in many of the wooded areas of central and eastern United States and also in eastern Canada.[37,38] Tremetol is the toxic compound, which becomes toxic after its metabolic activation by hepatic cytochrome P-450 enzymes. Tremetol is a cumulative poison; thus, it is not uncommon to see toxicosis occurring after repeated exposure to small amounts over a prolonged period.[39] The toxin is excreted in the milk more rapidly than by any other route, which often results in toxicosis in nursing animals without or early before maternal toxicity. The mechanism by which tremetol causes toxicity remains unknown; however, it has been suggested that tremetol inhibits the tricarboxylic acid cycle resulting in dysfunction of mitochondrial oxidative phosphorylation.[37,38]

The onset of clinical signs is often slow to develop and not particularly distinctive at first. Poisoned horses develop trembles, unsteady gait, sweating, and swallowing difficulties. Cardiac changes include arrhythmias, jugular distention, and ventral edema. Increased aspartate aminotransferase, lactate dehydrogenase, and creatine kinase serum enzyme activities are also seen.[1]

Lesions of white snakeroot poisoning can be acute or chronic in nature depending on the duration and the level of exposure. On postmortem examination, pale white to tan areas and linear streaks throughout the myocardium are seen. Microscopically, lesions include multifocal myocardial degeneration and necrosis with vacuolation of myocardial cytoplasm, loss of cross-striation, fragmentation of rhabdomyocytes, and cytoplasmic hypereosinophilia with nuclear pyknosis and karyolysis. Diagnosis depends on history of repeated exposure to white snakeroot and clinical signs and pathologic lesions.[25]

Other plants causing gross myocardial lesions in horses include cottonseed (*Gossypium* spp) and senna or coffee senna plant (*Cassia occidentalis* or *C obtusifolia*).

TOXINS AFFECTING THE GASTROINTESTINAL SYSTEM
Bister Beetle (Cantharidin) Toxicosis

The Meloidae family of blister beetles contains more than 200 species of beetles within North America, which contain the toxin cantharidin at different levels. Beetles are often killed and trapped within hay during harvesting.[40] Because beetles swarm for mating purposes, large numbers can be trapped with a single flake of hay. Cantharidin is produced by mature males and is passed to females during copulation, which later incorporates it into eggs to deter feeding by other insects. The minimum lethal oral dose of cantharidin in horses is estimated at 0.5 mg/kg bodyweight. It is known that males of *Epicauta funebris* can synthesize up to 17 mg of cantharidin representing 10% of their live weight, and thus the ingestion of 4 to 6 g of dried beetles can be fatal.[41]

Clinically, horses affected by this toxicosis have an acute onset of colic with restlessness, sweating, grunting, pawing, trembling, and an increased heart and respiratory rate. Frequent urination or straining to urinate small volumes can be seen. The urine can be red and may even contain blood clots. Serum calcium and magnesium are often decreased and help differentiate this toxicosis from other causes of equine colic. Mortality can be 50%.[42]

Cantharidin is corrosive to surface epithelial cells causing inflammation, necrosis, and ulceration of the mucosa of the GI tract and acantholysis and vesicle formation after contact with skin or mucous membranes.[43] Gross lesions of blister beetle toxicosis reflect the irritant nature of cantharidin and range from hyperemia to necrosis and hemorrhage within the esophagus, stomach, intestine, urinary bladder, and ureters. Myocardial necrosis can also be seen.[25]

Diagnosis is often based on history of hay consumption; clinical signs of colic with decreased serum calcium and magnesium; lesions within the GI system, the urinary system, and the heart; and the chemical detection of cantharidin in GI contents, urine, or serum.[41,42]

Nonsteroidal Anti-inflammatory Drugs

Nonsteroidal anti-inflammatory drugs (NSAIDs) are commonly used in horses because of their anti-inflammatory, antipyretic, and analgesic properties. NSAIDS are used to treat a variety of conditions including colic, endotoxemia, and musculo-skeletal disorders. Because of their narrow therapeutic range, NSAID toxicosis may occur in horses administered excessive doses. The risk of toxicity is exacerbated in horses with sepsis or dehydration even when therapeutic doses are administered.

The mechanism by which NSAIDs exert their therapeutic and toxic effects is related to their ability to inhibit the cyclooxygenase enzyme (COX) resulting in decreased prostaglandin synthesis. Two isoforms of COX have been identified: COX-1 and COX-2.[1] Because COX-1 is constitutively expressed, its main role is related to maintaining physiologic homeostasis. In contrast to COX-1, the expression of COX-2 is inducible and is found in many inflammatory and other cell types during inflammation. It has been hypothesized that NSAIDS that nonselectively inhibit both COX-1 and COX-2 have greater toxic potential because they not only decrease prostaglandins mediating inflammation, but also prostaglandins necessary for physiologic homeostasis.[44] NSAIDS that are selective inhibitors of COX-2 are thought to be less toxic; nonetheless, most of the NSAIDS used in horses are nonselective inhibitors of the COX enzyme, which increases the risk of adverse effects associated with their use. Although the nonselective inhibition theory is still valid, recent evidence suggests that this theory is overly simplistic. COX-1 is actually partially inducible and may play a role in inflammation and COX-2 can be induced in physiologic conditions without the presence of inflammation.[45,46] Thus, other factors not necessarily related to COX may also play a role in toxicity.

Common targets for NSAID toxicity include the GI tract and the kidney.[47] NSAID toxicity is known to cause ulceration anywhere within the GI tract. Two syndromes related to NSAID administrate are recognized to occur within the GI tract of horses: gastric ulceration and right dorsal ulcerative colitis. The inhibition of COX within the stomach is thought to decrease bicarbonate and mucous secretion while increasing acid output, impairing vasodilation, and diminishing epithelial restitution eventually leading to gastric ulceration.[48] Within the GI tract, the inhibition of COX-1 activity is thought to cause impairment of mucosal circulation leading to hypoxia and thrombosis resulting in mucosal epithelial ulceration.[25] It is unknown why the right dorsal colon is most commonly affected. In the kidney, prostaglandins are part of the vasodilative autoregulatory response to renal hypoperfusion; thus, hypovolemia, severe hemorrhage, and renal disease may increase the risk of renal toxicosis caused by NSAID administration.[25] The lesion is primarily seen within the renal papilla (renal papillary necrosis) and may lead to loss of urine concentration ability and renal failure and may predispose to nephrolithiasis or ureterolithiasis.

Clinical signs in horses with dorsal ulcerative colitis include colic, diarrhea, and weight loss and often appear days to weeks after NSAID administration making diagnosis a challenge. Hypoproteinemia and hypoalbuminemia are often present presumably from loss of protein through inflamed and ulcerated GI mucosa. Horses with oral ulceration may have difficulty in mastication and hypersalivation. Esophageal ulceration may result in pain and difficulty during swallowing evidenced by groaning and neck stretching.[1] Diagnosis of NSAID toxicity can be made based on history of NSAID administration with appropriate clinical signs and pathologic lesions.

REFERENCES

1. Gupta RC. Veterinary toxicology basic and clinical principles. 1st edition. Amsterdam; Boston: Elsevier; Academic Press; 2007.
2. Robles M, Choi BH, Han B, et al. Repin-induced neurotoxicity in rodents. Exp Neurol 1998;152(1):129–36.

3. Tukov FF, Anand S, Gadepalli RS, et al. Inactivation of the cytotoxic activity of repin, a sesquiterpene lactone from *Centaurea repens*. Chem Res Toxicol 2004;17(9):1170–6.

4. Tukov FF, Rimoldi JM, Matthews JC. Characterization of the role of glutathione in repin-induced mitochondrial dysfunction, oxidative stress and dopaminergic neurotoxicity in rat pheochromocytoma (PC12) cells. Neurotoxicology 2004; 25(6):989–99.

5. Cheng CH, Costall B, Hamburger M, et al. Toxic effects of solstitialin A 13-acetate and cynaropicrin from *Centaurea solstitialis L.* (Asteraceae) in cell cultures of foetal rat brain. Neuropharmacology 1992;31(3):271–7.

6. Young S, Brown WW, Klinger B. Nigropallidal encephalomalacia in horses caused by ingestion of weeds of the genus *Centaurea*. J Am Vet Med Assoc 1970; 157(11):1602–5.

7. Young S, Brown WW, Klinger B. Nigropallidal encephalomalacia in horses fed Russian knapweed–*Centaurea repens* L. Am J Vet Res 1970;31(8):1393–404.

8. Dickson DW, Braak H, Duda JE, et al. Neuropathological assessment of Parkinson's disease: refining the diagnostic criteria. Lancet Neurol 2009;8(12):1150–7.

9. Chang HT, Rumbeiha WK, Patterson JS, et al. Toxic equine parkinsonism: an immunohistochemical study of 10 horses with nigropallidal encephalomalacia. Vet Pathol 2012;49(2):398–402.

10. Voss KA, Smith GW, Haschek WM. Fumonisins: toxicokinetics, mechanism of action and toxicity. Animal Feed Science and Technology 2007;137(3–4):299–325.

11. Doko MB, Canet C, Brown N, et al. Natural co-occurrence of fumonisins and zearalenone in cereals and cereal-based foods from eastern and southern Africa. J Agric Food Chem 1996;44(10):3240–3.

12. Wang E, Norred WP, Bacon CW, et al. Inhibition of sphingolipid biosynthesis by fumonisins. Implications for diseases associated with *Fusarium moniliforme*. J Biol Chem 1991;266(22):14486–90.

13. Wang E, Ross PF, Wilson TM, et al. Increases in serum sphingosine and sphinganine and decreases in complex sphingolipids in ponies given feed containing fumonisins, mycotoxins produced by *Fusarium moniliforme*. J Nutr 1992;122(8): 1706–16.

14. de Barros CS, Driemeier D, Pilati C, et al. *Senecio* spp poisoning in cattle in southern Brazil. Vet Hum Toxicol 1992;34(3):241–6.

15. Odriozola E, Campero C, Casaro A, et al. Pyrrolizidine alkaloidosis in Argentinian cattle caused by *Senecio selloi*. Vet Hum Toxicol 1994;36(3):205–8.

16. Johnson AE, Molyneux RJ. Toxicity of threadleaf groundsel (*Senecio douglasii var longilobus*) to cattle. Am J Vet Res 1984;45(1):26–31.

17. Johnson AE, Molyneux RJ, Stuart LD. Toxicity of Riddell's groundsel (*Senecio riddellii*) to cattle. Am J Vet Res 1985;46(3):577–82.

18. Molyneux RJ, Johnson AE, Olsen JD, et al. Toxicity of pyrrolizidine alkaloids from Riddell groundsel (*Senecio riddellii*) to cattle. Am J Vet Res 1991;52(1):146–51.

19. Candrian U, Luethy J, Schmid P, et al. Stability of pyrrolizidine alkaloids in hay and silage. J Agric Food Chem 1984;32(4):935–7.

20. Johnson AE, Smart RA. Effects on cattle and their calves of tansy ragwort (*Senecio jacobaea*) fed in early gestation. Am J Vet Res 1983;44(7):1215–9.

21. Nobre D, Dagli ML, Haraguchi M. *Crotalaria juncea* intoxication in horses. Vet Hum Toxicol 1994;36(5):445–8.

22. Stegelmeier BL. Pyrrolizidine alkaloid-containing toxic plants (*Senecio, Crotalaria, Cynoglossum, Amsinckia, Heliotropium,* and *Echium* spp.). Vet Clin North Am Food Anim Pract 2011;27(2):419–28, ix.

23. Fu PP, Xia Q, Lin G, et al. Pyrrolizidine alkaloids: genotoxicity, metabolism enzymes, metabolic activation, and mechanisms. Drug Metab Rev 2004;36(1):1–55.
24. Stegelmeier BL, Gardner DR, James LF, et al. Pyrrole detection and the pathologic progression of *Cynoglossum officinale* (houndstongue) poisoning in horses. J Vet Diagn Invest 1996;8(1):81–90.
25. Maxie M. Jubb, Kennedy & Palmer's pathology of domestic animals. 5th edition. Philadelphia: Elsevier Saunders; 2007.
26. Walter KM, Moore CE, Bozorgmanesh R, et al. Oxidant-induced damage to equine erythrocytes from exposure to *Pistacia atlantica*, *Pistacia terebinthus*, and *Pistacia chinensis*. J Vet Diagn Invest 2014;26(6):821–6.
27. Agrawal K, Ebel JG, Altier C, et al. Identification of protoxins and a microbial basis for red maple (Acer rubrum) toxicosis in equines. J Vet Diagn Invest 2013;25(1):112–9.
28. George LW, Divers TJ, Mahaffey EA, et al. Heinz body anemia and methemoglobinemia in ponies given red maple (Acer rubrum L.) leaves. Vet Pathol 1982; 19(5):521–33.
29. Alward A, Corriher CA, Barton MH, et al. Red maple (Acer rubrum) leaf toxicosis in horses: a retrospective study of 32 cases. J Vet Intern Med 2006;20(5): 1197–201.
30. Morgan SE, Johnson B, Brewer B, et al. Sorghum cystitis ataxia syndrome in horses. Vet Hum Toxicol 1990;32(6):582.
31. Van Kampen KR. Sudan grass and sorghum poisoning of horses: a possible lathyrogenic disease. J Am Vet Med Assoc 1970;156(5):629–30.
32. Adams LG, Dollahite JW, Romane WM, et al. Cystitis and ataxia associated with sorghum ingestion by horses. J Am Vet Med Assoc 1969;155(3):518–24.
33. Knight PR. Equine cystitis and ataxia associated with grazing of pastures dominated by sorghum species. Aust Vet J 1968;44(5):257.
34. Plumlee KH. Clinical veterinary toxicology. St Louis (MO): Mosby; 2004.
35. Zachary JF, McGavin MD. Pathologic basis of veterinary disease + veterinary consult. St Louis (MO): Mosby Inc; 2011.
36. Smith BP. Large animal internal medicine. 3rd edition. St Louis (MO): Mosby; 2002.
37. Panter KE, James LF. Natural plant toxicants in milk: a review. J Anim Sci 1990; 68(3):892–904.
38. Sharma OP, Dawra RK, Kurade NP, et al. A review of the toxicosis and biological properties of the genus *Eupatorium*. Nat Toxins 1998;6(1):1–14.
39. Beier RC, Norman JO. The toxic factor in white snakeroot: identity, analysis and prevention. Vet Hum Toxicol 1990;32(Suppl):81–8.
40. Schmitz DG. Cantharidin toxicosis in horses. J Vet Intern Med 1989;3(4):208–15.
41. Edwards WC, Edwards RM, Ogden L, et al. Cantharidin content of two species of Oklahoma blister beetles associated with toxicosis in horses. Vet Hum Toxicol 1989;31(5):442–4.
42. Helman RG, Edwards WC. Clinical features of blister beetle poisoning in equids: 70 cases (1983-1996). J Am Vet Med Assoc 1997;211(8):1018–21.
43. Ray AC, Kyle AL, Murphy MJ, et al. Etiologic agents, incidence, and improved diagnostic methods of cantharidin toxicosis in horses. Am J Vet Res 1989; 50(2):187–91.
44. Lees P, Toutain PL. Pharmacokinetics, pharmacodynamics, metabolism, toxicology and residues of phenylbutazone in humans and horses. Vet J 2013; 196(3):294–303.
45. Ricciotti E, FitzGerald GA. Prostaglandins and inflammation. Arterioscler Thromb Vasc Biol 2011;31(5):986–1000.

46. Ehmke H, Kurtz A. Deciphering the physiological roles of COX-2. Am J Physiol Regul Integr Comp Physiol 2003;284:R486–7.
47. Rotting AK, Freeman DE, Constable PD, et al. Effects of phenylbutazone, indomethacin, prostaglandin E2, butyrate, and glutamine on restitution of oxidant-injured right dorsal colon of horses in vitro. Am J Vet Res 2004;65(11):1589–95.
48. Peskar BM. Role of cyclooxygenase isoforms in gastric mucosal defense and ulcer healing. Inflammopharmacology 2005;13(1–3):15–26.

Neurologic Diseases in Horses

Raquel Rech, DVM, MSc, PhD[a],*, Claudio Barros, DVM, PhD[b]

KEYWORDS

- Equine disease • Brain • Spinal cord • Gross lesions • Diagnosis

KEY POINTS

- Location of the lesion based on a thorough neurologic examination, gross examination of the nervous system, and adequate tissue collection and preservation are important steps toward the definitive diagnosis of neurologic diseases in horses.
- The most common diagnostic tools for neurologic diseases include histopathology, viral isolation, fluorescent antibody test, polymerase chain reaction, immunohistochemistry, and bacterial and fungal culture.

INTRODUCTION

Neurologic diseases are often fatal and are one of the most common reasons for euthanasia in horses. Necropsy is needed to confirm the clinical diagnosis and/or differential diagnoses. One of the most challenging and demanding tasks for a practitioner is to perform a field necropsy in cases of equine neurologic disease that requires removal of the brain, spinal cord, ganglia, and peripheral nerves. Sampling the nervous system of a horse takes the same amount of time than evaluating all other organs during a necropsy. However, it is almost impossible to diagnose a neurologic disease unless the nervous system is examined, with the possible exception of hepatic encephalopathy (HEP) when the pathologist can infer the brain lesion from the lesions observed in the liver.

Despite the general concern about how fast postmortem (PM) changes set in the central nervous system (CNS) tissue, the brain and spinal cord are relatively protected from PM autolysis and putrefaction when compared with other organs such as those of the gastrointestinal tract. The CNS is further away from the ports of entry of PM proliferated bacteria; being encased by a relatively thin osseous case, almost deprived of adipose and other insulating tissues, it can disperse heat and remain cooler than

[a] Department of Veterinary Pathobiology, College of Veterinary Medicine & Biomedical Sciences, Texas A&M University, 402 Raymond Stotzer Parkway, College Station, TX 77843, USA;
[b] Laboratory of Anatomic Pathology, College of Veterinary Medicine & Animal Husbandry, Federal University of Mato Grosso do Sul, Avenida Senador Filinto Müller 2443, Campo Grande, Mato Grosso do Sul 79074-460, Brazil
* Corresponding author.
E-mail address: rrech@cvm.tamu.edu

Vet Clin Equine 31 (2015) 281–306
http://dx.doi.org/10.1016/j.cveq.2015.04.010
0749-0739/15/$ – see front matter © 2015 Elsevier Inc. All rights reserved.

other organs. Brain and spinal cord sampled from a horse dead from 24 to 36 hours will still have useful information.

This article is divided in 3 topics: (1) gross examination of the CNS, (2) main neurologic diseases approached by the affected neuroanatomic site, and (3) recommended diagnostic methods for definitive diagnosis of neurologic diseases (**Table 1**).

Removal of the Brain and Spinal Cord

The removal of the brain was already covered elsewhere in this issue by Chad Frank and colleagues. Sampling the entire spinal cord is necessary for the diagnosis of many neurologic diseases in horses because lesions are often located in this area. Although a laborious process, the easiest way to take a spinal cord from a horse in the field is to use a human spinal cord remover (Mopec, Oak Park, MI) (**Fig. 1**A). First, with a handsaw, cut the vertebral column in segments of 40 to 50 cm each (see **Fig. 1**B). Next, grasp the dura mater using a rat tooth forceps (see **Fig. 1**C) and insert the spinal cord remover in the epidural space on each lateral side of the spinal cord to cut the nerve rootlets off. Then, pull the spinal cord covered by dura mater out of the spinal canal. Because multiple segments of the spinal cord will be collected, an effective way to properly label each segment is to write the location of the spinal cord segment on a paper towel and wrap around the spinal cord segment and place in formalin (see **Fig. 1**D). Using a hatchet or an axe to cut off the lateral processes of the vertebral column is an alternative way to access the whole length of spinal cord of adult horses; however, it should be performed by trained personnel. Proper sampling of the brain, spinal cord, and to less extent ganglia, nerves, and associated muscle is critical for the accurate diagnosis of neurologic diseases.

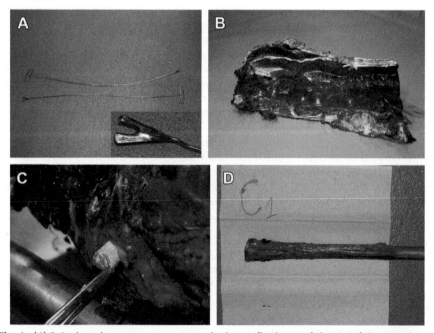

Fig. 1. (A) Spinal cord remover. Inset: Note the butterfly shape of the tip of the spinal cord remover that enables cuting off the nerve rootlets. (B) Section of spinal column from a horse cut with a handsaw. (C) Exposed segment of the spinal cord by grasping the dura mater with a rat tooth forceps. (D) Portion of a section of fresh spinal cord with appropriate labeling.

Table 1
Diagnosis of neurologic diseases in horses

Disease/Condition	Age	Presentation	Gross Lesions	Diagnosis
Hepatic encephalopathy	Any	Signs of hepatic failure that may include icterus	Diffuse hepatic necrosis or fibrosis. None in the brain	1. Increase in serum activity of hepatic enzymes 2. Gross lesions in the liver 3. Microscopic lesions: Alzheimer type II astrocytes in the brain
Leukoencephalomalacia	Mainly adult	Horses fed corn; abrupt onset and acute clinical course	Edema and malacia of the white matter of the cerebrum	1. Gross lesions in the brain 2. Feed analysis
Nigropallidal encephalomalacia	Mainly young (usually <2 y)	Chronic disease. Loss of weight, faulty prehension of feed, yawning, chewing movements	Bilateral symmetric malacic foci in the globus pallidus and/or substantia nigra	1. Gross lesions in the brain 2. Evidence of ingestion of yellow star thistle or Russian knapweed
Arboviral encephalomyelitides (EEE, WEE, VEE, WNV)	Nonvaccinated horses	Cases in late fall and early summer	Hemorrhage in the brainstem and spinal cord (WNV)	1. CSF: neutrophilic pleocytosis (EEE) 2. Microscopic lesions: neutrophilic (EEE) to nonsuppurative encephalomyelitis (WEE, VEE, WNV) 3. IHC 4. PCR 5. Viral isolation
Rabies	Any	Variable (usually spinal cord deficits); short clinical course	Hemorrhagic malacia in the spinal cord	1. Fluorescent antibody testing of the brain from accredited state laboratory
Equine protozoal myeloencephalitis	Any	Asymmetrical muscle atrophy, cranial nerve deficit	Hemorrhagic malacia in the brainstem and spinal cord	1. Microscopic lesions: nonsuppurative to granulomatous myeloencephalitis with intralesional merozoites 2. IHC
Cervical vertebral stenotic myelopathy	Young	Wobbling	Narrowing of the cervical spinal canal	1. Radiographs of the cervical vertebral column 2. Gross lesions in the spinal canal and vertebra 3. Microscopic lesions in the spinal cord

(continued on next page)

Table 1
(continued)

Disease/Condition	Age	Presentation	Gross Lesions	Diagnosis
Herpesvirus-1 encephalomyelopathy	Adult (usually female)	Respiratory disease and abortions in the farm	Hemorrhage in the spinal cord	1. PCR from blood, nasal swabs, spinal cord 2. Virus isolation 3. Microscopic lesion: CNS vasculitis and thrombosis
Polyneuritis equi	Adult	Urinary incontinence, hind limb incoordination	Thickening of the caudal spinal roots (cauda equina)	1. Biopsy of the sacrocaudalis dorsalis lateralis muscle 2. Gross lesions 3. Microscopic lesions: granulomatous polyradiculoneuritis
Dysautonomia	Young adult	Grazing horse with colic, gastrointestinal stasis and ileus	None in the CNS or PNS	1. Full-thickness ileal biopsy 2. Microscopic lesions: neuronal degeneration of celiac ganglia, the myenteric, and the submucosal ganglia
Laryngeal hemiplegia	Young adult	Racing thoroughbred horses with roaring	Atrophy of the LCLM	1. Transnasal endoscopy for laryngeal function 2. Ultrasonography of the LCLM
Stringhalt	Any	High-stepping gait of the hind limb	None	Clinical signs
Botulism	Any	Flaccid paralysis associated with recent wounds	None	Clinical signs
Tetanus	Any	Spastic paralysis associated with recent wounds	Occasionally hemorrhage in the psoas muscle, none in the CNS or PNS	Clinical signs

Abbreviations: CSF, cerebrospinal fluid; EEE, eastern equine encephalitis; IHC, immunohistochemistry; LCLM, left cricoarytenoideus lateralis muscle; PCR, polymerase chain reaction; PNS, peripheral nervous system; VEE, Venezuelan equine encephalitis; WEE, western equine encephalitis; WNV, West Nile virus.

GROSS EXAMINATION OF THE CENTRAL NERVOUS SYSTEM

After removal from the *calvarium* and the spinal canal respectively, the brain and spinal cord should be examined macroscopically searching for possible alterations. Five descriptive parameters should be analyzed: distribution, color, consistency, form, and size. These aspects are very important in the examination of the CNS because sometimes they define the diagnosis. In order to properly evaluate these parameters, an understanding of the basic aspects and anatomic landmarks of the brain and spinal cord (**Fig. 2**) is necessary.

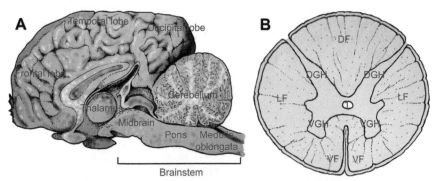

Fig. 2. Diagram of the longitudinal section of the horse brain (*A*) and cross section of the spinal cord (*B*) depicting main anatomic landmarks. Gray matter of the brain is found as a more or less thin layer on the cerebral surface (cortical gray matter) and cerebellum and in clusters of neuronal cell bodies (nuclei) in the brainstem. In the spinal cord, gray matter is the butterfly-shaped structure named as dorsal gray horn (DGH) and ventral gray horn (VGH) around the central canal (1) and surrounded by white matter funiculi: dorsal funiculi (DF), ventral funiculi (VF), and lateral funiculi (LF).

Distribution refers to the spatial arrangement of the lesions. In this context, lesions can be focal, multifocal, diffuse, segmental, or symmetric (eg, see **Fig. 11**), involving either the gray or white matter (eg, see **Fig. 9**) or both. Color is one of the main aspects of the gross examination. Redness denotes excess blood in the tissue, either caused by hyperemia or congestion (usually diffuse) or caused by hemorrhage (**Fig. 3**) and

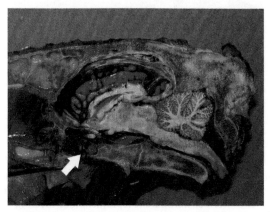

Fig. 3. Subdural hemorrhage around the entire brain caused by fracture of the basisphenoid bone (*arrow*).

thrombosis/infarction (usually focal or multifocal). Yellow indicates edema, necrosis (eg, see **Fig. 9**), or inflammatory exudate.

The most striking gross change in consistency of the brain or spinal cord is caused by malacia (softening) (eg, see **Fig. 9**). Cerebral abscesses usually contain a semisolid or fluid yellow exudate (**Fig. 4**). When the lesion is firm and organized, it will likely be a granulomatous inflammation (**Fig. 5**) or neoplasm. Primary tumors involving the brain of horses are rare. Melanoma is a common dermal neoplasm in gray horses that can occasionally become malignant and metastasize to the brain. Form and size are particularly important in cases of congenital defects and neoplasms. The brain structures are normally equally represented in number and size on both sides of the midline (symmetry). Lack of symmetry in the CNS usually reflects severe lesions. Swelling indicates edema, abscess, tumor, or hematoma is in the tissue. If a lack of tissue is appreciable, hypoplasia or atrophy is probably the case.

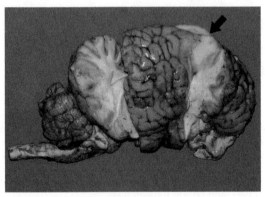

Fig. 4. Yellow fluid exudate from an abscess in the cerebrum (*arrow*). Most common cause of cerebral abscesses in horses is *Streptococcus equi*.

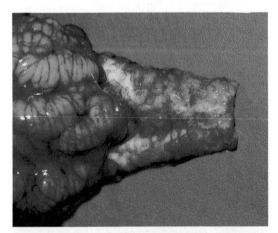

Fig. 5. Granulomatous meningitis caused by *Cryptococcus neoformans*. Note the granular, firm appearance of the granulomatous inflammation in the leptomeninges covering the brainstem (compare with normal transparent leptomeninges covering the cerebellum). In this case, impression smears were performed during necropsy; many cryptococcal yeasts were readily visible on microscopic examination.

Normal structures should not be erroneously interpreted as lesions in the CNS of horses. The pineal gland is a structure situated dorsally at the brainstem between the *colliculus rostralis* of the mesencephalic tectum and the thalamus. In horses, it is usually pigmented and could be mistaken for a neoplasm (**Fig. 6**). Some lesions of little or no significance, such as the cholesterol granuloma or cholesteatoma are found in 15% to 20% of older horses. Those are located in the choroid plexus of the lateral ventricles (see **Fig. 6**) and less frequently in the lateral apertures of the fourth ventricle, in the cerebellopontine angle. They vary in size and most of the time are considered an incidental finding with no clinical implications. However, they can become quite large and expand the lateral ventricles, filling the ventricular space, and cause atrophy of the periventricular white matter. Some affected horses may present with seizures, but these are unusual cases.

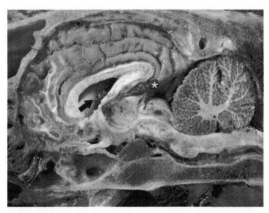

Fig. 6. Cholesterol granuloma (*arrow*) in the lateral ventricle and pigmented appearance of the pineal gland (*asterisk*).

DISEASES BY NEUROANATOMIC LOCATION
Diseases of the Brain

Hepatic encephalopathy
Horses are particularly prone to develop neurologic disturbances when associated with diffuse, acute, or chronic hepatic disease leading to liver failure. This syndrome is referred to as HEP. One important cause of hepatic disease associated with HEP in horses is the ingestion of hepatotoxic plants, mainly the ones containing pyrrolizidine alkaloids, such as *Crotalaria* spp (rattlebox), *Senecio* spp (groundsels), *Amsinckia* spp (fiddle neck), and *Cynoglossum officinale* (hound's tongue). Infectious diseases, portosystemic shunts (congenital or acquired), cholelithiasis, liver tumors, hepatic lipidosis, and hemochromatosis are also reported causes.[1,2]

It is generally accepted that the pathogenesis of HEP is associated with compromise in the liver detoxification of ammonia. The excess of ammonia is toxic for the nervous tissue when it is metabolized by brain astrocytes into glutamine.[2] Although hyperammonemia caused by liver failure is an important part of the pathogenesis in this syndrome, several other mechanisms have been theorized to participate in HEP.[1]

Clinical signs include stupor, head pressing, disorientation, loss of motor control, and constant pacing. Signs of liver failure, such as icterus and photosensitization, could support the clinical diagnosis of HEP in the horse; but those are not consistently present. Serum samples should be analyzed for the activity of liver enzymes, mainly of gamma-glutamyl-transferase, which seems to be consistently increased. Because of technical difficulties in sample preservation and instability of ammonia in the blood, the determination of serum ammonia levels is problematic.

There are no gross lesions in the CNS, but there is always evidence of severe diffuse liver disease at necropsy. One important histologic feature of HEP in horses is swollen astrocytes with large nuclei and a clear center, referred to as Alzheimer type II astrocytes. They can occur solitarily but are more commonly observed as small groups of 2 to 6 cells throughout the gray-white matter interface, particularly in the cerebral cortex and basal nuclei (**Fig. 7**).[2] In the authors' experience, spongy degeneration (*status spongiosus*) is much more common in cattle and rarely seen in horses.

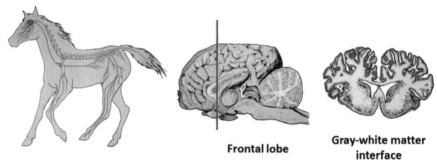

Frontal lobe

Gray-white matter interface

Fig. 7. The distribution of lesions (*red dots*) associated with HEP in the brain of the horse.

Leukoencephalomalacia

This disease is an acute fatal neurologic disease of horses, donkeys, and mules caused by prolonged ingestion (approximately 1 month or more) of moldy corn or corn products containing metabolites of *Fusarium* spp mainly *F verticillioides*. These fungi produce toxins (fumonisin B1, B2, B3) that inhibit the ceramide synthase and cause disruption of sphingolipid synthesis with accumulation of sphingosine, which is toxic to the white matter. In addition, fumonisin B1 has been shown to alter the permeability of endothelial cells, which could explain the protein exudation and edema that occurs at the early changes of the disease. Horses of any age, sex, and breed are affected. The mean morbidity rate is 18% (ranging from 4% to 100%), and the fatality rate is nearly 100%. Cases begin abruptly and can occur all year around but are more frequent in the winter and early spring. Outbreaks affecting several horses may occur in a farm.[3]

Clinical signs may appear up to 12 days after the withdrawal of the corn from the horse's diet. Common clinical signs include anorexia, somnolence, hyperexcitability, impaired food prehension and chewing, ataxia, tremors, head pressing, circling, dullness, unilateral or bilateral blindness, and recumbency. The clinical course is typically acute and varies from 2 to 72 hours. Most affected horses die within 6 to 24 hours of the onset of signs. There are anecdotal reports of horses that become dummies.[3]

The hallmark lesion of the disease is softening (malacia) mainly of the subcortical telencephalic (encephalon) white matter (leuko) (**Fig. 8**). One telencephalic hemisphere is usually asymmetrically enlarged with flattened gyri. Softness may be detected by palpating the telencephalic cortex. On a cut surface, these areas consist of soft, pulpy, gray areas of malacia in the white matter surrounded by numerous small hemorrhages and a yellow halo (**Fig. 9**). Lesions are usually located in centrum semiovale and

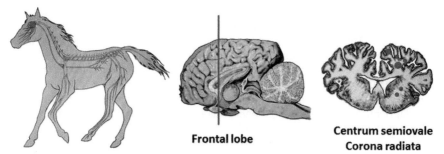

Frontal lobe

**Centrum semiovale
Corona radiata**

Fig. 8. The distribution of lesions (*red dots*) associated with mycotoxic leukoencephaloma-lacia in the brain of the horse.

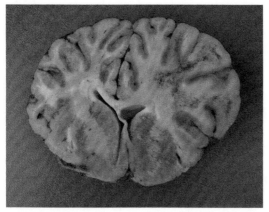

Fig. 9. Horse brain. Mycotoxic leukoencephalomalacia. Yellow areas of softening and cavitation in the white matter of the cerebrum are typical of this disease.

corona radiata of the cerebral hemispheres. They can be unilateral or bilateral but never symmetric. Internal capsule or thalamus may also be affected. Yellowish or hemorrhagic areas are occasionally observed in the colliculi, cerebellar peduncles, pons, and medulla oblongata. Necropsy lesions of leukoencephalomalacia are typical enough for diagnosis. Cerebrospinal fluid (CSF) examination is of no practical help. A clinically presumptive diagnosis is made when an acute neurologic disease occurs in horses that are fed corn (>1 kg/d for more than 1 month). Determination of fumonisin levels in the feed should be sought; but its presence is not, by itself, diagnostic if the typical lesions are missing.[3]

Nigropallidal encephalomalacia

Nigropallidal encephalomalacia (NPEM) is a toxic neurologic disorder of horses caused by prolonged ingestion (more than 1 month) of large quantities of either *Centaurea solstitialis* (yellow star thistle) or *Rhaponticum repens* (Russian knapweed), which are known poisonous plants. The toxic principle remains uncertain; repin, a sesquiterpene lactone present both in *C solstitialis* and *R repens*, interferes with striatal dopamine release. The destruction of the nigrostriatal pathways of the extrapyramidal system leads to dopamine deficiency, which is probably responsible for the neurologic signs.[4]

Affected horses are usually young (56% of the horses are ≤2 years of age), but 4-month-old to 8-year-old horses were reportedly affected. There is no sex or breed predisposition. The occurrence is sporadic, with only few cases occurring at particular farm. Clinical signs appear abruptly and consist of difficulty in prehending food or drinking water, which results in death by starvation or dehydration or intercurrent disease. Continuous chewing motions and yawning occur frequently.[5] The disease is nearly always fatal. The disease is so named because the discrete foci of necrosis (malacia) occur in the encephalon (encephalomalacia) mainly in the *substantia nigra* (nigro) and in the *globus pallidus* (pallidal) (**Figs. 10** and **11**). They are typically found in any of these 4 sites in the brain (**Box 1**). Lesions seem to always be of the same

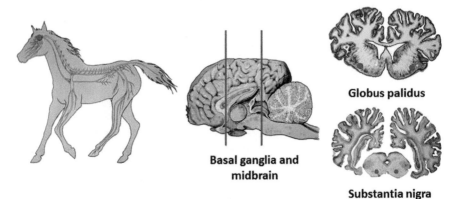

Globus palidus

Basal ganglia and midbrain

Substantia nigra

Fig. 10. Diagram of the distribution of the lesions (*red dots*) associated with nigropallidal encephalomalacia in the brain of the horse. *Substantia nigra* and *globus pallidus* are both components of the nigrostriatal tract of the extrapyramidal system. The corpus striatum consists of several basal nuclei (located in the ventral part of the telencephalon), of which the *globus pallidus* is a component. The *substantia nigra* is located in the basal portion of the mesencephalon in between the tegmentum and cerebral peduncles. These nuclei are important in regulating muscle tonus and stabilizing voluntary movements.

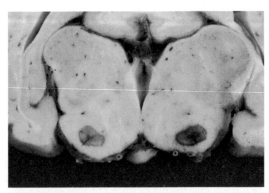

Fig. 11. Gross features of nigropallidal encephalomalacia in a 2-year-old colt caused by the ingestion of *Rhaponticum repens*. Well-demarcated, somewhat depressed, bilaterally symmetric foci of discoloration (malacia) in the *substantia nigra*. (*From* Elliott CR, McCowan CI. Nigropallidal encephalomalacia in horses grazing *Rhaponticum repens* [creeping knapweed]. Aust Vet J 2012;60:153; Copyright © 1999–2015 John Wiley & Sons, Inc, with permission.)

Box 1
Lesion distribution by anatomic sites in 133 horses affected by nigropallidal encephalomalacia

- Bilateral lesions in both *globus pallidus* and *substantia nigra* (4 affected sites) occurred in 58% of the horses.

- Bilateral symmetric lesions in the *substantia nigra* (2 sites affected) occurred in 26% of the horses.

- Bilateral symmetric lesions in the *globus pallidus* (2 sites affected) occurred in 11% of the horses.

- Unilateral asymmetrical malacic foci in both nuclei (2 sites affected) or odd numbers of nuclei affected (eg, just one nucleus affected bilaterally and the other one unilaterally) occurred in the remaining 5% of the horses.

Adapted from Cordy DR. Centaurea species and equine nigropallidal encephalomalacia. In: Keeler RF, Van Kampen KR, James LF, editors. Effects of poisonous plants on livestock. New York: Academic Press; 1978. p. 327–36.

---

age in each individual case.[4] Once formed, they apparently do not increase in size; however, within the limits of the lesion, changes occur and represent a continuum of liquefaction and removal of dead tissue within the malacic foci.[5]

A presumptive diagnosis of NPEM is made based on the characteristic clinical history of long-term access to large quantities of *C solstitialis* or *R repens*. The typical gross lesions in the brain are the standard method of making a tentative diagnosis.

Diseases of the Brainstem and Spinal Cord

Arboviral encephalomyelitides
Main arthropod-borne viral (arboviral) diseases affecting horses in North America are alphaviruses (eastern equine encephalitis [EEE], western equine encephalitis [WEE], and Venezuelan equine encephalitis [VEE]), flaviviruses (mainly West Nile virus [WNV]), and, to a lesser extent, bunyaviruses.[6] Horses are dead-end hosts of these diseases, except for epizootic viruses of VEE whereby horses can be amplifiers.[7] Transmission cycle for arboviruses is mosquito-avian (EEE, WEE, WNV) or mosquito-rodent (VEE), and clinical disease is often associated with peak activity of the mosquitoes (ie, mid to late summer).[6]

Clinical signs related to EEE are usually acute with fever, rapid deterioration of mentation, and death. Affected horses are usually young and not vaccinated.[6] Gross lesions are usually limited, self-induced trauma. Areas of yellow (necrosis) to dark red (hemorrhage) discoloration may be grossly apparent in the cerebral cortex. Microscopic lesions include polioencephalitis and leptomeningitis, more prominent in the cerebral cortex and thalamus (see **Fig. 12**), with neuronophagia (phagocytosis of dead neurons), infiltration of lymphocytes, neutrophils, macrophages, and occasional vasculitis.[8]

Morbidity in epizootics cases of VEE in horses is around 40% to 60%, and mortality rates are 50% to 90%. The meningoencephalitis in VEE is a mixture of lymphocytes and neutrophils. The cerebral cortex is most severely affected, but other parts of the brain can be affected. Lymphoid necrosis is a common feature in horses infected with VEE virus.[9]

Clinical signs caused by WEE infection are usually milder and more subacute than EEE and VEE; horses usually recover from infection, with mortality rates of 20% to 40%. Nonsuppurative meningoencephalomyelitis is more prominent in the basal ganglia and thalamus.[9]

Neuroinvasive disease caused by WNV occurs more frequently in older horses, but it can occur at any age. Moderate to severe ataxia, weakness, and rear limb incoordination are the most consistent clinical signs related to brainstem and spinal cord lesions. The mortality rate is usually around 35% to 45%. Grossly, multifocal areas of hemorrhage, mainly petechiae, are observed in the gray matter of the brainstem and ventral horns of the spinal cord. Varying degrees of lymphocytic polioencephalomyelitis in the brainstem (more prominent in the medulla oblongata and pons) and ventral horns of the thoracic and lumbar spinal cord (**Fig. 12**) are observed microscopically.[10]

Diagnosis of arboviral encephalitis is based on clinical history, histopathologic findings, virus isolation, polymerase chain reaction (PCR), and immunohistochemistry (IHC). Virus isolation, PCR, and IHC for WNV is challenging because of the low viral load in the CNS of infected horses, as opposed to EEE infection whereby infected horses have a high viral load in the brain. Virus isolation is more successful when the CNS is not frozen. Analysis of the CSF is a reliable tool for antemortem diagnosis in EEE cases with neutrophilic pleocytosis. In WEE and WNV, when pleocytosis is present, it is caused by mononuclear cells.[6]

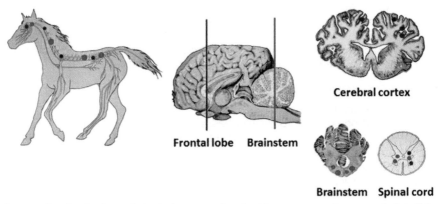

Cerebral cortex

Frontal lobe   Brainstem

Brainstem   Spinal cord

Fig. 12. The distribution of the lesions associated with eastern equine encephalitis (*blue dots*) and West Nile infection (*red dots*) in the brain and spinal cord of the horse.

Rabies

Rabies is a fatal zoonotic infection caused by a neurotropic RNA virus of the genus *Lyssavirus*, family Rhabdoviridae. It affects all mammals and occurs worldwide. Common clinical signs are progressive paralysis and behavioral changes (**Box 2**). Although clinical signs in horses are variable, and rabid horses may be presented with colic, they frequently include spinal cord deficits as pelvic limb lameness progression to loss of proprioception in hock joints, followed by ataxia and eventually pelvic limb paralysis.[11] Pruritus may develop at the site of viral inoculation.

Lesions at necropsy are usually absent or are secondary to the neurologic signs, such as self-induced trauma and urinary bladder atony. However, there are few reports of gross lesions involving the spinal cord of rabid horses, such as congestion, hemorrhage, and poliomyelomalacia; indeed hemorrhagic lesions of the spinal cord seem to be a consistent lesion in rabid horses (**Fig. 13**). The histologic feature is polioencephalomyelitis, particularly of the spinal cord and to a lesser extent of the brainstem (**Fig. 14**), characterized by perivascular mononuclear cuffs and glial nodules.[11]

> **Box 2**
> **Clinical presentation of rabies**
>
> - It may occur in 3 clinical forms: dumb, furious, and paralytic.
> - Spinal cord neurologic deficits are a common presentation in horses.
> - The incubation period is variable but was demonstrated to be approximately 15 days (mean) in experimental cases.
> - Clinical courses are always fatal and range from 5 to 10 days.

Clinical signs of rabies are nonspecific and can be misleading because there is no comparable disease of CNS in horses with so vast and diverse manifestation of neurologic signs such as rabies. To complicate matters further, there is no antemortem test to confirm suspected cases. Suspicion of rabies can be confirmed by the typical microscopic lesions associated with eosinophilic inclusion bodies in the cytoplasm of neurons, the so-called Negri bodies. Negri bodies are observed in approximately only half of the cases in horses and even so are more frequently found in the spinal cord, which underlines the importance of sampling the cord in suspected rabies cases.[11,12]

Rabies is often a differential diagnosis for neurologic animals. In order to achieve a definitive diagnosis, it is critical to follow the Centers for Disease Control and Prevention's guidelines for rabies sampling. This protocol was developed because viral spread may also be unilateral, especially in larger animals. The preferred sample is a transverse section of the cerebellum (containing vermis and cerebellar hemispheres) and the underlying brainstem (midbrain and pons) submitted unfixed. A negative finding for rabies can be made only if a complete cross section of the brain stem is examined.[13] To officially confirm a suspect case of equine rabies, fresh samples of the brain should be submitted to a state-accredited laboratory for the detection of viral antigen in the brain by direct fluorescent antibody test (FAT).

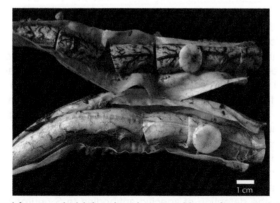

Fig. 13. Spinal cord from a rabid (*above*) and a normal horse for control. The dura mater is cut open in both spinal cords. Note marked hyperemia of leptomeninges and foci of malacic hemorrhage in the gray matter of the spinal cord from the affected horse. Those changes are absent in the cord of the nonaffected horse below. (*Courtesy of* Dr David Driemeier, Section of Veterinary Pathology, Federal University of Rio Grande do Sul, Brazil.)

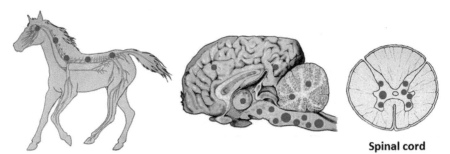

Spinal cord

Fig. 14. The distribution of the lesions (*red dots*) associated with rabies in the brain and spinal cord of the horse.

Equine protozoal myeloencephalitis

Equine protozoal myeloencephalitis (EPM) is caused by the protozoan *Sarcocystis neurona*.[14] Other protozoan parasites (eg, *Neospora hughesi* and *N caninum*) have been reported as the causative agent in a small number of horses with a similar disease.[15] Clinical EPM infections in horses have been reported from the United States and Canada, Brazil, and Panama.[14] Some evidence suggests the occurrence of a few cases in Europe. The prevalence of serologic-positive horses to *S neurona* in the United States varies from 10% to 60%, indicating a high rate of exposure to the organism; however, the development of clinical disease occurs in less than 1% of infected horses. The disease occurs in one or a few horses on a particular farm and does not develop as outbreaks affecting several animals.[15] All ages, breeds, and sexes are susceptible. Cases are described in horses of both sexes, with ages varying from 2 months to 24 years (mean 4.4 years).

Epidemiologically important is that *S neurona* has a 2-host life cycle, the opossum being the definitive host and the horse an intermediate aberrant host.[14]

The parasite induces inflammatory multifocal lesions in the CNS, and the clinical signs develop accordingly to the anatomic site of infection. Typically, there are asymmetrical spinal cord and cranial nerve manifestations of muscle atrophy, ataxia, dysphagia, muscle weakness, stumbling, and head tilt. Frequently, atrophied muscles are gluteal (half of the cases), temporalis, and masseter. Cases with symmetric signs and cerebrocortical signs are less frequent.[15]

Lesions appear as discolored red (hemorrhagic) necrotic foci of variable sizes throughout the neuraxis (**Fig. 15**) but mostly in the cervical and lumbar intumescences of the spinal cord (**Fig. 16**). The brain is less often involved; when it is, the lesions tend to be confined to the brainstem.[14] Microscopic lesions affect both gray and white matter with necrosis, hemorrhage, and inflammatory reaction consisting of lymphocytes, macrophages, neutrophils, eosinophils, and a few multinucleated giant cells. Intracellular merozoites can be observed in neurons, giant cells, neutrophils, or macrophages or extracellularly in cysts within the neuropil.[15]

The antemortem diagnosis of EPM is challenging, should be considered tentative, and depends on a detailed clinical examination, ruling out other neurologically similar diseases, and on the detection of specific antibodies to *S neurona* in the serum or CSF. However, none of these parameters is conclusive. The Western blotting technique for the detection of *S neurona*–specific antibodies in CSF is very helpful but by no means definitive because many neurologically normal horses have been found to have antibodies to *S neurona* in their serum and even in their CSF.[15] PM diagnosis

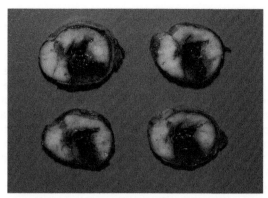

Fig. 15. The normal architecture of this horse's spinal cord is disrupted by multifocal and extensive areas of hemorrhage and softening (malacia) confined to right-ventral quadrant of the cord, involving the gray and white matter. The entire gray matter is replaced by a cavity.

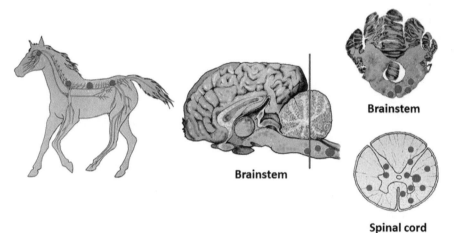

Brainstem

Brainstem

Spinal cord

Fig. 16. The distribution of the lesions (*red dots*) associated with equine protozoal myeloencephalitis in the brain and spinal cord of the horse.

can be confirmed by demonstrating the parasites by IHC associated with the characteristic histologic lesions.[14]

Diseases of the Spinal Cord

Cervical vertebral stenotic myelopathy

Cervical vertebral stenotic myelopathy (CVSM) of horses is characterized by narrowing of the vertebral canal with resultant compression of the spinal cord. The rather nonspecific term *wobbler*, when applied to this condition, refers to the clinical signs of incoordination.[16]

The disease occurs worldwide in sporadic form. Young, tall, male thoroughbred horses with long necks seem to be predisposed. There is no recovery, but death caused by this condition is unlikely. Clinical signs are generally insidious. The first sign appears as an uncoordinated gait in the form of symmetric ataxia. The horse tends to avoid moving in order to avoid pain. The signs may be progressive for weeks and then remain static.[16]

Two forms of CVSM are recognized in the horse: (1) cervical static stenosis and (2) cervical vertebral instability or dynamic stenosis. In cervical static stenosis, there is excessive vertebral bone formation over an extended period of time with permanent narrowing of the vertebral canal; this results in compression of the spinal cord regardless of the position of the horse's head. Horses from 1 to 4 years old are affected, and the spinal cord is compressed at C5-C7. In dynamic stenosis, the narrowing of the spinal canal is caused by vertebral subluxation and occurs during flexion of the neck. Horses from 8 to 18 months of age are affected, and the spinal cord is usually compressed at C3-C5.[16]

Besides obvious narrowing of the cervical spinal canal in the static form or on neck ventroflexion in the dynamic form, multiple cross sections of the spinal cord in the site of the narrowing should be performed, looking for softening (malacia) and hemorrhage (**Fig. 17**). In chronic cases, the only change may be a slight depression on the contour of the spinal cord. Microscopically, degeneration of both gray and white matter is observed at the site of compression.[16]

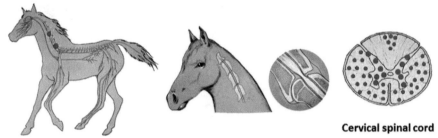

Cervical spinal cord

Fig. 17. The location and distribution of the lesions (*red dots*) in the cervical vertebral stenotic myelopathy, at the site of the compression. The narrowing of the spinal canal in the static and dynamic forms is at C5-C7 and C3-C5, respectively. Lesions are segmental areas of hemorrhagic softening in the white and gray matter of the spinal cord, better appreciated in cross sections.

Equine degenerative myeloencephalopathy and equine motor neuron disease

Equine degenerative myeloencephalopathy (EDM) and equine motor neuron disease (EMND) are neurodegenerative conditions of horses. Low levels of dietary vitamin E (alpha-tocopherol) with resultant oxidative damage to selected neurons are thought to participate in the pathogenesis of these conditions.[17]

The clinical course is chronic and progressive for both disorders. Clinical signs in EDM include obtunded mentation, weakness, ataxia, tremors, wide-based stance, muscle atrophy, sweating, and apparent pain.[18] Prolonged weight loss, acute trembling, and frequent lying down that progresses to permanent decubitus have been reported in horses with EMND.[17]

Unfortunately, the definitive diagnosis of both EDM and EMND relies on PM examination and microscopic examination of the selected nuclei of the brainstem and segments of the spinal cord (**Box 3, Fig. 18**). Biopsy of the *sacrocaudalis dorsalis medialis* muscle is an alternative way for antemortem diagnosis of EMND.[19]

Box 3
Comparison between EDM and EMND

Disease	EDM	EMND
Age	Young (6–12 mo)	Adult (2–25 y)
Sex predisposition	No	No
Breed	Quarter horse, paint, Appaloosa, Haflinger, standardbred, thoroughbred, Lusitano, Andalusian, Morgan, Paso Fino, Arabian, Tennessee walking horse, Norwegian fjord, Mongolian wild horses, Pony of the Americas, American miniature horse, Welsh ponies	All breeds (frequent in quarter horse)
Hereditary basis	Yes (Morgan, Appaloosa, Lusitano)	No
Gross lesions	No	Marked muscle wasting, mostly in *triceps brachii* and *vastus intermedius*
Microscopic lesions	Degeneration of neurons (vacuolation) and their axons (axonal spheroids) in the lateral (accessory) cuneate, medial cuneate, and *gracilis* nuclei, dorsal and ventral spinocerebellar tracts, and ventromedial funiculi of the cervicothoracic spinal cord (see **Fig. 18**)	Degeneration of motor neurons in the ventral horn of the spinal cord and in the hypoglossal, facial, trigeminal motor nuclei, and nucleus ambiguous (see **Fig. 18**) • Neurogenic muscle atrophy • Lipopigments in the retina

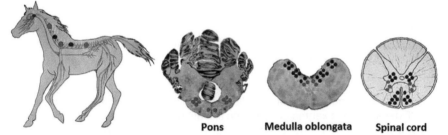

Pons   Medulla oblongata   Spinal cord

Fig. 18. The distribution of the microscopic lesions in equine degenerative myeloencephalopathy (*blue dots*) and equine motor neuron disease (*red dots*).

Equine herpesvirus-1 myeloencephalopathy

Equine herpesvirus-1 (EHV-1) infection causes a paralytic disease in horses and is often referred to as equine herpesvirus myeloencephalopathy (EHM). Infection by EHV-1 occurs in the first weeks or months of life with initial replication in the respiratory epithelium, which may be asymptomatic or accompanied by clinical respiratory disease. The virus infects T lymphocytes; a cell-associated viremia that usually persists for approximately 14 days leads to endothelial infection of the CNS and uterus and may lead to myeloencephalopathy and abortion, respectively. Abortion usually occurs in the last trimester of gestation. Fever is the most consistent initial clinical indication of recent infection. Reactivation from latency in the trigeminal ganglia or lymphoid tissue may lead to nasal shedding and transmission to susceptible hosts or viremia and the possibility of subsequent abortion or neurologic disease.[20,21]

Typically 10% of the horses develop myeloencephalopathy and are usually females and older animals (>3 years of age). Although all EHV-1 strains are capable of developing neurologic disease, recent molecular studies have shown that a single nucleotide polymorphism (A[2254]/G[2254]) in the genome region of the open reading frame 30, which results in an amino acid variation (N[752]/D[752]) of the EHV-1 DNA polymerase, is strongly associated with equine myeloencephalopathies. The interval between the first detection of fever and the development of neurologic signs typically ranges from 4 to 9 days.[21]

Common neurologic signs are ataxia, hind limb paralysis, sensory deficits in the perineal area, and urinary bladder atony with passive dribbling of urine. Affected horses usually progress to recumbency and death. Neurologic signs correlate with damage to the endothelial cells in the CNS, leading to vasculitis, microthrombosis, and local hemorrhage.[17,21] The caudal spinal cord (thoracic, lumbar, and sacral) is more commonly affected. The brainstem is infrequently affected.[17]

Gross lesions consist of focal areas of hemorrhage within cross sections of the spinal cord, following a linear radiating pattern from the surface into the white matter (wedge-shaped lesions) (**Fig. 19**) that correlates with the areas of vasculitis, thrombosis, ischemia, and mononuclear perivascular cuffing following affected blood vessels on microscopic examination. The lesion is usually focal, and careful examination of multiple segments of the spinal cord is undoubtedly important to achieve a definitive diagnosis.[17]

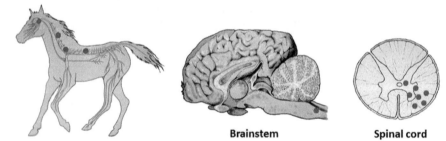

Brainstem   **Spinal cord**

Fig. 19. The distribution of the lesions (*red dots*) in EHV-1 myeloencephalopathy in the CNS of the horse.

Antemortem diagnosis of EHM is challenging and not always conclusive. Analysis of the CSF demonstrates xanthochromia with elevation of protein concentration. Laboratory diagnosis of EHM is currently based on at least one of the following criteria: detection of EHV-1 in nasal swabs or blood by PCR, virus isolation, serologic testing (virus neutralization), and PM examination. Serologic tests are hard to interpret because of the cross-reactivity between EHV-1 and EHV-4 infections. Also, by the time of the development of the neurologic disease, both nasal swabs and blood samples may be EHV-1 negative because neurologic disease occurs days after viremia.[20,21]

Diseases of Ganglia and Nerves

Polyneuritis equi

Polyneuritis equi (PNE) or neuritis of the cauda equina or cauda equina syndrome is a rare chronic idiopathic disease in horses. The disease is often characterized by perineal anesthesia, urinary incontinence, urinary bladder atony with sabulous cystitis, fecal retention, tail paralysis, and hind limb incoordination caused by lesions in the sacral and coccygeal nerves. It also may affect the cranial nerves; in such cases, the horse may develop Horner syndrome. Because of the widespread distribution of lesions in the peripheral and cranial nerves, the term *PNE* is favored over neuritis of the cauda equina or cauda equina syndrome (**Fig. 20**).[22]

The cause and pathogenesis of PNE are unknown.[22] *Halicephalobus gingivalis* has been reported as a cause in one case of PNE.[23] Persistent herpesvirus-1 infection and adenovirus infection have been implied on inciting an immune-mediated inflammatory reaction. Results of CSF cytologic analysis in PNE are variable and nonspecific.[22] Unfortunately, the definitive diagnosis of PNE is only possible through PM evaluation of the cauda equina and other peripheral nerves.

Grossly, the most severe lesion of PNE is irregular thickening of the extradural sacral and caudal spinal roots forming a fibrotic mass (**Fig. 21**). Intradural nerve segments and cranial nerves are affected to a less extent. Histologically, granulomatous polyradiculoneuritis (inflammation of multiple nerve roots) with marked extradural fibrosis is observed in the spinal nerves and occasionally into the intramuscular nerve branches in the hypaxial muscles.[17] The inflammation spares the muscles, which exhibit secondary changes of neurogenic atrophy. Recently, biopsy of the base of the tail musculature (*sacrocaudalis dorsalis lateralis muscle*) has been an aid in the antemortem diagnosis of PNE.[24]

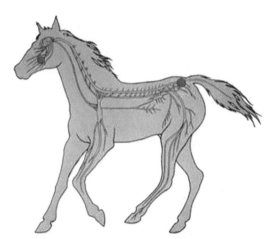

Fig. 20. The distribution of the lesions (*red dots*) in PNE affecting cauda equina and, to a lesser extent, the cranial nerves.

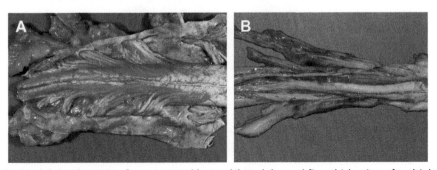

Fig. 21. (*A*) Cauda equina from a normal horse. (*B*) Nodular and firm thickening of multiple nerve roots of the cauda equina is the typical gross lesion of polyneuritis equi.

Dysautonomia

Equine dysautonomia or equine grass sickness (EGS) is a debilitating and often fatal disease of grazing horses, ponies, and donkeys. It is highly prevalent in Great Britain and northern European countries. Isolated cases have been reported in Australia, the United States, and South America, especially the Patagonia region where it is known as *mal seco*. EGS has a peak of incidence in young adult horses (2–7 years old) with low serum antibody levels to *Clostridium botulinum* type C and *Clostridium novyi* type A surface antigens and *C botulinum* type C toxoid. Horses that have had cograzed with a horse that had EGS may acquire immunity and are less prone to develop the disease. Environmental risk factors associated with the increased incidence of EGS include increased soil nitrogen, pasture disturbance with construction or increased numbers of horses, and cooler, drier weather. Although many risk factors have been associated with EGS, a definitive cause still remains obscure. All factors are considered together; a resilient soil-borne agent that, in certain climate conditions, produces a neurotoxin to which the horse may mount an immune response may be a plausible hypothesis.[25]

Clinical disease can be classified as acute (<2 days), subacute (2–7 days), or chronic (>7 days). Clinicopathological findings reflect dysfunction of the autonomic nervous system, especially of the gastrointestinal tract. Clinical signs include colic, dysphagia, nasogastric reflux with linear ulcers in the in the distal esophagus, gastric and small intestinal fluid-filled dilation, colonic impaction, sweating, and muscle tremors.[26] Death occurs from gastric rupture. In chronic cases, bilateral ptosis with ventral deviation of eyelashes, rhinitis sicca, mucus-coated hard feces, and weight loss are the most common clinical signs; horses would die of emaciation.[27]

Presumptive diagnosis in live animals relies on clinical history, clinical signs, epidemiology, and ruling out other causes. The only highly sensitive and specific test for a definitive diagnosis of EGS in live animals is full-thickness ileal biopsies obtained at exploratory celiotomy. Rectal biopsies are not reliable for antemortem diagnosis of EGS.[26] Typical histologic changes include neuronal degeneration mostly in neurons of the autonomic (eg, celiac) ganglia (**Fig. 22**), of the myenteric and submucosal ganglia, and, to a lesser extent, from the brain and spinal cord.[25,26]

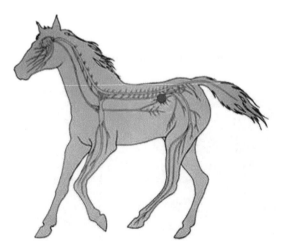

Fig. 22. Diagram of the distribution of the lesions (*red dot*) in equine dysautonomia affecting the celiac ganglion.

Laryngeal hemiplegia

Recurrent laryngeal neuropathy (RLN) is a common idiopathic disease of young adult horses (2–12 years) with a tall and long neck phenotype. Racing thoroughbred horses are the most commonly affected by RLN.[28] The cause of RLN still remains obscure, and a hereditary basis has been suspected. The underlying lesion is degeneration of the left recurrent laryngeal nerve, most prominent in the distal segment of the nerve (distal axonopathy). A lesser degree of involvement is seen on the right recurrent laryngeal nerve. Long peripheral nerves (common, deep, and superficial peroneal and tibial nerves) may also be affected. Clinical signs relate to upper airway dysfunction. Because of the dorsal cricoarytenoid muscle paralysis, the *rima glottidis* cannot be totally opened during inspiration, restricting the airflow; an audible sound (roaring) is produced.[29] Affected horses also demonstrate poor performance and exercise intolerance. Grossly, there is denervation atrophy of the laryngeal adductor muscles as compared with the abductors, especially of the left adducting *cricoarytenoideus dorsalis* muscle (**Fig. 23**).[17] Transnasal endoscopy at rest or during exercise for observation of the laryngeal function is the best way to make the diagnosis of RLN, which reveals asymmetry of the glottis.[28] Recently, ultrasonography of the *cricoarytenoideus lateralis* muscle has been an aid in the diagnosis of RLN, because it is the first muscle to undergo neurogenic atrophy in RLN, and is histologically the most severely affected.[29]

Nonidiopathic unilateral laryngeal paralysis is usually caused by guttural pouch mycosis. Bilateral laryngeal paralysis occurs more frequently in ponies, and it is linked to HEP and general anesthesia.[28]

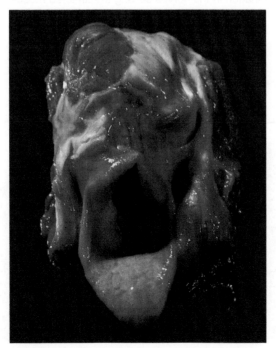

Fig. 23. The left *cricoarytenoideus dorsalis* muscle is diffusely pale and attenuated (left-sided denervation laryngeal muscular atrophy). (*Courtesy of* Dr Brian Porter, DVM, Texas A&M University, United States.)

Stringhalt

Stringhalt or equine reflex hypertonia is an ancient disease of horses reported worldwide. Affected horses have a high stepping gait with varying degrees of hyperflexion and delayed protraction of the hind limbs (**Fig. 24**). Markedly affected horses will kick the ventral abdomen, thorax, and elbow during gait and in extreme cases develop a peculiar bunny-hopping gait.[30]

Two epidemiologic presentations are known: Australian stringhalt occurs as outbreaks in late summer and autumn, generally in horses on poor-quality pastures, and has been associated with the ingestion of toxic-related plants, such as flat weed (*Hypochaeris radicata*), dandelion (*Taraxacum officinal*), and cheese weed (*Malva parviflora*).[30,31] The disease has been reproduced in horses by feeding *H radicata*.[31] Other than Australia, this form of stringhalt has been described in several countries.[31] Estimated morbidity is reportedly 17%; lethality is close to zero; spontaneous recovery is possible; however, some owners will opt for euthanasia because of the decrease in the horse's performance.[30]

The second form, the conventional stringhalt, has sporadic occurrence and no known cause, although several hypothesis have been suggested. The recovery without surgical intervention is uncommon for this type of the disease.[30]

No laboratory test is useful to confirm a diagnosis of stringhalt, but the clinical picture is so characteristic that it warrants a clinical definitive diagnosis. Muscle atrophy can be detected on the clinical examination and/or at necropsy. There are no specific gross lesions.[30,31]

Histopathologic and ultrastructural changes have been reported for Australian-type stringhalt[3], characterized by distal axonopathy caused by repeated bouts of demyelination and remyelination in the nerves serving the affected muscles.[31]

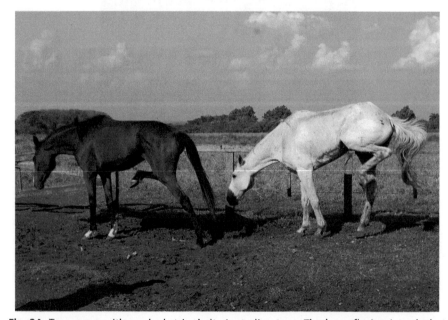

Fig. 24. Two mares with marked stringhalt, Australian type. The hyperflexion is such that the right pelvic limb of both mares almost kicks the abdomen. (*Courtesy of* Dr Paulo Bandarra, Section of Veterinary Pathology, Federal University of Rio Grande do Sul, Brazil.)

Diseases of the Neuromuscular Junction

Botulism and tetanus

These are sporadic diseases in horses caused by toxins produced by gram-positive anaerobic bacteria: *Clostridium tetani* (tetanus) and *Clostridium botulinum* (botulism). Tetanus toxins act at several sites within the CNS, including peripheral motor end plates, spinal cord, and brain, and in the sympathetic nervous system synapses, inhibiting the release of gamma-aminobutyric acid (the inhibitory protein at the interneuron) causing the characteristic spastic paralysis (tetany). Botulism toxin blocks neurotransmitter (acetylcholine) exocytosis vesicles in the peripheral myoneural synapses causing bilateral symmetric flaccid paralysis. There is no gross or histologic-specific lesions observed in either of these two diseases, but clinical signs are sufficiently characteristic.[32]

Tetanus can be observed 5 to 21 days (mean 9 days) after *C tetani* spores infect deep penetrating wounds, such as those of castration, metritis, injection, and sole infrequently. Clinical disease runs a course of 5 to 7 days and is fatal in 77% of the cases. Clinical signs in tetanus result from the action of the toxin in skeletal and smooth muscle. Most cases progress to diffuse symmetric tetanic spasm of muscles. Hyperesthesia and prolapse of the third eyelid are consistent signs, and bloat occurs because of spasm of smooth muscle of the gastrointestinal tract. Muscle rigidity leads to the classic sawhorse stance of tetanus. Although no specific lesions are reported, the authors have observed hemorrhages in the psoas muscle in horses that die of tetanus **(Fig. 25)**. These hemorrhages are probably caused by muscle exertion.[32]

Equine botulism can be produce by 3 mechanisms: (1) ingestion of preformed toxin from the environment (the most common); (2) elaboration of toxin from *C botulinum* infection in wounds; and (3) ingestion of *C botulinum* spores, which produce toxin within the gastrointestinal tract. Clinical signs are diffuse, symmetric flaccid paralysis with normal mentation and absence of CNS signs. Signs develop from 12 hours to 10 days after ingestion of the toxin. The lethality is high after a clinical course that may be acute (12 hours to 2 days), subacute (3–7 days), or chronic (up to 30 days).[32]

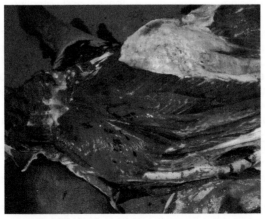

Fig. 25. Hemorrhage and edema (*yellow area*) in the psoas muscle of a horse that died of tetanus. (*Courtesy of* Dr David Driemeier, Section of Veterinary Pathology, Federal University of Rio Grande do Sul, Brazil.)

For diagnosis of tetanus or botulism, the practitioner would be better off relying on the history and the characteristic clinical signs. The absence of specific necropsy and histopathologic findings is further evidence to support the clinical diagnosis. Identification (by culture or smears of the infected wounds) of the characteristic gram-positive tennis racket–shape bacteria also supports the clinical diagnosis of tetanus.

There is a mouse bioassay for the detection of botulism toxin in the serum of affected animals; however, because of the high susceptibility of horses to develop botulism, the amounts of toxin able to produce disease in horses will not induce disease in mice, thus giving high numbers of false negatives. The bioassay results are more confusing than helpful; however, a positive test, although rare, is confirmatory.[32]

SUMMARY

The main purpose of the necropsy of a neurologic horse is to elucidate the cause of the neurologic signs. The diagnosis of these diseases is important because some occur as outbreaks, such as HEP associated with ingestion of hepatotoxic plants, and/or have zoonotic implications, such as rabies and arboviral encephalomyelitides. Sampling of the brain and at least 3 segments of the spinal cord (cervical, thoracic, and lumbar) are always needed for a definitive diagnosis. Practicing sampling the brain in any equine necropsy is still the best way to be skilled on this task, making the process less laborious when needed.

ACKNOWLEDGMENTS

The authors are deeply grateful for the medical illustrations by Dr Mario Francisco de Assis Neto.

REFERENCES

1. Hurcombe S. Equine hepatic encephalopathy. In: Furr M, Reed F, editors. Equine neurology. 2nd edition. Oxford (United Kingdom): Blackwell Publishing; 2008. p. 257–68.
2. Vandevelde M, Higgins RJ, Oevermann A. Metabolic encephalopathy. In: Veterinary neuropathology. Essentials of theory and practice. Oxford (United Kingdom): Wiley-Blackwell; 2012. p. 122–4.
3. Riet-Correa F, Meireles M, Barros C, et al. Equine leukoencephalomalacia in Brazil. In: Garland TC, Barr C, editors. Toxic plants and other natural toxicants. Wallingford (CT): CABI Publishing; 1998. p. 479–82.
4. Cordy DR. Centaurea species and equine nigropallidal encephalomalacia. In: Keeler RF, Van Kampen KR, James LF, editors. Effects of poisonous plants on livestock. New York: Academic Press; 1978. p. 327–36.
5. Fowler ME. Nigropallidal encephalomalacia in the horse. J Am Vet Med Assoc 1965;147:607–16.
6. Long MT. West Nile virus and equine encephalitis viruses: new perspectives. Vet Clin North Am Equine Pract 2014;30(3):523–42.
7. Taylor KG, Paessler S. Pathogenesis of Venezuelan equine encephalitis. Vet Microbiol 2013;167(1–2):145–50.
8. Silva ML, Galiza GJ, Dantas AF, et al. Outbreaks of eastern equine encephalitis in northeastern Brazil. J Vet Diagn Invest 2011;23(3):570–5.
9. Steele KE, Twenhafel NA. Pathology of animal models of alphavirus encephalitis. Vet Pathol 2010;47(5):790–805.

10. Cantile C, Del Piero F, Di Guardo G, et al. Pathologic and immunohistochemical findings in naturally occurring West Nile virus infection in horses. Vet Pathol 2001; 38(4):414–21.
11. Boone AC, Susta L, Rech RR, et al. Pathology in practice: poliomyelitis with intraneuronal Negri bodies. J Am Vet Med Assoc 2010;237(3):277–9.
12. Stein LT, Rech RR, Harrison L, et al. Immunohistochemical study of rabies virus within the central nervous system of domestic and wildlife species. Vet Pathol 2010;47(4):630–3.
13. Centers for Disease Control and Prevention. Protocol for postmortem diagnosis of rabies in animals by direct fluorescent antibody testing. Available at: http://www.cdc.gov/rabies/pdf/rabiesdfaspv2.pdf. Accessed February 14, 2015.
14. Dubey JP, Lindsay DS, Saville WJA, et al. A review of Sarcocystis neurona and equine protozoal myeloencephalitis (EPM). Vet Parasitol 2001;95:89–131.
15. Furr M. Equine protozoal myeloencephalitis. In: Furr M, Reed F, editors. Equine neurology. 2nd edition. Oxford (United Kingdom): Blackwell Publishing; 2008. p. 197–212.
16. Zacchary JF. Cervical stenotic myelopathy. In: Zacchary JF, McGavin MD, editors. Pathologic basis of veterinary disease. 5th edition. St Louis (MO): Elsevier; 2012. p. 833–5.
17. Summers BA, Cummings JF, De Lahunta A. Veterinary neuropathology. St Louis (MO): Mosby; 1995. p. 527.
18. Finno CJ, Higgins RJ, Aleman M, et al. Equine degenerative myeloencephalopathy in Lusitano horses. J Vet Intern Med 2011;25:1439–46.
19. Bedford HE, Valberg SJ, Firshman AM, et al. Histopathologic findings in the sacrocaudalis dorsalis medialis muscle of horses with vitamin E–responsive muscle atrophy and weakness. J Am Vet Med Assoc 2013;242:1127–37.
20. Lunn DP, Davis-Poynter N, Flaminio MJ, et al. Equine herpesvirus-1 consensus statement. J Vet Intern Med 2009;23:450–61.
21. Pusterla N, Hussey GS. Equine herpesvirus-1 myeloencephalopathy. Vet Clin Equine 2014;30:489–506.
22. Furr M. Disorders of the peripheral nervous system. In: Furr M, Reed F, editors. Equine neurology. 2nd edition. Oxford (United Kingdom): Blackwell Publishing; 2008. p. 334–5.
23. Johnson JS, Hibler CP, Tillotson KM, et al. Radiculomeningomyelitis due to Halicephalobus gingivalis in a horse. Vet Pathol 2001;38(5):559–61.
24. Aleman M, Katzman SA, Vaughan B, et al. Antemortem diagnosis of polyneuritis equi. J Vet Intern Med 2009;23:665–8.
25. Pirie RS, Jago RC, Hudson NP. Equine grass sickness. Equine Vet J 2014;46(5): 545–53.
26. Mair TS, Kelley M, Pearson GR. Comparison of ileal and rectal biopsies in the diagnosis of equine grass sickness. Vet Rec 2011;168:266.
27. MacKay R. Neurodegenerative disorders. In: Furr M, Reed F, editors. Equine neurology. 2nd edition. Oxford (United Kingdom): Blackwell Publishing; 2008. p. 235–55.
28. Dixon PM, McGorum BC, Railton DI, et al. Laryngeal paralysis: a study of 375 cases in a mixed-breed population of horses. Equine Vet J 2001;33(5):452–8.
29. Chalmers HJ, Yeager AE, Cheetham J, et al. Diagnostic sensitivity of subjective and quantitative laryngeal ultrasonography for recurrent laryngeal neuropathy in horses. Vet Radiol Ultrasound 2012;53(6):660–6.
30. Hahn C. Equine reflex hypertonia. In: Furr M, Reed F, editors. Equine neurology. 2nd edition. Oxford (United Kingdom): Blackwell Publishing; 2008. p. 366–7.

31. Araújo JA, Curcio B, Alda J, et al. Stringhalt in Brazilian horses caused by Hypochaeris radicata. Toxicon 2008;52:190–3.
32. Furr M. Clostridial neurotoxins: botulism and tetanus. In: Furr M, Reed F, editors. Equine neurology. 2nd edition. Oxford (United Kingdom): Blackwell Publishing; 2008. p. 221–9.

Respiratory Disease

Diagnostic Approaches in the Horse

Joanne Hewson, DVM, PhD*, Luis G. Arroyo, DVM, DVSc, PhD

KEYWORDS

- Respiratory • Equine • Endoscopy • Tracheal aspirate • Bronchoalveolar lavage
- Guttural pouch • Cytology • Pathogen

KEY POINTS

- Localization of pathologic lesions to the upper versus lower respiratory system is a key factor in determining the initial diagnostic approach in horses with suspected respiratory disease.
- Patient status must be considered during the selection of diagnostic tests applied to horses with respiratory compromise. Struggling during procedures can precipitate patient deterioration or death in some cases.
- The method of sample collection and sample handling may impact test results, such as viral testing and airway cytology.

INTRODUCTION

As with other body systems evaluated in equine medicine, diagnostic evaluation of the respiratory system starts first with a detailed and targeted patient history and a thorough physical examination. Historical information that may reflect pathologic lesions of the respiratory system includes details of mentation, appetite, presence of abnormal ocular or nasal discharge or cough, alterations in respiratory rate or character, and changes in performance.[1] Altered posture or gait may also reflect thoracic pain or reduced respiratory capacity. Taking the time to fully understand the description of signs is crucial to determining the diagnostic path that follows.

Details about patient housing (location in the barn, proximity to feed or bedding storage areas or arenas, air quality and flow) and specific feeding information (including types of feed, feed quality, how the feed is provided) are important in generating potential differential diagnoses as well as in treatment planning for many respiratory

Disclosures: The authors have nothing to disclose.
Department of Clinical Studies, Ontario Veterinary College, University of Guelph, 50 Stone Road East, Guelph, ON N1G2W1, Canada
* Corresponding author.
E-mail address: jhewson@uoguelph.ca

Vet Clin Equine 31 (2015) 307–336
http://dx.doi.org/10.1016/j.cveq.2015.04.008
0749-0739/15/$ – see front matter Crown Copyright © 2015 Published by Elsevier Inc. All rights reserved.
vetequine.theclinics.com

diseases. Similarly, details of recent travel, barn activity by other horses, and knowledge of geographic disease trends also can influence the diagnostic process when evaluating the respiratory system. Data on infectious disease trends can be solicited from local diagnostic laboratories or through online resources. For example, unified efforts to report and track animal diseases are emerging (eg, http://www.wormsandgermsmap.com/), and these should be consulted by practitioners when investigating herd outbreaks.

CLINICAL EVALUATION OF THE RESPIRATORY SYSTEM

Before working with the patient, the clinician should observe respiratory function at rest, including the respiratory rate, effort to breathe, and the presence of any respiratory sounds audible without a stethoscope. Character of respiration may include observations of any head extension, nostril flare, abnormal posture or gait, presence of any ocular or nasal discharge, or increased expiratory effort seen over the external abdominal oblique musculature. During the routine physical examination, additional procedures to assess the respiratory system should include percussion of the sinuses, palpation of the submandibular and retropharyngeal lymph nodes, and lung auscultation. A complete respiratory cycle (one full inspiration and expiration) should be evaluated by auscultation at each intercostal site over both hemithoraces. As such, a complete and thorough examination of lung sounds may take approximately 5 minutes to complete; this time invested in careful auscultation can greatly help the practitioner to determine the next steps in the diagnostic process by localizing and characterizing the respiratory pathologic abnormality.

In a healthy adult horse at rest, lung sounds may not be audible. Increasing ventilation by altering the depth of respiration aids in hearing lung sounds, and this may be achieved through use of a rebreathing bag placed over the horse's nose to increase respiratory drive as carbon dioxide accumulates. Finesse is required for a rebreathing bag to be used successfully; the technique is described in Box 1. The examiner should also note whether the patient achieves deep respiration during use of the rebreathing bag; horses with restrictive lung disease or pleural pain may develop rapid, shallow breathing to compensate in lieu of taking deep breaths. On removal of the rebreathing bag, the examiner should note the number of breaths taken to return to resting respiration as an indication of recovery rate, and the development of any cough induced by deep breathing. The trachea should also be ausculated at several levels, to detect variation in intensity of abnormal sounds originating from the upper versus lower airways. Movement of mucus within the trachea may be appreciated. Referred lung sounds (particularly wheezes) may be audible in the lower trachea as well, and stimulation of the trachea by firm rubbing or compression may elicit a series of coughs if the trachea is hyperreactive.

When abnormal sounds are appreciated, they should be described in terms of type of sound (eg, crackle, wheeze, pleural friction rub, stridor), stage of respiratory cycle (inspiratory vs expiratory), and location where they are heard loudest (eg, upper trachea, ventral lung field). These descriptive characteristics help to interpret the sounds in the context of potential respiratory diseases. For example, stridor heard during inspiration and loudest in the upper trachea is characteristic of upper airway obstruction, such as with enlarged retropharyngeal lymph nodes during *Streptococcus equi* subsp *equi* infection (strangles). In contrast, wheezes audible over the distal trachea and lungs during expiration is a finding often associated with inflammatory airway disease (IAD) or recurrent airway obstruction (RAO, "heaves").

Percussion of the thorax can be used to detect pleural effusion, areas of altered lung density (such as pulmonary abscesses), or an expanded lung field (as occurs with chronic lower airway obstruction and inflammation in heaves). Percussion can be accomplished using a plexor and a spoon nestled in the intercostal space or can be performed using simply the examiner's fingers.

ANCILLARY DIAGNOSTIC TESTS TO EVALUATE THE RESPIRATORY SYSTEM

Once the patient history and clinical findings have directed the practitioner to suspect a condition of the respiratory system, further diagnostic testing that may be performed will depend on the location and nature of suspected disease. The various diagnostic tests available to assess the respiratory system are described here.

During test selection, the practitioner must consider carefully the patient's temperament and respiratory status. If the patient is intractable or likely to struggle during a particular test, this may exacerbate respiratory distress and can cause death in extreme instances.

Other factors that may dictate the diagnostic path include costs, timeliness of results to alter the course of workup or treatment of the patient, and any need for diagnostic information that addresses the population as a whole, such as during disease outbreaks.

Evaluation of the Upper Respiratory Tract

Field diagnostic tests focused on evaluating the upper respiratory tract most commonly include upper airway endoscopy and sampling for pathogen testing.

UPPER AIRWAY ENDOSCOPY AT REST

Airway endoscopy is routinely performed under field conditions and in referral centers for in-depth examination of the respiratory tract of the horse. Direct visualization of the upper airways allows the clinician to assess dynamic or static abnormalities of sport horses referred for poor performance evaluation. In such cases, endoscopy is performed initially at rest without any patient sedation in order to assess the functional integrity of upper airway structures known to interfere with athletic performance, such as the arytenoid cartilages and soft palate. Sedation may alter laryngeal function to a degree that false positive diagnoses are otherwise made. Following assessment of laryngeal function, the patient may be sedated for more detailed endoscopic examination of static lesions if necessary.

During upper airway endoscopy of patients with nasal discharge, swelling in the retropharyngeal or throatlatch region, or periodic epistaxis, it may be indicated to enter the guttural pouches. Flexible endoscopes can be introduced into the pouches using biopsy forceps as a guidewire over which the endoscope is passed into each guttural pouch. The technique is described in Box 2 and **Fig. 1**. Although this technique does require practice to master, it is a procedure that can easily be executed in the field and serves as a valuable diagnostic aid to evaluating horses with nasal discharge or epistaxis. In particular, the retropharyngeal lymph nodes are located caudal to the medial compartment and may drain purulent material into the guttural pouch when abscess formation occurs as a result of *S equi* infection (strangles). Additional lesions that may be identified through guttural pouch endoscopy include such conditions

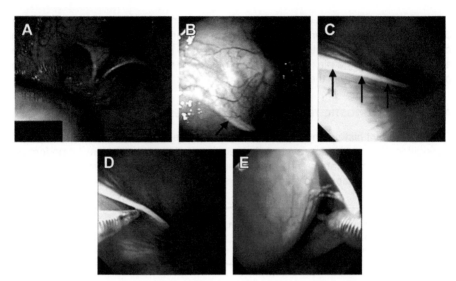

Fig. 1. (A) Endoscopic image of the pharynx. Both guttural pouch slits are seen opening during swallowing. (B) Endoscopic image of the pharynx. The right guttural pouch opening (*arrow*) is seen on the lateral pharyngeal wall. (C) Endoscopic image of the pharynx. To facilitate entry into the right guttural pouch, the endoscope has been rotated so that the guttural pouch opening (*arrows*) is seen ventrally when viewed through the endoscope. (D) Endoscopic image of the pharynx. The biopsy forceps (held closed at all times) are advanced through the biopsy channel of the endoscope and slid into the right guttural pouch opening. (E) Endoscopic image of the pharynx. Twisting the endoscope causes the guidewire (biopsy forceps) to open the guttural pouch slit so that the endoscope can be advanced into the pouch.

as mycotic plaques, temporohyoid osteopathy, guttural pouch tympany, and chondroid formation.

UPPER AIRWAY ENDOSCOPY DURING EXERCISE

Upper airway endoscopy during exercise is indicated for horses exhibiting exercise intolerance or poor performance, or respiratory noise during exercise, and to further assess abnormal endoscopic finding at rest in some instances. Endoscopic evaluation of the larynx during high-speed treadmill exercise was historically used to identify various functional airway conditions that endoscopic examination at rest was unable to identify. Poor sensitivity of high-speed treadmill endoscopy stemmed from the artificial conditions under which intense performance was evaluated. More recently, dynamic endoscopy has evolved and allows the examination of horses of multiple sport disciplines exercising under natural conditions and in their normal working environments, overcoming the main drawback of treadmill endoscopy. Portable wireless endoscopes that can be safely attached to the horse's saddle or harness have been designed to allow video recording of the upper airways of horses at rest or while exercising. The video recording is transmitted wirelessly to a hand-held monitor.

Emerging literature suggests that there are differences in the frequency of diagnosis of upper airway conditions between high-speed treadmill endoscopy and dynamic endoscopy, but the reasons for these discrepancies are currently not well characterized.[2-5] Variables such as lack of standardization of the exercise tests, shorter training distances, and an inability to re-create racing conditions have been proposed.

SAMPLING OF THE UPPER AIRWAYS FOR PATHOGEN TESTING

Common viruses that can cause infections and clinical signs associated with the upper respiratory tract in horses include equine influenza virus (EIV), equine herpesviruses (EHV) 1 and 4, equine rhinitis A and B viruses (ERAV, ERBV), and equine viral arteritis virus. The clinical signs associated with these viruses are not specific to the particular virus and resemble many other infectious and noninfectious conditions of the upper respiratory tract in horses. The clinical diagnosis of any of these suspected viral infections should therefore be confirmed by laboratory diagnostic testing. Laboratory diagnosis of equine respiratory viruses often requires combined testing through virus isolation, viral nucleic acid or antigen detection, and serology.[6] Many veterinary diagnostic laboratories offer test panels for virus isolation or polymerase chain reaction (PCR) that include most of the respiratory viral and bacterial pathogens of horses.

Appropriate sample collection and submission is an integral part of getting a successful diagnosis. The ideal sample and method of collection are dictated by the intended test. For example, nasal swabs are the best sample to detect EHV shedding using conventional or quantitative PCR analysis; however, if the objective is virus isolation, whole blood or pharyngeal swabs may be more appropriate samples.

Cotton, polyester, or rayon swabs can be used to collect samples for detection of viruses associated with respiratory infections in horses. Synthetic swabs (polyester-tipped) are preferred over cotton swabs because viruses may adhere to cotton fibers, which may affect the isolation of the virus, or these may contain substances that are inhibitory to enzymes used in PCR reactions. Flocked synthetic swabs (Copan Diagnostics, Murrieta, CA, USA) seem to be more absorbent and elute samples more efficiently.

Sampling the pharyngeal region can be achieved by using commercially available double-guarded, 33-inch-long culture swabs. Horses usually dislike the passage of the swabs through the nose; therefore, adequate patient restraint with a nose twitch, and in some cases sedation, is required. Once the swab reaches the pharyngeal area, the swab is advanced out of the casing and gently pushed against the walls of the pharynx. A rotational motion or back-and-forth maneuvers help ensure good contact with the mucosa and adequate sample collection. The tip of the swab should appear discolored (ie, yellowish, reddish, or dirty), indicating that adequate sample material was obtained from the pharyngeal mucosa.

If viral isolation is desired, one sample swab should be dedicated specifically for this purpose. On collection, the swab should be placed in a sterile tube containing virus transport media and placed in ice. If virus transport media are not available at the time of sampling, the swab may be placed in sterile isotonic saline and placed on ice for shipping; bacterial culture media should not be substituted for transporting these samples.

VIRAL ISOLATION

Nasal or pharyngeal swabs are suitable for virus isolation. Different respiratory viruses have differing growth requirements (eg, embryonated eggs, varying cell culture lines); therefore, the diagnostic laboratory may either offer an equine diagnostic panel that covers these alternatives or request information on which virus or viruses are suspected in order to appropriately set up conditions for successful virus isolation. For the clinician, disadvantages of virus isolation include the need to submit samples to specialized laboratories, high cost, and the fact that the time delay in obtaining results is too slow for impacting the management of clinical cases. Nevertheless, virus isolation from cases sampled during disease outbreaks is highly recommended, because it is critical for epidemiologic investigations to determine genetic changes of viral pathogens (antigenic drift/shift) and to guide future vaccine development. Virus isolation in cell culture is the gold standard for diagnosing EHV-1/4 as well, and it is more sensitive than immunofluorescence (IF) and PCR assay in clinical samples.[7]

ANTIGEN DETECTION

Antigen capture enzyme-linked immunosorbent assay (ELISA) has been used to detect EIV proteins with good sensitivity.[8,9] Immunofluorescence is also a rapid test to detect EHV antigens in nasal or pharyngeal swab samples with acceptable sensitivity and specificity.[7]

ANTIBODY DETECTION

The role of the practitioner is to provide the diagnostic laboratory with paired sera for antibody detection, ensuring that the acute sample was collected from the patient sufficiently early in the infection to provide meaningful results. Diagnosis of respiratory viral infection requires evidence of an increasing antibody titer over the 2 to 4 weeks following exposure to the virus. Patients sampled after the onset of clinical signs often fail to show seroconversion because their acute sample was collected after an antibody response had already been initiated. As such, it is the goal of the practitioner to sample early or at-risk cases for serology—those exposed to sick animals that have not yet or are only just starting to show clinical signs. The acute serum is harvested and stored frozen until a convalescent sample can be collected from the same animal or animals 2 to 4 weeks later. Acute and convalescent samples from individual animals are run simultaneously as pairs to avoid intra-assay variability impacting test results.

The diagnostic laboratory will need to use a variety of serologic tests in order to assess for all common equine respiratory viruses. Tests used to detect EIV antibodies include hemagglutination inhibition, virus neutralization, complement fixation, single radial hemolysis (SRH), and ELISA immunoassays. Hemagglutination inhibition and SRH are sensitive tests, with SRH shown to be more reproducible and sensitive, although more labor intensive.[10]

EHV antibodies can be measured by complement fixation, virus neutralization, and enzyme immunoassays (ie, ELISA). Immunoglubulin G antibody levels can be detected by 8 to 10 days after infection, peaking between 30 and 40 days and remaining increased for several months after infection.[11] Complement fixation and virus neutralization are not able to distinguish between EHV-1 and EHV-4, whereas ELISA is capable of differentiating between these 2 viruses.

Virus neutralization assay is use to detect ERAV- and ERBV-specific antibodies in serum samples. Although ELISA tests have been developed and provide a more rapid, high-throughput assay for detecting ERAV and ERBV, they appear less sensitive.[12]

POLYMERASE CHAIN REACTION

PCR-based techniques are becoming the most rapid and sensitive diagnostic method. PCR can detect as few as 10 to 100 copies of the target viral DNA of EHV,[13] and quantitative real-time PCR has been used to estimate the viral load. Fresh whole blood, nasopharyngeal swabs, or nasal swab samples can be used for PCR analysis for all equine viruses that affect the upper respiratory tract. Nasal swab samples appear to yield a higher number of PCR-positive results (at least in the case of EHV).[14]

BACTERIAL TESTING

Bacterial culture of pharyngeal swabs or washes, purulent discharge collected from an abscess, or guttural pouch lavage fluid remains the gold standard to detect organisms such as *S equi* subsp *equi*.[15]

The technique for sampling the guttural pouch endoscopically has been described earlier in this article. Blind sampling of the guttural pouches can also be performed when an endoscope is not available or when it is desirable to limit exposure of clinic equipment to infectious cases during herd outbreaks. The guttural pouches can be blindly catheterized for sampling using a Chambers catheter. The natural curve of the Chambers catheter allows it to be passed through the ventral meatus and blindly slid into the guttural pouch opening directly when the catheter end is moved laterally by the operator. However, when a sterile Chambers catheter is not immediately available, a sterile uterine insemination pipette with the tip bent to an angle of 60° may also serve as a substitute catheter to enter the guttural pouch. The technique differs from that of the Chambers catheter and is described in Box 3 and **Fig. 2**.

In addition to bacterial culture of guttural pouch wash fluid, PCR is a rapid and sensitive assay that identifies the DNA sequence of the SeM gene encoding the antiphagocytic M protein of *S equi*. Although PCR is more sensitive than bacterial culture, clinicians should be aware that PCR does not distinguish between live and dead *S equi* organisms and thus cannot be used to diagnose active infection with the organism. A recent study reported a sensitivity of 84% for PCR versus 39% for culture, and a combined (culture + PCR) sensitivity of 91% when used on samples from confirmed

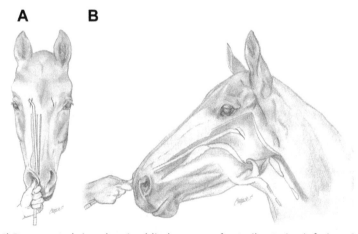

Fig. 2. (*A*) Dorsoventral view showing blind passage of a sterile uterine infusion pipette into the right guttural pouch. Once the pipette has been passed to the level of the lateral canthus of the eye, the operator's hand is moved dorsomedially as much as possible in order to push the tip against the lateral wall of the pharynx. The tip of the pipette is rotated laterally (clockwise when attempting to enter the right guttural pouch). (*B*) Lateral view showing blind passage of a sterile uterine infusion pipette into the right guttural pouch. The guttural pouch opening is approximately level with the lateral canthus of the eye. (*Courtesy of* Dr Carina Cooper, University of Guelph, Guelph, ON; with permission.)

strangles cases.[16] PCR is particularly useful for the detection of carriers or shedding from healthy animals.

Evaluation of the Lower Respiratory Tract

Field diagnostic tests focused on evaluating the lower respiratory tract most commonly include ultrasonography, bronchoscopy, and sampling by tracheal aspiration or bronchoalveolar lavage (BAL) for cytology and pathogen testing. Thoracocentesis may also be performed to sample fluid within the pleural space. Less commonly, lung biopsy is performed for diagnostic and prognostic purposes in chronic lung disease.

THORACIC ULTRASONOGRAPHY

Ultrasonography of the thorax can be performed using most common ultrasound units and transducers available in private practice. A high-frequency, linear transducer can effectively screen the lung of both adult horses and foals. Lower frequencies may be desirable to obtain more detailed images of pathologic areas. The technique is briefly described in Box 4, whereas a detailed description including video examples of abnormal findings has been published online.[17] A limitation to this diagnostic technique is that abnormal lung tissue can only be visualized if the lesion extends to the lung surface; lesions that lie deep to normal, aerated lung will not be seen because of air interference with the ultrasound beam.

Key indications for thoracic ultrasonography are to assess the lung for pneumonia, abscessation, atelectasis, or neoplasia; the lung surface for fibrin; and the chest cavity for abnormal fluid accumulation or pneumothorax. Given the noninvasive, rapid nature of this diagnostic test, the simplicity of screening for pulmonary lesions or pleural effusion, and immediacy of results, thoracic ultrasound examination provides valuable information to the practitioner regarding diagnosis, prognosis, and management of many lung conditions in horses. It should therefore be viewed as a technique used by the general practitioner during evaluation of all cases of lower respiratory tract disease.

BRONCHOSCOPY AND SAMPLING OF THE LOWER RESPIRATORY TRACT

Sampling of the lower airways is indicated when disorders of the lung are suspected and there is a need to characterize the type, degree, and origin of inflammation. Most commonly, this is accomplished through either tracheal aspirate (TA) or BAL.

The decision of whether to perform sampling via TA versus BAL depends on the suspected diagnosis; thus, it is important to have thoroughly investigated the patient history and clinical findings before sampling. BAL samples a discrete portion of the lung; therefore, it is more applicable to use for sampling conditions that cause diffuse lung disease (ie, sampling anywhere will yield similar cytology results) or when the precise location of lung inflammation can be identified and can dictate where the endoscope is wedged for BAL (such as when an obvious trail of purulent debris from a specific bronchus is seen on endoscopy). In contrast, tracheal aspiration provides a sample of cell types that have originated from throughout the lung and have traveled forward to the tracheal puddle via mucociliary clearance—although cellular morphology is less well preserved, inflammation from a focal site will be represented in this sample, whereas it could have been missed if BAL was done in a different site in the lung.

Other considerations for choosing how to collect the sample include patient respiratory status and temperament. A patient that is in moderate respiratory distress may not tolerate sedation for endoscopy but may stand well for percutaneous TA. Young animals or those unfamiliar with handling may struggle excessively during restraint for endoscopy and may collapse if they exceed their respiratory capacity; these interventions could precipitate deterioration or death in such patients. A decision tree is included to demonstrate how aspects of the clinical history and examination of the respiratory system may impact choice between the 2 sampling methods (**Fig. 3**).

Endoscopy of the lower airways requires use of an endoscope that has been sterilized; otherwise, iatrogenic contamination may occur, leading to serious infection of the lung.

Practitioner's tip

Iatrogenic infection or injury of the lung can occur if both the exterior and the interior surfaces of the endoscope are not properly cleaned and disinfected. All aspects of the endoscope should be rinsed again before use for airway sampling as well.

Endoscope care includes thorough cleaning and disinfection of the exterior surface, biopsy channel, air and water channels, as well as the water bottle and stopcock extension set. Cleaning involves an enzymatic detergent that breaks down organic debris, followed by brushing the biopsy channel with an endoscope channel cleaning brush. The enzymatic detergent and all debris are thoroughly rinsed away using sterile water, after which a disinfectant chemical such as glutaraldehyde is used to disinfect the endoscope. Personal protective equipment and adequate ventilation are required during endoscope disinfection. The disinfectant chemical is extremely irritating to mucous membranes; thus, it must be fully removed by copious flushing of all channels and rinsing the exterior surfaces of the endoscope with sterile water after the prescribed disinfecting period has elapsed. The final step in endoscope cleaning is to flush all channels with alcohol, followed by air, to facilitate thorough drying of the endoscope. The endoscope should be hung in a vertically straight position to further facilitate drainage, because residual moisture in the endoscope channels may lead to bacterial growth between uses. Specific instructions on how to perform this cleaning and disinfecting process should be obtained from the manufacturer at the time of purchase. Unfortunately, proper endoscope cleaning, disinfection, and storage are commonly neglected aspects of veterinary endoscopy as practitioners add this technique to their clinical tool kit.

Practitioner's tip

Clinic personnel should be fully trained on proper cleaning and disinfection of the endoscope when performing sampling of the airways. This includes training on PPE (personal protective equipment) and working conditions when using the chemicals for cleaning and sterilization of the endoscope.

TRACHEAL ASPIRATION

Tracheal aspiration may be performed percutaneously via a through-the-needle catheter inserted into the trachea between 2 tracheal rings or through the biopsy channel of an endoscope.

Percutaneous tracheal aspiration is easily performed in horses, particularly in foals, using the technique described in Box 5. Potential complications are summarized in **Box 6**; these should be discussed with the owner before the procedure so that informed consent can be obtained.

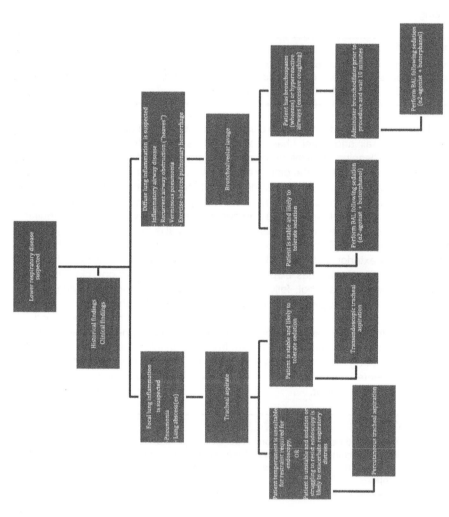

Fig. 3. A decision tree demonstrating factors influencing sampling method for the lower respiratory tract.

Box 6
Possible complications of percutaneous tracheal aspiration

- The catheter tip may flip retrograde (proximally) in the trachea during patient coughing, resulting in inability to retrieve a sample from the tracheal puddle.

- The needle may transect the catheter (the lost portion of catheter will ultimately be coughed up by the animal or may be retrieved endoscopically if appropriate in the patient).

- A subcutaneous abscess may develop at the site of needle entry through the skin, requiring drainage and treatment.

- Subcutaneous emphysema or cellulitis may develop, which can become severe and life-threatening.

In horses where endoscopy is appropriate to perform (accounting for patient stability, temperament, and available equipment for the procedure), TA can also be done transendoscopically during visual assessment of the airways. The technique is described in Box 7 and **Fig. 4**. Potential complications of transendoscopic tracheal aspiration are minimal and are described in **Box 8**.

BRONCHOALVEOLAR LAVAGE

When diffuse lung inflammation is suspected, such as with IAD or RAO (heaves), a BAL is more appropriate. Patients must be stable for tolerating endoscopy and sedation. If bronchospasm is present, based on detection of audible wheezes during lung auscultation, it is prudent to pretreat the horse with a bronchodilator before initiating endoscopy and BAL.

The technique of transendoscopic BAL is described in Box 9 and **Fig. 5**. This procedure is slightly more invasive than tracheal sampling, but the cytology results are better correlated with pulmonary disease than TA cytology. The potential complications described in **Box 10** (although uncommon) should be discussed with the owner before the procedure.

It is important to monitor the horse for at least 48 hours after a BAL for early detection of pneumonia. This monitoring should include observation of patient mentation, appetite, and respiratory effort as well as determining rectal temperature twice daily. Return to prior exercise activities may be resumed if no complications are detected after 48 hours.

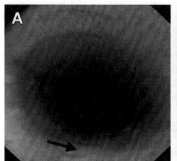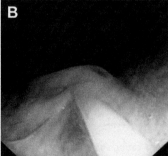

Fig. 4. (*A*) Endoscopic image of the trachea. Tracheal debris is noted (*arrow*). (*B*) Endoscopic image of the trachea. Transendoscopic TA is performed to sample the debris via a sterile catheter passed through the biopsy channel of the endoscope. The end of the endoscope is not allowed to contact the tracheal debris during sampling in order to prevent false positive culture results resulting from upper airway contamination of the sample during collection.

A transient, very mild increase in rectal temperature may be noted after routine BAL, whereas actual fever accompanied by depressed mentation and decreased appetite signals the need for reassessment and possible treatment of lung infection.

Box 8
Possible complications of transendoscopic tracheal aspiration

- Upper airway contamination of the endoscope may contaminate the sample (this risk is minimized by using a catheter passed through the biopsy channel for sampling).

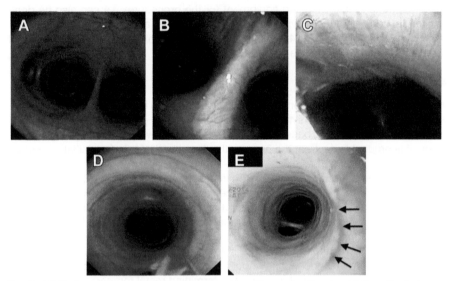

Fig. 5. (*A*) Endoscopic image of the distal trachea. The carina (tracheal bifurcation) shown here has the normal appearance of being a sharp septum. (*B*) Endoscopic image of the distal trachea. The carina (tracheal bifurcation) shown here is abnormally thickened due to bronchospasm and edema/inflammation. (*C*) Endoscopic image of the distal trachea. Topical instillation of dilute (0.3%) lidocaine is performed through the biopsy channel of the endoscope in order to desensitize cough receptors at the carina before advancing the endoscope into the lung. (*D*) Endoscopic image of bronchi. Topical instillation of dilute (0.3%) lidocaine is performed through the biopsy channel of the endoscope at each bronchial bifurcation in order to desensitize cough receptors before advancing the endoscope deeper into the lung. (*E*) Endoscopic image of the distal airways. Successful wedge of the endoscope is seen as slight tissue pucker (*arrows*) around the margin of the endoscopic image.

Box 10
Possible complications of transendoscopic bronchoalveolar lavage

- Upper airway contamination of the endoscope may contaminate the sample or lead to iatrogenic infection in the lung.
- Pre-existing focal pneumonia may become more diffuse if spread throughout the lung during lavage with large amounts of saline.

BAL can also be performed blindly, using a commercially available, cuffed, flexible nasotracheal catheter (8–13-mm outer diameter). The technique varies mildly from transendoscopic BAL and is described in Box 11. This technique provides an affordable, quick, and easy method to obtain lower airway samples in practices that cannot justify the expense of purchasing endoscopy equipment based on practice demographics.

INTERPRETATION OF TRACHEAL ASPIRATE CYTOLOGY

The TA reflects all cellular and noncellular debris that is carried forward from the lower airways via the mucociliary clearance mechanism of the lungs. It is not uncommon to see macrophages, neutrophils, other cell types, mucus, and occasional bacteria in the TA cytology. Transendoscopic tracheal aspiration has a higher risk of sample contamination with commensals from the upper respiratory tract, and bacterial proliferation in the sample may occur when the fluid is not promptly chilled after collection. Low numbers of bacteria inhabiting the lower trachea have also been documented in horses without lung inflammation.[18] It is therefore necessary to also interpret the findings of TA cytology in consideration of the patient history, clinical findings, as well as the sample handling that occurred before processing. For instance, cytology results may include both extracellular and intracellular bacteria and degenerate neutrophils; the clinician must determine whether true lung infection is present versus sample contamination during collection combined with improper handling and delay in sample processing after collection. A decision tree demonstrating this is given in **Fig. 6**.

INTERPRETATION OF BRONCHOALVEOLAR LAVAGE CYTOLOGY

BAL cytology requires evaluation of both cellular and noncellular components. As such, full interpretation of a sample should include gross inspection as well as microscopic viewing of both direct smear and a cytospin slide preparation. The gross inspection is done by holding the container up to a bright light and gently swirling the fluid; characteristics such as color, turbidity, presence of surfactant (white foam), and any flocculant debris or larvae within the sample should be recorded on the sample submission form. Describing these characteristics of the sample allows the clinical pathologist to interpret the cytologic findings in a more meaningful manner. Because of potential issues associated with any delay in sample processing (bacterial growth, loss of cellular morphology), it is useful to prepare slides within the first 4 to 8 hours after collection, in advance of shipping the sample (Box 12 and **Fig. 7**). Although the BAL fluid needs to remain chilled for transport and should be packed within icepacks for shipping, the slides must remain at room temperature; chilling the slides can damage cellular morphology. Therefore, packaging slides separately from the BAL fluid is recommended for shipping to the laboratory.

Interpretation of BAL cytology is no simple task, and advanced training and experience in this skill are needed. Although it is tempting to perform microscopic analysis of the BAL fluid in-house, it is highly recommended that BAL samples be sent to a diagnostic laboratory instead. Not all laboratories routinely evaluate BAL cytology, and practitioners are encouraged to become familiar with the methods used by local laboratories to process and report on BAL samples.

Many laboratories will perform a total nucleated cell count on the BAL fluid as part of the sample analysis. In general, the total nucleated cell count is noted but is not a key aspect of sample interpretation. Although reference ranges for the total cell count can be found in the literature, use of this parameter for BAL interpretation remains controversial; variable dilution of the sample occurs depending on how much of the lung is

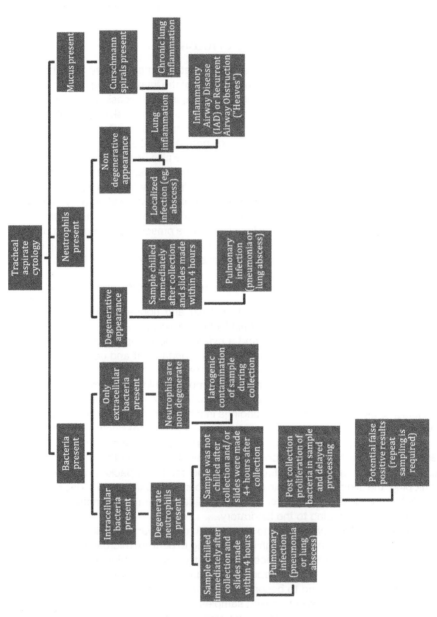

Fig. 6. A decision tree demonstrating factors that influence interpretation of TA cytology.

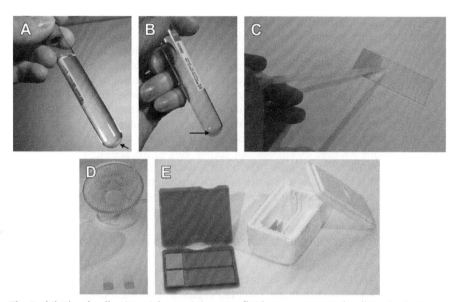

Fig. 7. (*A*) Blood collection vial containing BAL fluid. A concentrated pellet of cells is seen (*arrow*) at the base of the vial following centrifugation of the BAL fluid sample. (*B*) Blood collection vial containing BAL fluid. The supernatant fluid has been removed by gently inverting the tube and decanting the fluid as waste. The concentrated cellular pellet is then resuspended in the very small volume of residual fluid (*arrow*), by either gently tapping the vial or using a pipette to mix the sample. (*C*) A pipette is used to transfer a drop of the concentrated cellular pellet onto a glass slide. A direct smear is then made. This is accomplished by using a second slide, laid at a 45° angle against the drop of fluid, to draw the fluid across the slide. Avoid drawing the fluid across the entire slide, because the slide end typically does not get adequately stained when an automated staining method is used by the diagnostic laboratory. (*D*) Very rapid drying of the direct smears is needed in order to preserve cellular morphology. A desktop fan is the preferred method to rapidly dry the slides as soon as the smears are made. (*E*) Direct smear slides should be packaged safely for shipping to the diagnostic laboratory. Shipping containers should prevent crushing damage to the slides as well as any contact with the slide surfaces. Slides should be shipped at room temperature.

lavaged. Using a consistent volume of infusate (300–500 mL of saline) and retrieving approximately 50% of that fluid may somewhat standardize the degree of sample dilution.[19]

A thorough cytologic report of BAL fluid analysis should include both a differential cell count and a description of cellular morphology and a comment as to whether noncellular components were present in the sample. Cytospin preparations are useful to expedite performing the differential cell count, because adequate numbers of cells can be quickly and efficiently assessed. However, aspects of cytospin preparation can alter the results; in particular, mucus may be missed when pipetting of the sample is done during preparation of the cytospin slides. Therefore, examination of the noncellular components of the BAL fluid is best performed on the direct smear. The direct smear will generally show cells along the feathered edge. Mucus strands may be seen across the slide, and these should be evaluated for a predominance of specific cell types (such as neutrophils) trapped within the mucus. Mast cell granules may also be appreciated trapped within the mucus if degranulation has occurred.

The differential cell count is a key factor to identifying the type and degree of lung inflammation that is present. In general, 400 to 500 cells should be counted to ensure a representative sample has been evaluated. The clinical pathologist will count each cell that they see sequentially in order to avoid bias from counting abnormal cell types ahead of others. For cell types of low proportions, such as eosinophils and mast cells, this differential cell counting method may spuriously report these types depending on the cellular density of the slide. Therefore, recent recommendations are to perform a 5-field cell count at ×500 magnification regardless of the cellularity of the slide.[20] This approach yields more reliable counts of these uncommon cell types. Established reference ranges for BAL differential cell counts vary in the literature, but typically reflect 50% to 70% macrophages, 30% to 50% lymphocytes, less than 5% neutrophils, less than 2% mast cells, and less than 0.1% eosinophils in clinically normal horses at rest.[21] Detailed descriptions of each cell type present in BAL fluid have been published online.[22]

PATHOGEN TESTING IN TRACHEAL ASPIRATE/BRONCHOALVEOLAR LAVAGE FLUID SAMPLES

BAL fluid may also be submitted for bacterial culture or viral testing. Although PCR to test for EHV-5 and EHV-2 has been reported in cases of equine multinodular pulmonary fibrosis (EMPF), false positives may occur because many unaffected horses may also test positive for these gammaherpesviruses without developing nodular pulmonary lesions. As such, a combination of PCR on lung tissue, obtained by biopsy, plus characteristic lesions on histopathology, is preferred to confirm this diagnosis.[23,24]

THORACOCENTESIS

When excess fluid is noted within the pleural space on ultrasonography, sampling is indicated in order to characterize the nature of the thoracic pathologic lesions. The procedure for thoracocentesis is described in Box 13 and **Fig. 8**. Analysis of pleural effusion should include gross appearance, total nucleated cell count, and differential cell count as well as a description of cellular morphology. In addition, biochemical parameters can be used to estimate the likelihood of bacterial infection while awaiting cytology results. Sample pH, lactate, and glucose concentrations can be compared with a venous blood sample. Pleural effusion with a lower pH, higher lactate concentration, and lower glucose concentration compared with venous blood suggests that these parameters have been altered by bacterial metabolism, indicating bacterial pleuritis. Pleural fluid should be cultured, both aerobically and anaerobically. Whole fluid should be sent as well as swabs in appropriate bacterial transport media. If anaerobic culturettes are not available, then completely filling a blood collection tube (without anticoagulant) with the fluid, to exclude all air, will allow the sample to be used for anaerobic culture by the laboratory. Samples should be shipped chilled to the laboratory within hours of sampling. Neoplastic processes within the chest may also be detected through cytologic analysis of pleural effusion in some cases. A high proportion of a specific cell type or abnormal cellular appearance may suggest neoplasia. Not all thoracic neoplasms shed cells into the effusion, and therefore, lack of abnormal cell morphology does not exclude a diagnosis of neoplasia.

THORACIC RADIOGRAPHY

Thoracic radiography in adult horses is limited to referral centers and requires multiple images in order to capture the entire lung field. In contrast, thoracic radiography may

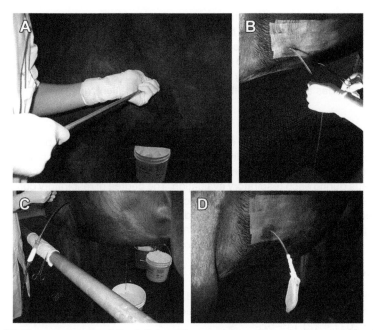

Fig. 8. (*A*) Thoracocentesis of the left hemithorax. A large-bore chest drain is used when large volumes of fluid are to be removed. The operator places one hand several centimeters from the end of the drain when passing it through the intercostal muscles and parietal pleura, to avoid overzealous penetration of the thorax. (*B*) Thoracocentesis of the left hemithorax. The operator must be ready to clamp off the drain at all times to avoid pneumothorax when effusion is no longer draining from the tube. (*C*) Thoracocentesis of the left hemithorax has been performed, and a unidirectional Heimlich valve has been attached to the drain to prevent pneumothorax. The opposite hemithorax is also being drained simultaneously. Pleural effusion should be drained into buckets, as shown here, in order to limit environmental contamination as well as to record the volume obtained from each side of the chest. (*D*) Indwelling chest drain in the left hemithorax. A finger from a sterile glove is used to create unidirectional flow of fluid, to prevent pneumothorax. A small slit in the end of the finger permits effusion to continue to drain, whereas the finger collapses closed during each inspiration.

be attempted on young foals using portable field equipment if screening for pulmonary abscessation (*Rhodococcus equi*) is needed. The procedure for performing and interpreting thoracic radiography is described in detail in an online veterinary article[25] and includes multiple examples of lung pathologic abnormality for reference for the equine practitioner.

LUNG BIOPSY

The diagnostic utility of lung biopsy is limited to a few respiratory disorders of the lung. Nodular pulmonary masses that appear cellular on ultrasound examination may be sampled by lung biopsy. Lung biopsy may therefore assist with the diagnosis of EMPF and provides a sample for histopathology and viral PCR testing for EHV-5 in such cases.[26,27] Biopsy of lung in patients with chronic and severe RAO may be done as well to characterize the degree of pulmonary fibrosis that is present. This information may allow the practitioner to understand what degree of respiratory improvement may be anticipated following careful management of environmental factors exacerbating heaves, versus residual lung impairment that exists from increased collagen deposition and cannot be reversed.[28] In most cases, this information may help owners to make end-of-life decisions in horses in which considerable effort has been invested into controlling heaves signs without achieving remission to a degree that provides adequate quality of respiration for patient well-being.

SUMMARY

Multiple diagnostic aids exist for evaluating the upper and lower respiratory tract of equine patients under field conditions. Detailed investigation of the patient history and thorough clinical examination are critical to determining the appropriate diagnostic steps during each respiratory evaluation. The degree of respiratory compromise and patient temperament should also be considered during selection of diagnostic tests, because struggling may precipitate deterioration of the patient during invasive sampling procedures. Finally, understanding how sample selection, collection, and handling can impact test results is a key element to achieving an accurate diagnosis.

REFERENCES

1. Wasko AJ, Barkema HW, Nicol J, et al. Evaluation of a risk-screening questionnaire to detect equine lung inflammation: results of a large field study. Equine Vet J 2011;43(2):145–52.
2. Allen KJ, Franklin SH. Assessment of the exercise tests used during overground endoscopy in UK Thoroughbred racehorses and how these may affect the diagnosis of dynamic upper respiratory tract obstructions. Equine Vet J Suppl 2010;(38):587–91.
3. Allen KJ, Franklin SH. Comparisons of overground endoscopy and treadmill endoscopy in UK Thoroughbred racehorses. Equine Vet J 2010;42:186–91.
4. Kelly PG, Reardon RJ, Johnston MS, et al. Comparison of dynamic and resting endoscopy of the upper portion of the respiratory tract in 57 Thoroughbred yearlings. Equine Vet J 2013;45:700–4.
5. Trope G. Dynamic endoscopy of the equine upper airway—what is significant? Vet Rec 2013;172:499–500.
6. Diaz-Mendez A, Viel L, Hewson J, et al. Surveillance of equine respiratory viruses in Ontario. Can J Vet Res 2010;74:271–8.
7. Slater J. Equine herpesviruses. In: Sellon DC, Long T, editors. Equine infectious diseases. 2nd edition. St Louis (MO): Saunders Elsevier; 2014. p. 151–68.
8. Livesay GJ, O'Neill T, Hannant D, et al. The outbreak of equine influenza (H3N8) in the United Kingdom in 1989: diagnostic use of an antigen capture ELISA. Vet Rec 1993;133:515–9.
9. Ji Y, Guo W, Zhao L, et al. Development of an antigen-capture ELISA for the detection of equine influenza virus nucleoprotein. J Virol Methods 2011;175: 120–4.
10. Gibson CA, Wood JM, Mumford J, et al. A single-radial haemolysis technique for measurement of antibody to influenza virus neuraminidase in equine sera. J Virol Methods 1985;11:299–308.
11. Stokes A, Corteyn AH, Murray PK. Clinical signs and humoral immune response in horses following equine herpesvirus type-1 infection and their susceptibility to equine herpesvirus type-4 challenge. Res Vet Sci 1991;51:141–8.
12. Horsington J, Lynch SE, Gilkerson JR, et al. Equine picornaviruses: well known but poorly understood. Vet Microbiol 2013;167:78–85.

13. Elia G, Decaro N, Martella V, et al. Detection of equine herpesvirus type 1 by real time PCR. J Virol Methods 2006;133:70–5.
14. Pusterla N, Mapes S, Wilson WD. Diagnostic sensitivity of nasopharyngeal and nasal swabs for the molecular detection of EHV-1. Vet Rec 2008;162:520–1.
15. Sweeney CR, Timoney JF, Newton JR, et al. Streptococcus equi infections in horses: guidelines for treatment, control, and prevention of strangles. J Vet Intern Med 2005;19(1):123–34.
16. Lindahl S, Båverud V, Egenvall A, et al. Comparison of sampling sites and laboratory diagnostic tests for S. equi subsp. equi in horses from confirmed strangles outbreaks. J Vet Intern Med 2013;27:542–7.
17. Reef VB. Ultrasonography. In: Lekeux P, editor. Equine respiratory diseases. Ithaca (NY): International Veterinary Information Service; 2006. p. 1–12. B0306.0106. Available at: www.ivis.org.
18. Hewson J, Viel L. Streptococcus in the trachea: is it merely a contaminant?. In: Ainsworth DM, McGorum BC, Viel L, et al, editors. Third world equine airways symposium. Ithaca (NY): International Veterinary Information Service; 2005. p. 1–3. P2119.0705. Available at: www.ivis.org.
19. Couëtil LL, Hoffman AM, Hodgson J, et al. Inflammatory airway disease of horses. J Vet Intern Med 2007;21(2):356–61.
20. Fernandez NJ, Hecker KG, Gilroy CV, et al. Reliability of 400-cell and 5-field leukocyte differential counts for equine bronchoalveolar lavage fluid. Vet Clin Pathol 2013;42(1):92–8.
21. Hoffman AM. Bronchoalveolar lavage: sampling technique and guidelines for cytologic preparation and interpretation. Vet Clin North Am Equine Pract 2008; 24(2):423–35.
22. Hewson J, Viel L. Sampling, microbiology and cytology of the respiratory tract. In: Lekeux P, editor. Equine respiratory diseases. Ithaca (NY): International Veterinary Information Service; 2002. p. 1–16. B0308.0602. Available at: www.ivis.org.
23. Torfason EG, Thorsteinsdottir L, Torsteindottir S, et al. Study of equid herpesvirus 2 and 5 in Iceland with a type-specific polymerase chain reaction. Res Vet Sci 2008;85:605–11.
24. Fortier G, van Erck E, Pronost S, et al. Equine gammaherpesviruses: pathogenesis, epidemiology and diagnosis. Vet J 2010;176:148–56.
25. Sande RD, Tucker RL. Radiology of the equine lungs and thorax. In: Lekeux P, editor. Equine respiratory diseases. Ithaca (NY): International Veterinary Information Service; 2004. p. 1–18. B0305.0104. Available at: www.ivis.org.
26. Wong DM, Belgrave RL, Williams KJ, et al. Multinodular pulmonary fibrosis in five horses. J Am Vet Med Assoc 2008;232(6):898–905.
27. Schwarz B, Klang A, Bezdekova B, et al. Equine multinodular pulmonary fibrosis (EMPF): five case reports. Acta Vet Hung 2013;6(3):319–32.
28. Setlakwe EL, Lemos KR, Lavoie-Lamoureux A, et al. Airway collagen and elastic fiber content correlates with lung function in equine heaves. Am J Physiol Lung Cell Mol Physiol 2014;307(3):L252–260.

APPENDIX

Box 1
Procedure for use of a rebreathing bag

Note: Use of a rebreathing bag is intended to increase the rate and depth of respiration such that lung sounds become audible during auscultation of the thorax. This procedure is therefore contraindicated (and unnecessary) in patients with an elevated respiratory rate or showing signs of respiratory distress.

Supplies needed:

- Medium-sized (50–75 L approximate capacity) plastic garbage bag
- Two to 3 people (3 is ideal)
- Stethoscope

Method:

1. The size of the bag opening should be reduced by tying one corner of the bag opening into a knot. This makes it easier for the people holding the bag to prevent additional air from leaking into the bag during the procedure.

2. Three people are ideally required to perform respiratory auscultation during use of a rebreathing bag, although it can be done with only 2 people if necessary. One person restrains the horse and also helps to hold the bag. A second person holds the bag, and the third person performs lung auscultation.

3. The 2 people holding the bag should stand on either side of the horse's head. Avoid standing in front of the horse, because occasionally they will toss their head, which could lead to personal injury.

4. Fill the bag with air and then slowly slide the bag over the mouth and nares of the horse. Gather the edges of the bag opening so that it fits snugly around the nose. Each person holding the bag should tent their side of the bag up over the nostril—this is to ensure that the bag does not flatten over either nostril and acutely obstruct inspiration. (If this occurs, the horse will usually panic and toss their head, causing the bag to fall off and terminating the procedure. It is typically difficult to replace the bag on the horse's nose a second time after this has occurred.)

5. The bag is maintained over the horse's nose for 1 to 2 minutes, during which time the horse will begin to breathe more deeply, and respiratory rate will increase in response to the elevation in carbon dioxide within the inspired air from the bag. If deep inspiration causes the bag to fully collapse, a small amount of additional fresh air may be introduced into the bag in order to accommodate the increased tidal volume during respiration (one person lifts the edge of the bag opening off of the nose slightly to create a small gap for fresh air to enter; do not fully remove the bag to do this, because you want the horse to continue inspiring deeply).

6. Lung auscultation over the entire lung field on one side of the horse is performed while the rebreathing bag is held in place, noting any regions where abnormal lung sounds are heard or suspected. The trachea should also be auscultated for any referred wheezes or mucus movement. Once the entire lung field has been assessed, the operator should return to any suspected regions for final lung auscultation as the bag is removed, because this is when abnormalities are most likely to be detected (as the horse takes several deep breaths after bag removal).

7. After removing the bag from the horse's nose, the operator should note how many breaths are required for the horse to return to their previous rate and depth of respiration (recovery rate). Most horses will require 4 to 6 breaths to recover, whereas prolonged recovery may be noted in horses with impaired lung function. Any cough induced by deep inspiration is also noted.

8. The bag is then replaced over the horse's nose, and the other side of the chest is auscultated similarly.

Box 2
Procedure for endoscopically entering the guttural pouch

Supplies needed:

- Patient sedation

- Nose twitch

- Water-soaked gauze squares

- Flexible endoscope

- Endoscopic biopsy forceps

- Sterile saline (30 mL) in a syringe

- Sterile sample collection vials (without anticoagulant)

Method:

1. Sedate and appropriately restrain the patient (a nose twitch is commonly required in addition to sedation).

2. Clean the external nares using a water-soaked gauze square.

3. The endoscope is inserted through the ventral meatus of the ipsilateral nostril to the pouch to be catheterized and is advanced until the guttural pouch openings are visualized in the nasopharynx (**Fig. 1A, B**).

4. At this stage, rotate the endoscope so that the lateral wall of the pharynx is seen ventrally on the endoscope image, with the end of the endoscope situated just proximal to the guttural pouch opening (see **Fig. 1C**).

5. The biopsy forceps are fed through the biopsy channel of the endoscope and gently advanced into the guttural pouch opening several centimeters to serve as a guidewire over which the endoscope will be passed (see **Fig. 1D**). Do not excessively feed the forceps into the pouch, in particular when pathologic processes such as mycosis are suspected. Also, keep the biopsy forceps closed at all times during this procedure to avoid inadvertent damage to structures within the guttural pouch!

6. As a result of the peripheral location of biopsy channel on the end of the endoscope, rotating the endoscope will manipulate the pouch to open due to the guidewire (see **Fig. 1E**). As the endoscope is rotated, it is also slowly advanced to slide into the pouch over the guidewire. The ability to accomplish this does take practice, and persistence is required to successfully enter the guttural pouches on occasion.

7. Once in the guttural pouch, the internal structures can be visualized while avoiding direct contact as much as possible. The stylohyoid bone divides the guttural pouch cavity into a medial and lateral compartment. Both compartments should be examined for any discharge, chondroids, plaques, or abnormal appearance to the mucosal lining. External structures such as swollen lymph nodes pressing in on the guttural pouch wall are noted as well.

8. Regardless of whether discharge is present, if strangles is suspected from the patient history or physical examination, a lavage should be performed to collect a sample. A sterile catheter is passed through the biopsy channel of the endoscope into the guttural pouch. Avoid contact by the catheter with the mucosal lining of the pouch in order to not cause iatrogenic injury. Sterile saline is infused through the catheter and then is retrieved. The sample should be submitted for bacterial culture as well as PCR testing for *S equi*. Keep the samples chilled during submission to the diagnostic laboratory.

9. It is possible to enter both guttural pouches with the endoscope from a single nostril, particularly when using a small-diameter endoscope, which is easier to manipulate and requires just a small opening to enter the pouch. However, in general, it is much easier to remove the endoscope and pass it up the other nostril when attempting to enter the second guttural pouch.

Box 3
Procedure for blind catheterization of the guttural pouch to obtain a diagnostic sample (or to perform therapeutic lavage)

Supplies needed:

- Patient sedation
- Nose twitch
- Water-soaked gauze squares
- Sterile uterine infusion pipette
- Sterile saline (30 mL) in a syringe
- Sterile sample collection vials (without anticoagulant)

Method:

1. Sedate and appropriately restrain the patient (a nose twitch is commonly required in addition to sedation).

2. Clean the external nares using a water-soaked gauze square.

3. While the uterine infusion pipette is still in its sterile casing, create a bend (60°) in the pipette approximately 5 cm from the tip. Also, premeasure it against the horse's head to the level of the lateral canthus of the eye.

4. Remove the sterile casing. Then insert the pipette through the ventral meatus of the ipsilateral nostril to the pouch to be catheterized, with the bent tip facing ventrally.

5. Once the tip of the pipette reaches the approximate level of the lateral canthus of the eye, the operator's hand is moved medially as much as possible at the nose in order to push the pipette tip against the lateral wall of the nasopharynx (**Fig. 2**A).

6. The pipette is then rotated 90°, moving the bent tip from a ventral to a lateral position; this lifts and opens the fibrocartilaginous guttural pouch opening.

7. Once the pipette tip enters the pouch opening, the operator can feel the pipette easily slide into the pouch cavity (see **Fig. 2**B). Several attempts may be required to successfully pass the catheter.

8. Once in the guttural pouch, sterile saline is infused through the pipette and then retrieved for pathogen testing. The sample should be submitted for bacterial culture as well as PCR testing for *S equi*. Keep the samples chilled during submission to the diagnostic laboratory.

9. More saline may be infused for lavage to remove debris as necessary while the pipette is in the guttural pouch. The infusate should be collected in a bowl for disposal rather than allowing the saline to drain onto the ground in order to limit environmental contamination with infectious material during guttural pouch lavage.

Box 4
Lung ultrasonography

Supplies needed:

- Ultrasound and transducer
- Alcohol

Method:

1. It is not necessary to clip the hair over the site of interest, provided that copious alcohol is applied to the hair coat to remove any air trapped within the hair. The quality of the image may not be ideal in unclipped animals, however; therefore, clipping the hair is recommended if high-quality images are desired for assessment in some cases.

2. Place the ultrasound probe on the chest wall midthorax, where the lung is easily seen in order to first adjust the image depth and contrast for performing the examination. Holding the probe still while watching the horse breathe allows the practitioner to identify the lung surface as it slides from side to side on the ultrasound image. A normal lung will appear as a consistently smooth, bright hyperechoic line, running parallel to the skin surface. A very small amount of pleural fluid lubricates the lung movement within the chest; this may be appreciated as a very thin, anechoic line between the lung surface and the parietal pleura/intercostal muscles. Set the image depth so that the lung surface is midscreen on the ultrasound unit, optimizing the ultrasound image of the lung.

3. The transducer should be oriented so that it sits slightly angled, within the intercostal space and parallel to the ribs. Keep the probe within a single intercostal space while the probe is moved from a dorsal to ventral position over the chest. Always move the ultrasound transducer in the direction of the hair in order to avoid introducing air into the hair coat, which will disrupt the image quality.

4. A systematic examination of the entire lung on each side of the chest is performed. Starting at the 16th intercostal space at the transverse processes of the thoracic vertebrae, the lung underlying each intercostal space is sequentially examined from dorsal to ventral until the diaphragm is observed, marking the end of the lung field in that location. (Cranially, the heart will signal the ventral landmark for lung ultrasonography on each side.)

5. On reaching the ventral landmark of the lung at an intercostal space, the probe is then advanced cranially to the next intercostal space and the process is repeated, always running from dorsal to ventral.

6. If a site of interest is identified that requires more thorough re-examination, the probe should be lifted off the body, moved more dorsal than the site, and then slid ventrally until the site is reached; the probe should not be moved in a ventral-to-dorsal direction because this disturbs the hair coat and will introduce air into the hair, interfering with imaging the lung.

Box 5
Procedure for tracheal aspirate (percutaneous)

Supplies needed:

- Hair clippers or shaving razor
- Sterile/surgical preparation materials
- 1 mL lidocaine 2%, 25-gauge needle (for skin desensitization)
- Sterile gloves
- 14-gauge, 1.5-inch needle
- 30-cm length of sterile polypropylene catheter (dog urinary catheter) or commercial aspirate set
- 20 mL sterile saline drawn up in a sterile syringe
- Sample containers (1 vial without anticoagulant, 1 EDTA vial)

Method:

1. Clip and surgically prepare a 10 cm × 10 cm square on the ventral aspect of the trachea (approximately 10 cm from the thoracic inlet).
2. Instill 1 mL of lidocaine subcutaneously to desensitize the area.
3. Don sterile gloves.
4. Insert a 14-gauge needle between the tracheal rings, with the bevel facing caudally.
5. Once inserted, angle the needle to point caudally down the trachea. Keep it in this position throughout the procedure to avoid traumatizing the tracheal mucosa.
6. Insert the sterile polyethylene catheter into the trachea through the needle and pass it approximately 15 cm distally in the trachea.
7. Have an assistant attach the syringe and slowly instill 20 mL of sterile saline.
8. Have the assistant withdraw the fluid sample using the same syringe. It may be necessary for you to slowly withdraw the catheter as they apply negative pressure to the syringe in order to locate the tracheal puddle.
9. Once adequate sample has been collected (note: you will not likely retrieve your entire original volume), remove the catheter from the needle and then remove the needle from the trachea. It is important to remove the catheter and needle following this sequence because if the catheter and needle are removed simultaneously, contaminated contents within the catheter may be deposited in the tissue layers and cause local infection.
10. Place the sample into a sterile container (for culture) as well as an EDTA tube (for cytology).
11. Keep the TA samples chilled (in a refrigerator or in a container of iced water) until submitted to the laboratory (within 4–8 hours of collection). Direct smears should also be made and shipped at room temperature.

Box 7
Procedure for tracheal aspirate (transendoscopic)

Supplies needed:

- Sedation (α_2-agonist plus butorphanol)
- Nose twitch
- Water-soaked gauze to clean nares
- Sterilized and rinsed endoscope
- Sterile polypropylene catheter (that fits within the biopsy channel) with a needle inserted at one end
- 20 mL sterile saline drawn up in a sterile syringe
- Sample containers (1 vial without anticoagulant, 1 EDTA vial)

Method:

1. Sedate and appropriately restrain the patient (a nose twitch is commonly required in addition to sedation).

2. Clean the external nares using a water-soaked gauze square.

3. Pass the endoscope through the nasopharynx and into the proximal trachea. Do NOT administer lidocaine in the proximal trachea! Gravity will drain such fluid distally in the trachea, contaminating the tracheal puddle and potentially causing false positive culture results.

4. Slowly advance the endoscope to the level of midtrachea. Discharge may be seen along the length of the trachea, or a "tracheal puddle" may be visible: do not contact this area with the endoscope to avoid contamination by upper respiratory tract microflora (**Fig. 4A**)!

5. Advance a sterile polypropylene catheter through the biopsy channel of the endoscope (you will need to remove the extension set or cap from the biopsy channel to do this). Either wear sterile gloves to handle the catheter or avoid contacting the distal 20 cm as you pass it into the biopsy channel.

6. Pass the catheter beyond the end of the endoscope and into the region of the tracheal puddle. Manipulate the endoscope to avoid scraping the catheter along the tracheal mucosa as you do this.

7. Directly aspirate any discharge present through the catheter (see **Fig. 4B**). If minimal or no discharge is seen, administer 20 mL of sterile saline through the catheter. Avoid allowing the end of the endoscope to contact the puddle of saline. Use a small amount of air to clear the catheter and then collect the sample from the tracheal puddle using the same catheter.

8. Once an adequate sample has been collected, remove the catheter from the endoscope and then remove the endoscope from the patient.

9. Place the sample into a sterile container (for culture) as well as an EDTA tube (for cytology).

10. Keep the TA samples chilled (in a refrigerator or in a container of iced water) until submitted to the laboratory (within 4–8 hours of collection). Direct smears should also be made and shipped at room temperature.

Box 9
Procedure for bronchoalveolar lavage (transendoscopic)

Supplies needed:

- Sedation (α_2-agonist plus butorphanol)
- Nose twitch
- Water-soaked gauze to clean nares
- Sterilized and rinsed endoscope
- 120 to 180 mL of dilute (0.3%) lidocaine[a] in sterile saline; drawn up as 60-mL aliquots in syringes and warmed to 37°C
- 300 to 500 mL of sterile saline, drawn up as 60-mL aliquots in syringes and warmed to 37°C
- Sample containers (1 vial without anticoagulant, 1 EDTA vial)

Method:

1. Sedate and appropriately restrain the patient (a nose twitch is commonly required in addition to sedation).
2. Clean the external nares using a water-soaked gauze square.
3. Pass the endoscope through the nasopharynx and into the proximal trachea. Do NOT administer lidocaine in the proximal trachea! Gravity will drain such fluid distally in the trachea, contaminating the tracheal puddle, and potentially causing false positive culture results if performed.
4. Note the presence of any debris, hyperemia, or hyperreactivity of the trachea.
5. Slowly advance the endoscope to the level of midtrachea. Collect any TA samples (Box 9) before allowing the endoscope to contact the tracheal puddle.
6. Advance the endoscope to visualize the carina. Note the character of the carina (crisp margin vs appearing blunted or thickened) (**Fig. 5A, B**). Do NOT touch the carina until it has been desensitized!
7. Spray 60 mL of 0.3% dilute lidocaine onto the carina through the biopsy channel of the endoscope (see **Fig. 5C**). Allow 20 to 30 seconds or longer for effect before advancing the endoscope further.
8. Sequentially pause to desensitize bronchi with dilute lidocaine as the endoscope is slowly advanced deeper into the lung (see **Fig. 5D**).
9. When resistance is encountered to further passage of the endoscope despite gentle pressure, or when a ring of tissue encircling the endoscope tip is visualized through the endoscope, the endoscope is "wedged" and no further advancement is needed (see **Fig. 5E**). Keep the endoscope gently at this location. Pinching the endoscope against the external nares is helpful to minimize inadvertent shifting of the endoscope during patient movement.
10. Instill 120 mL of sterile saline through the extension set of the biopsy channel. Clear the channel with 15 mL of air and then gently aspirate to retrieve the infusate. Discontinue suction when a continuous flow of infusate is no longer retrieved.
11. Instill an additional 60 mL of sterile saline, followed by 15 mL of air. Then gently aspirate.
12. Repeat until a total of 300 mL of sterile saline has been instilled and aspirated. Approximately 40% to 60% of the infusate should be retrieved for reliable cytology results. The retrieved sample should have a surface layer of foam (surfactant), indicating alveolar sampling.
13. Remove the endoscope from the patient, noting where the final endoscope placement was for the BAL.
14. Mix the BAL fluid samples gently. Place the combined sample into a sterile container (for culture) as well as an EDTA tube (for cytology).
15. Keep the sample chilled (in a refrigerator or in a container of iced water) until submitted to the laboratory (within 4–8 hours of collection). Direct smears should also be made and shipped at room temperature.

[a] Dilute (0.3% v/v) lidocaine solution: Aseptically add 100 mL of 2% lidocaine without epinephrine to a 500-mL bottle of sterile saline. This creates a stock solution of diluted (0.3%) lidocaine that can be stored and refrigerated for later use. Warm the solution to body temperature after drawing up the desired quantity into 60-mL syringes before a BAL procedure.

Box 11
Procedure for bronchoalveolar lavage (blind technique using nasotracheal catheter)

Supplies needed:

- Sedation (α_2-agonist plus butorphanol)

- Nose twitch

- Water-soaked gauze to clean nares

- Sterile nasotracheal catheter with cuffed end

- 6-mL syringe filled with air (to inflate cuff)

- 120 mL of dilute (0.3%) lidocaine[a] in sterile saline; drawn up as 60-mL aliquots in syringes and warmed to 37°C

- 300 to 500 mL of sterile saline, drawn up as 60-mL aliquots in syringes and warmed to 37°C

- Sample containers (1 vial without anticoagulant, 1 EDTA vial)

Method:

1. Check the cuff of the nasotracheal catheter to ensure that it is not leaking when filled with air. Deflate again before use.

2. Sedate and appropriately restrain the patient (a nose twitch is commonly required in addition to sedation).

3. Clean the external nares using water-soaked gauze square.

4. Pass the cuffed nasotracheal catheter through the nasopharynx and into the proximal trachea. It is helpful to extend the head at the time of passing the catheter through the larynx.

5. Advance the nasotracheal catheter down the trachea and into the lung. If an excessive cough response is elicited as the catheter passes the carina, 60 mL of dilute (0.3%) lidocaine can be administered at this site before proceeding. Wait 20 to 30 seconds after lidocaine is instilled before advancing the nasotracheal catheter further.

6. Advance the nasotracheal catheter slowly until you encounter resistance to gently passing the catheter any further. At this point, if you try to advance the catheter further and then let go of it, it will slide backwards slightly as another indicator of being wedged. Inflate the catheter cuff using 6 mL of air.

7. Instill 120 mL of sterile saline, followed by 15 mL of air to empty the catheter.

8. Gently aspirate to withdraw the sample. Discontinue suction when a continuous flow of infusate is no longer retrieved.

9. Instill an additional 60 mL of sterile saline, followed by 15 mL of air. Then gently aspirate.

10. Repeat until a total of 300 mL of sterile saline has been instilled and aspirated. Approximately 40% to 60% of the infusate should be retrieved for reliable cytology results. The retrieved sample should have a surface layer of foam (surfactant), indicating alveolar sampling.

11. Deflate the catheter cuff.

12. Remove the nasotracheal catheter.

13. Mix the BAL fluid samples gently. Place the combined sample into a sterile container (for culture) as well as an EDTA tube (for cytology).

14. Keep the sample chilled (in a refrigerator or in a container of iced water) until submitted to the laboratory (within 4–8 hours of collection). Direct smears should also be made and shipped at room temperature.

[a] Dilute (0.3% v/v) lidocaine solution: Aseptically add 100 mL of 2% lidocaine without epinephrine to a 500-mL bottle of sterile saline. This creates a stock solution of diluted (0.3%) lidocaine that can be stored and refrigerated for later use. Warm the solution to body temperature after drawing up the desired quantity into 60-mL syringes before a BAL procedure.

Box 12
Procedure for direct smear preparation

Supplies needed:

• Desktop centrifuge

• Blood collection tubes without anticoagulant

• Pipette

• Glass slides

• Packaging for shipping the slides to a laboratory

Method:

1. Place two 10-mL aliquots of sample into blood collection tubes (without any anticoagulant) and centrifuge them for 10 minutes at 600 to 800 g. This generates a concentrated pellet of cells at the bottom of each tube (**Fig. 7**A).

2. The supernatant fluid is gently poured out from the tubes as waste. The remaining pellet is resuspended in any residual fluid by gently tapping the side of the tube (see **Fig. 7**B).

3. A drop of the concentrated sample is placed on a glass microscope slide using a pipette (see **Fig. 7**C). As when preparing a blood smear, a second slide is used to spread the drop across the slide in a thin layer. Because cells will collect at the feathered edge, avoid spreading the drop the entire length of the slide, so that the cells remain in the field of view after staining.

4. It is essential that the slide is rapidly air-dried immediately, otherwise the cellular morphology becomes distorted and slide interpretation can be challenging. A desktop fan is useful to achieve rapid drying of the slides as they are made (see **Fig. 7**D).

5. Once several slides have been made from the pellet and are thoroughly dried, the slides are carefully packaged for transport, keeping them at room temperature (see **Fig. 7**E). Any fluid sample shipped along with the slides needs to be kept chilled; therefore, careful attention must be paid to avoid any chilling of the slides, because freezing or condensation resulting from temperature fluctuations may damage cell morphology on the slide preparations.

Box 13
Procedure for thoracocentesis

Supplies needed:

- Ultrasound (optional)
- Sedation (if appropriate based on patient respiratory status)
- Hair clippers or razor blade
- Surgical preparatory solutions (scrub, alcohol, solution) and gauze squares
- 2% lidocaine (12 mL in syringe, 18-gauge 1.5-inch needle)
- Sterile gloves
- Scalpel blade (no. 15)
- 14-gauge, 13.3-cm intravenous catheter or sterile teat cannula or large-bore chest drain
- Extension set and stopcock, with sterile 60-mL syringe attached for sample collection
- Collection vials (EDTA for cytology, sterile tubes without anticoagulant for culture)
- Skin suture (if placing a large bore chest drain)

Method:

1. Ultrasound guidance to select a ventrally located site for sampling, while avoiding the heart, is desirable. However, if ultrasound guidance is not available, then thoracocentesis at the sixth or seventh intercostal space, several centimeters above the lateral thoracic vein, is advised. Both sides of the thorax should be sampled independently.

2. Because of the potential hypotension associated with rapidly draining large volumes of fluid from the chest cavity, it is recommended that intravenous catheterization be performed and the patient be maintained on intravenous fluid replacement therapy during thoracic drainage.

3. Patient sedation is performed if medically appropriate.

4. The site (8 cm × 8 cm) should be clipped and prepared aseptically. Local anesthetic (approximately 10–12 mL) is infiltrated as well to desensitize the skin down to the parietal pleura, followed by a final preparation of the sterile site.

5. Sterile gloves should be donned at this stage.

6. If only a sample is required, a 14-gauge, 13.3-cm intravenous catheter may be used to perform the thoracocentesis. However, often sampling is combined with thoracic drainage of the excess fluid in order to simultaneously improve respiratory effort. As such, thoracocentesis is more commonly performed using a larger-bore chest drain (**Fig. 8**A) or sterile teat cannula. Both require that a stab incision be made through the skin and intercostal muscles before inserting the drain/cannula. This should be performed on the cranial margin of a rib in order to avoid the intercostal vessels located along the caudal border of each rib.

7. The drain/cannula is held approximately 4 cm from its tip during insertion, to avoid overzealous penetration of the chest cavity as pressure is applied to pass it through the parietal pleura. A change in resistance (pop) may be felt as the catheter/cannula passes through the parietal pleura.

8. Negative pressure should be present within the chest, and the catheter may suck air into the chest cavity if the tip of the catheter is not within the pleural effusion. Therefore, the practitioner should be prepared to clamp the catheter or block the end of the cannula at all times, to avoid pneumothorax during thoracocentesis (see **Fig. 8**B). Attaching an extension set to the catheter or cannula can facilitate easy clamping.

9. Pleural effusion is collected either through free flow or by applying very gentle suction on the extension set. Samples are immediately transferred to collection vials for laboratory submission as follows:

- EDTA tube for cytology
- Sterile collection tubes without anticoagulant for bacterial culture. Both aerobic and anaerobic culture should be requested.
    a. The sample for anaerobic culture should completely fill the collection tube to eliminate all air. A swab of pleural fluid inserted deeply into an anaerobic culture tube may also be submitted.

10. If a large volume of fluid was drained from the chest, it may be desirable to maintain an indwelling chest drain in the horse. The skin around the chest drain is closed using a purse-string suture pattern, and the drain is secured with the same suture. To avoid pneumothorax, the drain should be attached to a continuous portable suction apparatus, or a one-way valve should be configured from a Heimlich valve (see **Fig. 8**C) or by creating a makeshift valve; the finger from a sterile glove can be taped over the catheter end and a small slit in the finger tip allows fluid to continue draining (whereas the glove finger collapses closed during each inspiration by the horse) (see **Fig. 8**D). Maintaining a chest drain is challenging because of complications with the drain becoming kinked or blocked by fibrin. The challenges often necessitate transfer of such patients to a referral facility for more continuous monitoring and to optimize management of chest drainage.

Gastritis, Enteritis, and Colitis in Horses

Francisco A. Uzal, DVM, MSc, PhD[a],*, Santiago S. Diab, DVM[b]

KEYWORDS

- Enteritis • Gastritis • Colitis • Horse

KEY POINTS

- The most prevalent bacterial causes of enteritis/colitis include *Clostridium perfringens* type C, *Clostridium difficile*, *Clostridium piliforme*, *Salmonella* spp, *Rhodococcus equi*, *Ehrlichia risticii*, and *Lawsonia intracellularis*.
- Equine rotavirus and coronavirus are the most prevalent viral agents of enteric disease.
- *Cryptosporidium parvum* and strongyles are the most prevalent parasitic agents of enteric diseases in this species.
- Nonsteroidal antiinflammatory drugs are responsible for ulceration of most of the alimentary tract.

INTRODUCTION

There are a large variety of infectious and noninfectious inflammatory diseases that affect the gastrointestinal system of horses (**Table 1**).[1–8] For many years the percentage of these conditions in which a cause was found was low, but increased knowledge along with more and better laboratory diagnostic techniques now available for routine use in diagnostic laboratories has increased the number of cases with a confirmed cause. Nevertheless, there is a still a significant percentage of severe inflammatory conditions of the intestinal tract in which a cause is never found; this is frustrating for pathologists, clinicians, and owners. Frequently in the past and occasionally nowadays, severe, often fatal enteric inflammatory lesions of horses of unknown cause were referred to as colitis X. Because the name colitis X does not refer to a specific disease condition, but rather to a group of unknown causes that lead to a similar lesion and clinical outcome, it has been recommended that this term be no longer used. This recommendation is further supported by several enteric diseases of horses having been better characterized in recent years, and it has been shown that several different

[a] California Animal Health and Food Safety Laboratory, School of Veterinary Medicine, University of California Davis, 105 West Central Avenue, San Bernardino, CA 92409, USA; [b] California Animal Health and Food Safety Laboratory, School of Veterinary Medicine, University of California Davis, One Shields Avenue, Davis, CA 95616, USA
* Corresponding author.
E-mail address: fuzal@cahfs.ucdavis.edu

Vet Clin Equine 31 (2015) 337–358
http://dx.doi.org/10.1016/j.cveq.2015.04.006
0749-0739/15/$ – see front matter © 2015 Elsevier Inc. All rights reserved.

Table 1
Summary of clinical signs, pathologic changes, and diagnostic tools and criteria for the main causes of enteric disease in horses

Agent or Disease	Main Clinical Signs	Main Age Affected	Main Pathologic Findings	Diagnostic Tools/Criteria	
				Presumptive	Definitive
Gastric ulceration	Usually asymptomatic	All ages	Ulceration (mostly pars esophagea)	Clinical signs	Gastroscopy; gross changes
Clostridium perfringens type C	Diarrhea, colic, fever, sudden death	Neonates; adults may occasionally be affected	Enterotyphlocolitis, necrotizing	Clinical signs; gross and microscopic findings; isolation of C perfringens type C from feces/intestinal content	Detection of beta toxin in feces/intestinal content (ELISA)
Clostridium difficile	Diarrhea, fever, dehydration, colic	All ages	Enterotyphlocolitis, necrotizing; mucosal edema; volcano lesions	Clinical signs; gross and microscopic findings; isolation of toxigenic C difficile from feces/intestinal content	Detection of toxins A and/or B of C difficile in feces/intestinal content (ELISA)
Clostridium piliforme	Diarrhea, weakness, lethargy, anorexia, dehydration, fever, icterus	Foals	Colitis, hepatitis, myocarditis	Clinical signs; gross findings	Microscopic findings; PCR; culture of C piliforme in embryonated egg
Salmonella spp	Diarrhea, colic, fever	All ages	Enterotyphlocolitis, necrotizing	Clinical signs; gross and microscopic findings	Detection of Salmonella spp in feces/intestinal content by culture and/or PCR
Rhodococcus equi	Diarrhea, colic	Foals, up to 5 mo of age	Colitis, pyogranulomatous	Clinical signs; gross and microscopic findings	Detection of virulent strains of R equi in feces/intestinal content by culture and/or PCR

	Clinical signs	Age	Pathology	Diagnosis	Detection
Ehrlichia risticii	Diarrhea, colic, fever, anorexia, depression, leucopenia	All ages	Typhlocolitis, necrotizing	Clinical signs; gross and microscopic findings (including observation of organisms in silver-stained sections)	Detection of *E risticii* in feces/intestinal content by PCR
Lawsonia intracellularis	Diarrhea, fever, lethargy, hypoproteinemia, edema, weight loss	Weanling foals	Proliferative enteropathy	Clinical signs; gross and microscopic findings (including observation of organisms in silver-stained sections)	Detection of *L intracellularis* in feces/intestinal content by culture and/or PCR
Rotavirus	Diarrhea, fever, depression, anorexia, dehydration	Foals up to 3–4 mo of age	Liquid content in small and large intestine; villus atrophy	Clinical signs; gross and microscopic findings	Detection of equine rotavirus in feces/intestinal content by ELISA, latex agglutination assay, polyacrylamide electrophoresis, electron microscopy, RT loop-mediated isothermal amplification, and/or PCR
Coronavirus	Colic, diarrhea, fever, depression, anorexia. Occasionally, neurologic alterations	Adults	Necrotizing enteritis	Clinical signs; gross and microscopic findings	Detection of equine coronavirus in feces/intestinal content/intestinal tissues by PCR, immunohistochemistry, and/or electron microscopy

(continued on next page)

Table 1
(continued)

Agent or Disease	Main Clinical Signs	Main Age Affected	Main Pathologic Findings	Diagnostic Tools/Criteria	
				Presumptive	Definitive
Cryptosporidium spp	Diarrhea	Foals 5–6 wk old	Liquid content in small intestine and sometimes colon; villus atrophy	Clinical signs; gross findings	Genus: demonstration of oocysts in feces/intestinal content by Giemsa, modified Ziehl-Neelsen, auramine O, fluorescent antibody technique, ELISA; demonstration of oocysts in intestinal tissue by histology Species: PCR, loop-mediated isothermal DNA amplification
Large strongyles	Larvae: colic Adults: anemia, ill thrift	All ages	Larvae: endoarteritis; may produce colonic infarction Adults: nodules in subserosa of cecum or colon, loss of condition, anemia	Clinical signs; gross and microscopic findings; hyperbetaglobulinemia	Genus: large numbers of strongyle eggs in feces Species: larval culture
Small strongyles	Diarrhea, anorexia, weight loss, edema of ventral parts	All ages (more prevalent in horses up to 1 y old)	Nodules in cecal and colonic mucosa	Clinical signs; gross and microscopic findings	Genus: large numbers of strongyle eggs in feces Species: larval culture
NSAID intoxication	Diarrhea, colic, ulceration of upper alimentary system, hypoproteinemia, hypoalbuminemia	All ages	Ulceration of upper and lower alimentary tract (particularly right dorsal colon); renal papillary necrosis	Clinical signs; gross and microscopic findings; history of NSAID administration	No specific tests available

Abbreviations: ELISA, enzyme-linked immunosorbent assay; NSAID, nonsteroidal antiinflammatory drug; PCR, polymerase chain reaction; RT, reverse transcription.

agents can produce clinical signs and lesions that are similar or identical to those of the so-called colitis X.[8] This article discusses here the main inflammatory conditions of the gastrointestinal system of horses, with special emphasis on the diagnostic criteria.

GASTRITIS

Gastritis in horses is uncommon, except for those associated with gastric ulceration and parasitic causes.

Gastric Ulceration

Most cases of gastric ulceration in horses are nonspecific and are associated with stress related to diet, enteric disease, colonic impaction, ileus, surgery, nonsteroidal antiinflammatory drug (NSAID) therapy, or conditions that eventually produce duodenal reflux.[7–9] The most common ulcers are those of the pars esophagea and, although the pathogenesis is unclear, it has been suggested to be similar to that in swine. It has been proposed that abnormal fluid content associated with feeding patterns allows acids, enzymes, and bile reflux into the cranial portion of the stomach, where, when the pH decreases to levels less than ∼4.0, it damages the nonglandular gastric mucosa and leads to ulceration.[8] Reflux of acidic content into the cranial part of the stomach is also thought to occur as a consequence of gastric compression associated with exercise-induced increased intra-abdominal pressure.[10] This process would explain the high prevalence of ulceration of the pars esophagea seen in racehorses under intensive training.[8,11–13] For as-yet unexplained reasons, ulcers of the pars esophagea tend to be located close to the margo plicatus (Uzal and Diab, unpublished observation, 2015). These ulcers in racehorses are most often considered an incidental necropsy finding, with no clinical significance. However, in rare cases, very deep ulcers may lead to tearing of the stomach wall and gastric rupture.[7] Unlike what often happens in pigs, the ulcers of the pars esophagea in horses do not cause massive internal bleeding. Ulcers of the pars esophagea in horses tend to be chronic, multifocal to coalescing, variably sized (ranging from less than 1 cm to several centimeters), round to irregularly shaped, with elevated borders, and a dark red or pale ulcer bed (**Fig. 1**). The depth of the mucosal damage varies from superficial erosions or shallow ulcers to very deep ulcers. On rare occasions, the damage from deep ulcers can extend into the underlying submucosa, muscularis, and serosa and lead to tearing of the wall and even stomach perforation or rupture, especially if the animal develops gastric impaction or bloat for other reasons. Microscopically, subacute and chronic ulcers have an ulcer bed of granulation tissue of variable thickness and maturity, which is surrounded by an infiltrate of mixed inflammatory cell population. A thin layer of necrotic debris is usually observed overlying the ulcers.[8] Although ulcers of the glandular stomach are considered rare by many veterinarians (including the authors of this review), others suggest that they may be more common than is generally believed (Uzal and Diab, unpublished observation, 2015). These lesions have been associated with administration of NSAIDs.[7,8] The only way to establish a definitive diagnosis of gastric ulcers in the live horse is by gastric endoscopy.[10] In dead horses these ulcers are readily visible during postmortem examination.[8]

Parasitic Gastritis

Gasterophilus spp

Gasterophilus spp larvae (botflies) are the most common parasites of the stomach in horses.[8] The genus *Gasterophilus* comprises 6 species: *Gasterophilus intestinalis*, *Gasterophilus nasalis*, *Gasterophilus haemorrhoidalis*, *Gasterophilus pecorum*,

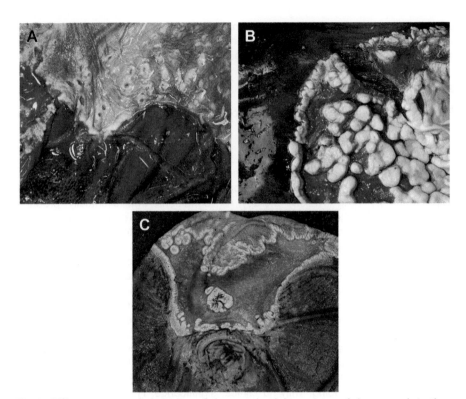

Fig. 1. Different stages of ulceration of the nonglandular mucosa of the stomach in thoroughbred racehorses. (*A*) Mild, multifocal, superficial erosion and ulceration close to the margo plicatus; (*B*) moderate, multifocal to coalescing, chronic ulceration adjacent to the margo plicatus, with tearing of the underlying submucosa; (*C*) severe, locally extensive, chronic ulceration of the nonglandular mucosa likely developing from prior multifocal coalescing ulcers.

Gasterophilus nigricornis, and *Gasterophilus inermis*. The first 2 are the most common.[7] In all cases, the flies lay eggs on the hairs of the face, intermandibular region, or of the ventral part of the body and legs. When the eggs hatch, the first-stage larvae penetrate the oral mucosa, molt, emerge, and migrate through the alimentary canal. *G intestinalis*, the most common species, attaches to the mucosa of the pars esophagea, most commonly close to the cardia but also in other parts of this region, where it completes the subsequent molts. *G nasalis* attaches to the pyloric mucosa and the duodenal ampulla. *G haemorrhoidalis* attaches to the rectal mucosa.[8,14] All of these parasites occasionally attach themselves to the pharynx and esophagus, but consequences to the host are minimal to none. The exception is *G pecorum*, which may cause pharyngitis. In the summer, after the deposition of the ova, the larvae leave the stomach and pass out in the feces to pupate.[8]

The clinical relevance of *Gasterophilus* spp infestation is generally assumed to be minimal, although bot larvae infestations have been associated with gastric ulceration, peritonitis, gastroesophageal reflux, splenitis, and pleuritis.[15,16] Grossly, the larvae can be seen attached to the alimentary tract mucosa. In the pars esophagea of the stomach, the area of attachment of the larvae is surrounded by a thin area of hyperplastic squamous epithelium (**Fig. 2**). Typically round and well-demarcated multifocal ulcers can be seen after the larvae detach from the mucosa.[8,14–16]

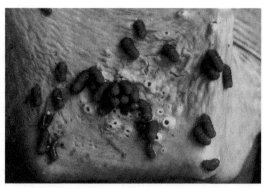

Fig. 2. Numerous larvae of *Gasterophilus* sp (horse bots) attaching to the nonglandular mucosa of the stomach. Note the multifocal, round ulcers with raised, hyperplastic margins left by the larvae on detachment.

Diagnosis of infection by *Gasterophilus* spp can be achieved by direct observation of the eggs on the hair, and larvae occasionally attached to the oral cavity of horses. Larvae attached to the lower alimentary tract can be visualized by endoscopy or by direct examination during necropsy. An enzyme-linked immunosorbent assay (ELISA) to detect *Gasterophilus* spp antigens has recently been developed.[17]

Draschia megastoma, Habronema majus, and Habronema muscae
These are spirurid nematodes that occasionally also parasitize the stomach of horses. The adult worms are between 1 and 2 cm long. The 2 *Habronema* spp mentioned earlier are not considered to cause significant gastric disease in horses. Draschia megastoma can produce large nodules by burrowing into the submucosa of the stomach, inciting a severe granulomatous reaction.[8,14] Grossly, these lesions appear as protrusions of ~5 cm in diameter with a small opening. The nodules are usually not clinically significant, although they can cause abscesses and even stomach perforation if infected with pyogenic bacteria.[8,14] Gross lesions and adult worms found during necropsy are diagnostic, as are eggs or larvae found in feces.

ENTERITIS AND COLITIS

Most inflammatory conditions of the small and large intestine in horses are of infectious origin, although there are a few noninfectious inflammatory conditions of importance that are discussed here (see **Table 1**). As stated earlier, a significant number of severe inflammatory lesions in the small or large intestine remain of undetermined cause.

Infectious Diseases

Bacterial disease
Infections by Clostridium perfringens type C and Clostridium difficile are considered the most common enteric clostridial diseases of horses. Although C perfringens type A has been, and sometimes still is, blamed for cases of enterocolitis in horses,[18–20] diagnostic criteria have not been established for this microorganism, mostly because type A can be found in the intestine of most healthy horses[21] (Uzal and Diab, unpublished observation, 2015) and mere isolation of this microorganism from a horse with enteric disease has no diagnostic significance. However, it is possible that certain strains of C perfringens type A carry virulence factors that are

not present in commensal strains. If that is the case, determining those virulence factors would help ascribing a pathogenic role to strains of this microorganism isolated from horses with intestinal disease. However, until such information is available, determining a pathogenic role to *C perfringens* type A is difficult, if not impossible.

Clostridium perfringens type C *C perfringens* type C disease occurs mostly in neonates, although cases in older foals and adult horses are occasionally seen. Foals can contract the disease as early as a few hours after birth and most cases occur in the first 2 weeks of life.[3,22] Isolates of *C perfringens* type C must carry the genes to encode for alpha and beta toxins, although individual isolates may also produce a variety of other so-called minor toxins.[23] Experimental evidence has clearly shown that the main virulence factor of *C perfringens* type C is beta toxin, a highly trypsin-labile protein.[24,25] Because of this, animals with low levels of trypsin activity in the intestine, such as neonatal individuals caused by the trypsin inhibitory effect of colostrum, are particularly susceptible to type C disease.[3] Trypsin inhibitors in the diet, such as those present in sweet potatoes, may also be involved in the pathogenesis of type C disease in some species,[25] but this does not seem to be an important predisposing factor in horses.[3,22]

The disease caused by *C perfringens* type C is clinically characterized by yellow to hemorrhagic diarrhea, colic, dehydration, and weakness, usually followed by death within 24 hours of onset. It tends to appear in small clusters of cases and it seems to be recurrent year after year in the same properties. Occasional cases of sudden death without any clinical signs may also occur.[3,26] On necropsy, the jejunum and ileum are most frequently affected (**Fig. 3**), although lesions are often also observed in the colon and cecum (**Fig. 4**). Gross findings include segmental to diffuse hemorrhagic and necrotizing enteritis, colitis, or typhlocolitis, with hyperemic intestinal wall and mesentery, and gray dull or diffusely bright red intestinal mucosa that may or may not be covered by a pseudomembrane. The intestinal contents are often fluid and bright or dark red (hemorrhagic) and may have strands of fibrin.[3,8] Gross lesions observed outside the intestinal tract are often the result of endotoxemia and include serous or serosanguineous fluid in the pericardium, multifocal hemorrhages of thoracic and abdominal serous membranes, subendocardial and epicardial hemorrhages, and pulmonary edema and congestion.[3,8]

A presumptive diagnosis of type C disease can usually be established based on the young age of the affected animals, coupled with compatible clinical signs and

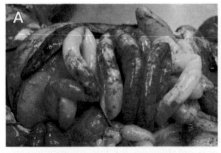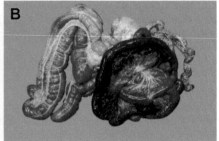

Fig. 3. *C perfringens* type C enteritis in foals. (*A*) The small intestine is dilated by gas and shows multifocal areas of transmural hemorrhage readily visible on the serosal surface. (*B*) A segment of the small intestine and mesentery is diffusely dark red as the result of severe necrosis, transmural congestion, and hemorrhage. (*Courtesy of* [*B*] Farshid Shahriar, DVM, PhD, DACVP, University of California Davis, San Bernardino, CA.)

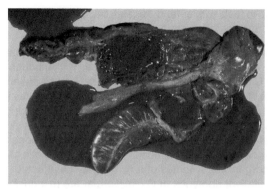

Fig. 4. *C perfringens* type C typhlocolitis in a foal. The large colon and cecum are filled with abundant bright red (hemorrhagic) fluid.

lesions.[3,8] However, the clinical, gross, and microscopic findings of foals with *C perfringens* type C disease may be similar to those produced by other enteric pathogens (notably *Salmonella* spp, *C difficile*, and *Ehrlichia risticii*). Therefore, a definitive diagnosis cannot be based on pathologic findings alone.[3,8] Confirmation of type C disease requires the detection of beta toxin in intestinal contents and/or feces, most frequently by ELISA.[27] However, a negative result does not preclude a diagnosis of *C perfringens* type C infection because this toxin is very sensitive to trypsin and it is frequently broken down if diagnostic samples are not readily collected and properly preserved. Freezing and/or adding trypsin inhibitor to intestinal content specimens preserve the lifespan of beta toxin for several weeks.[22] Isolation of *C perfringens* type C from intestinal contents or feces of animals with necrotizing enteritis is diagnostically significant because this microorganism is rarely found in the intestine of normal animals.[8] Typing is done by polymerase chain reaction (PCR), for which several protocols are available.[27] However, although at low prevalence, type C can be found in the intestine of healthy horses. Isolation of *C perfringens* type C from horses without intestinal disease is therefore of no diagnostic significance.[3] (Uzal and Diab, unpublished observation, 2015). Combined infections by *C perfringens* type C and *C difficile* have been described in foals in which the gross and microscopic findings were almost identical to those described in the diseases caused by each of the microorganisms individually (**Fig. 5**).[28] This observation stresses the need to perform a complete

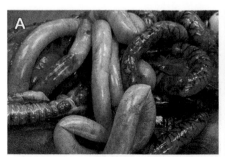 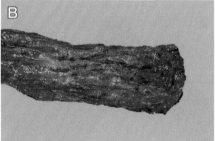

Fig. 5. Coinfection between *C perfringens* type C and *C difficile* in a foal. (*A*) The small intestine is dilated by gas and shows multifocal areas of transmural hemorrhage readily visible on the serosal surface. (*B*) The mucosa of the small intestine is diffusely necrotic and multifocally covered by a thin, yellow to orange pseudomembrane. (*Courtesy of* Pat Blanchard, DVM, PhD, DACVP, University of California Davis, Tulare, CA.)

diagnostic work-up in foals with enteric disease, because detection of one agent does not preclude the presence of others as well.

Clostridium difficile *C difficile* is a ubiquitous gram-positive rod that may be found in the soil and the intestine of many mammals and birds.[4,5,29] Although the major predisposing factors for *C difficile* infection for humans and horses are antibiotic treatment and hospitalization,[29] in the past few years there have been cases in people and animals that have not received antibiotics or been hospitalized; these are called community-associated cases.[4,5] In horses, *C difficile* infection seems to be most frequently associated with β-lactam antibiotics, but this is probably a consequence of the high prevalence of their use, because virtually any antibiotic can predispose disease by this microorganism.[29] Horses of any age may be affected.[4,5,29]

Because highly virulent ribotypes of *C difficile* that are responsible for human outbreaks (ie, 027 and 078) have been also found producing disease in horses and other animal species, it has been speculated that *C difficile* infection could be a zoonosis.[30] Although controversy still exists about the importance of the role of each of the toxins of *C difficile*–associated disease for the virulence of this microorganism, it is now well accepted that both main toxins of this microorganism (ie, toxin A [TcdA] and B [TcdB]) are important for the virulence of *C difficile*.[4,5,31,32]

Clinical signs of *C difficile*–associated disease in horses are highly variable, both in terms of type of signs and severity, and they are by not specific. The cardinal clinical sign is diarrhea, which may be accompanied by 1 or more of the following: colic, fever, red mucous membranes, fever, prolonged capillary refill time, tachycardia, tachypnea, dehydration, and abdominal distention.[4,5,8] The lethality rate in foals may vary between 0% and 42%. In older horses, the lethality seems to be lower, although no specific information is available in this regard.

The gross lesions of *C difficile* infections in young foals are usually restricted to the small intestine, but may also involve the cecum and/or colon (**Fig. 6**). A more caudal distribution of lesions is seen in older foals and adult horses, in which the colon and cecum are usually involved and the small intestine typically spared (**Fig. 7**). Exceptions to this age-related distribution of lesions may occur and therefore the disease cannot be ruled in or out based on lesion location only.[4,5,29] The lesions tend to be similar regardless of the localization within the gastrointestinal tract, and they include hemorrhagic and/or necrotic mucosa that may or may not be covered by a multifocal or diffuse pseudomembrane, mesenteric and serosal hyperemia, and hemorrhage. When the colon is affected, the wall is typically thickened by clear or hemorrhagic,

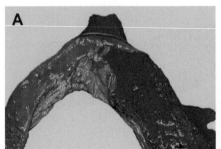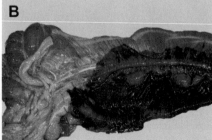

Fig. 6. *C difficile*–associated disease in foals. (*A*) Segment of the small intestine showing hemorrhagic content and a diffusely dark red mucosa. (*B*) The large colon of a foal with diffuse hemorrhagic necrosis of the mucosa. (*Courtesy of* [*A*] Francisco Carvallo, DVM, MSc, PhD, DACVP, University of California Davis, San Bernardino, CA.)

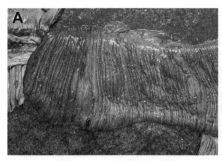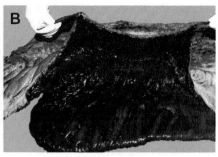

Fig. 7. *C difficile*–associated disease in adult horses. (*A*) The mucosa and submucosa of the large colon show diffuse, marked, clear, gelatinous edema and the colon contents are a mix of well-chopped green roughage and abundant green fluid. (*B*) A more hemorrhagic form of the disease shows similar mucosal and submucosal edema but the mucosa is diffusely dark red as the result of necrosis, hyperemia, and hemorrhage.

gelatinous, submucosal and mucosal edema. The small intestinal content in foals is most frequently hemorrhagic, but it may be yellow and pasty or green/brown and watery. In older foals and adults, the large intestinal contents may be hemorrhagic or composed of abundant green fluid. As in the case of infections by *C perfringens* type C, gross lesions outside the gastrointestinal may include hydropericardium, hemorrhages of serous membranes, subendocardial and epicardial hemorrhage, and pulmonary edema and congestion.[4,5,29]

A presumptive diagnosis of *C difficile*–associated disease can usually be established based on clinical and pathologic findings. However, because the clinical signs and gross and microscopic findings in *C difficile*–associated disease are nonspecific, a definitive diagnosis should be made by detection of toxins A, B, or both in intestinal content or feces. Several tests are currently available, but the ELISA test is the most frequently used.[4] Isolation of toxigenic strains *C difficile* from these specimens is also of moderate diagnostic significance because this microorganism is usually found at a low prevalence in the intestine of normal horses (usually <10%).[4] Typing of isolates is necessary because nontoxigenic strains exist and isolation of those is not diagnostically significant. Typing is routinely performed by PCR.[4,5,29]

Clostridium piliforme *C piliforme* is the agent of Tyzzer disease.[8] This microorganism is the only gram-negative species of the pathogenic clostridia. Young foals are usually affected.[33] The disease in many animal species has been traditionally characterized by clinical signs associated with a classic triad of lesions involving the heart, intestinal tract, and liver.[34] In horses, however, most cases present only with changes in the liver and present clinically as acute liver failure.[33] Alimentary manifestations of Tyzzer disease in foals are unusual, but, when present, they are clinically characterized by semiliquid diarrhea, which may or may not be combined with other clinical signs, including weakness, lethargy, anorexia, dehydration, fever, tachycardia, and icterus.[33] Gross and microscopic changes in the digestive tract include catarrhal to fibrinohemorrhagic colitis, with long, thin bacilli forming pick-up-sticks arrays in the cytoplasm of enterocytes.[8] Although these rods can be seen faintly in hematoxylin and eosin–stained tissue sections, they are better shown with silver stains or Giemsa.[8] In the liver, the typical lesion is multifocal, random foci of acute hepatocellular necrosis, with minimal inflammation and long and thin bacilli, arranged as described earlier, observed in the cytoplasm of hepatocytes at the periphery of the lesion.

Because *C piliforme* cannot be cultured in conventional media, the diagnosis is usually based on the characteristic microscopic lesions, coupled with the demonstration of intracellular bacilli with the classic morphology of this microorganism.[8] Culture in embryonated eggs and more recently PCR has also been used to detect the presence of this microorganism in tissues of affected foals.[33,35]

Salmonella spp The most common cause of salmonellosis in horses is *Salmonella enterica* subspecies *enterica* serovar Typhimurium but other serovars may also be responsible for cases of equine salmonellosis.[8] *Salmonella* spp can be found in the intestine of clinically healthy horses. Stress and antibiotic treatment are considered the main predisposing factors for clinical salmonellosis to occur. The former is particularly significant when antibiotic resistant strains of *Salmonella* spp are present in the intestine.[8,36–38]

Clinically, salmonellosis in horses may be peracute, acute, or chronic. The peracute form is usually septicemic, tends to occur in foals, and is beyond the scope of this article. The acute and chronic forms are primarily enteric and occur most frequently in older foals and adult horses. The disease may occasionally be seen in young foals with clinical and pathologic characteristics similar to those of older horses.[8,36] Clinical signs of acute salmonellosis include diarrhea and fever for 1 to 2 weeks; full recovery or death may be the outcome of this form of the disease. In chronic salmonellosis, the clinical signs may persist for weeks or months and include soft feces, anorexia, and loss of condition.[7,8]

The gross lesions of the enteric form of salmonellosis may be similar, if not identical, to those produced by other bacterial agents of enterocolitis, such as *C perfringens* type C and *C difficile*. They are characterized by diffuse and severe fibrinohemorrhagic to necrotizing inflammation of the cecum and colon, although the small intestine (**Fig. 8**) may also be affected. A tan, gray or red pseudomembrane is usually present loosely attached to the necrotic mucosa.[8] Chronic cases of enteric salmonellosis may have diffuse or multifocal, fibrinous or ulcerative lesions of the cecum and colon. Occasionally, lesions resembling button ulcers are seen, and edema of the submucosa is usually present.[8]

A presumptive diagnosis of salmonellosis can be based on clinical signs and gross and microscopic lesions. As stated earlier for *C perfringens* type C enterotoxemia and *C difficile*–associated disease, the clinical signs and lesions are nonspecific and

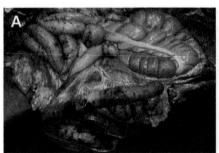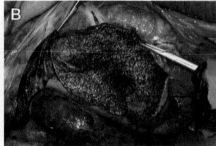

Fig. 8. Enteric salmonellosis in an adult horse. (*A*) A long segment of the small intestine (bottom of the image) shows thickening and multifocal transmural areas of hemorrhage and necrosis readily visible from the serosal surface. (*B*) The mucosa of the small intestine from image *A* is dull, thickened, and diffusely mottled light/dark brown as the result of fibrinonecrotizing enteritis. (*Courtesy of* Mark Anderson, DVM, PhD, DACVP, University of California Davis, Davis, CA.)

confirmation of the diagnosis should rely on demonstration of the organism in intestinal content and/or intestinal tissue by culture and/or PCR.[39] Serogrouping and serotyping of isolated strains provides specific identification of the isolated serovar.

Rhodococcus equi *Rhodococcus equi* is an intracellular gram-positive pleomorphic bacillus that may be part of the normal intestinal flora of horses and can be also found in the soil. *R equi* produces respiratory and, less frequently, intestinal disease in foals from a few weeks to ~5 months of age.[40] The strains isolated from foals carry a virulence plasmid named pVAPA1037, which is essential for disease in horses because it provides the microorganism with the capacity to replicate in macrophages.[40–42] *R equi* is traditionally associated with pneumonia in foals and approximately 50% of these cases may also develop enterotyphlocolitis, mesenteric lymphadenitis, abscesses, and/or peritonitis.[41] The development of enteric lesions in foals with pneumonia is thought to be a consequence of swallowing of respiratory exudate containing *R equi*.[8,40]

The gross lesions of enteric disease produced by *R equi* may occur in the small and large intestine, but are more common and most severe in the cecum, large colon, regional lymph nodes, and over Peyer patches in small intestine (**Fig. 9**). The intestinal and mesenteric lymph node lesions are characteristic and provide reasonable diagnostic certainty. The intestinal lesions consist mainly of many multifocal, elevated, and crateriform mucosal and submucosal nodules with a central ulcer. These ulcerated nodules range between 1 and 2 cm in diameter and are often covered by a pseudomembrane. Mesenteric lymph nodes are typically markedly enlarged and firm. Nodal lesions without concurrent enteric lesions are occasionally seen.[8,41]

Microscopically there are multifocal mucosal and submucosal pyogranulomas with variable numbers of gram-positive coccobacilli in the cytoplasm of macrophages. The presence of these intracellular bacteria is a useful diagnostic feature. Pyogranulomatous mesenteric lymphadenitis, often with intracellular bacteria, is another characteristic feature of the disease.[8,41]

Gross lesions are highly suggestive of *R equi* infection and, together with the microscopic detection of enteric and nodal pyogranulomas with intracellular bacteria, allow the establishment of a strong presumptive diagnosis. However, confirmation relies on isolation of *R equi* from tissues and/or intestinal content and determination of the virulence plasmid in isolated strains, because nonvirulent strains may also be present and are of no diagnostic significance.[7,8,40]

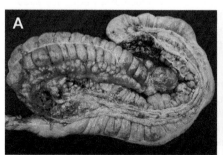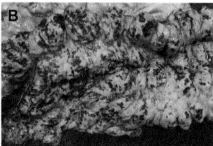

Fig. 9. *R equi* ulcerative colitis and mesenteric lymphadenitis in a foal. (*A*) Mesenteric lymph nodes along the mesocolon are diffusely markedly enlarged as a result of severe, pyogranulomatous lymphadenitis. (*B*) The mucosa of the colon from image *A* shows multifocal to coalescing, irregularly shaped, ulcerated mucosal and submucosal nodules, many of which are covered by a dark green pseudomembrane. (*Courtesy of* Peter Chu, DVM, PhD, University of California Davis, Davis, CA.)

Ehrlichia risticii *E risticii* is the causal agent of Potomac horse fever (equine monocytic ehrlichiosis, equine ehrlichial colitis, or equine neorickettsiosis). Horses of all ages can be affected. This disease is clinically characterized by diarrhea of not more than 10 days' duration, fever, anorexia, depression, and leucopenia; colic is occasionally seen.[7,8,43]

Grossly, there is congestion and ulceration of the mucosa of the cecum and colon, usually accompanied by enlargement of mesenteric lymph nodes. Microscopically, lesions are consistently found in the colon, although similar changes may be seen in the small intestine. The lesions consist of superficial epithelial necrosis, erosion, and fibrin effusion. With silver stains, the organisms can be seen as small clusters of dark dots (~1 μm in diameter) in the apical cytoplasm of crypt enterocytes and also in the cytoplasm of macrophages in the lamina propria.[8,44] Although a presumptive diagnosis is usually based on observation of necrotizing colitis and the presence of intracellular microorganisms on silver preparations, confirmation is achieved by demonstration of the agent in feces or peripheral buffy coat by PCR.[8,44,45]

Lawsonia intracellularis In horses, infection by *Lawsonia intracellularis* is infrequently observed and is called equine proliferative enteritis (EPE).[46–48] EPE affects mostly weanling foals and is clinically characterized by fever, lethargy, diarrhea, hypoproteinemia, edema, and weight loss.[49]

Grossly, there is thickening of the mucosa, mostly in the distal small intestine. Occasionally, gross lesions are not evident. In severe chronic cases, there can be marked irregular hyperplasia and thickening of the mucosa, which is covered by a fibrinonecrotic pseudomembrane and variable edema of the submucosa.[8] Intracellular curved bacteria can be seen microscopically in the apical cytoplasm of enterocytes using silver stains or by immunohistochemistry.[8]

A presumptive diagnosis of proliferative enteritis in any species can be based on typical gross and histologic lesions, and further supported by silver staining to visualize the intracellular bacteria.[8] Confirmation can be obtained by immunohistochemistry and/or by PCR.[8,48,50–52] Cultivation of *L intracellularis* is rarely attempted because it requires the use of tissue culture.[8]

Escherichia coli Although there are rare reports of enterotoxigenic *Escherichia coli* (ETEC) isolated from foals with diarrhea,[7] no evidence exists that this microorganism is responsible for disease, because inoculation of ETEC into foals failed to produce diarrhea or other clinical signs.[53] The other forms of colibacillosis frequently associated with enteric disease in other species have not been reported in horses. Current thinking is therefore that *E coli* has little significance in enteric disease of horses. Neonatal *E coli* septicemia may manifest with secondary nonspecific diarrhea in foals.[8]

Other bacterial agents of enteric disease in horses
Clostridium sordellii,[8] *Actinobacillus equuli*,[4,5] *Streptococcus equi*,[6] *Histoplasma* spp,[54] *Listeria monocytogenes*,[55,56] *Klebsiella pneumoniae*,[8] and others have been rarely associated with enteritis and/or colitis in horses, although definitive evidence of their role in enteric disease is therefore lacking.

Viral Diseases

Rotavirus
Rotavirus is considered a significant cause of diarrhea in foals up to 3 or 4 months of age, although an age-related resistance to diarrhea starts to develop at 2 to 3 weeks of age.[7,8,57] As in other animal species, the disease usually presents in the form of

outbreaks. Coinfections with equine coronavirus, *Salmonella* spp, and *Cryptosporidium* spp may also occur.[8] Clinically, infection by rotavirus is characterized by fever, depression, anorexia, diarrhea, and dehydration.[7,57] Mortality is rare.[8,57]

Gross changes are subtle and consist of liquid content within the small and large intestine. Pathologic changes are nonspecific and the diagnosis has to be confirmed by detecting the virus in intestinal contents or feces. A variety of tests are currently available for this purpose, including ELISA, latex agglutination assay, polyacrylamide electrophoresis, electron microscopy, reverse transcription (RT) loop-mediated isothermal amplification, and PCR.[7,58–60]

Coronavirus

Equine coronavirus is a betacoronavirus that has been associated with enteritis in adult horses in the United States and Japan, but likely occurs also in other countries. The disease usually affects individual horses, but outbreaks have also been reported.[61] Clinical signs are nonspecific and include colic, fever, diarrhea, depression, and anorexia. Occasionally, some horses may show neurologic alterations, which are thought to be a consequence of hyperammonemia associated with the severe intestinal alterations.[61]

Gross and microscopic changes consist of necrotizing enteritis, which may be subtle but is usually severe, especially if the animal died of the disease or was euthanized because of poor prognosis. Lesions outside the alimentary tract include the presence of Alzheimer type II astrocytosis in the cerebral cortex, which is speculated to be a consequence of colitis-associated hyperammonemia.[8,61]

As with many of the bacterial diseases, clinical, gross, and histologic signs are nonspecific and testing to detect coronavirus in intestinal contents and tissues is increasingly being included in the routine testing of horses with diarrhea and enteritis or enterocolitis. Equine coronavirus should be investigated, especially when horses showing compatible clinical signs and lesions test negative for other infectious agents of enteritis. The diagnosis is confirmed by detection of equine coronavirus in intestinal contents or feces by PCR, in tissues by immunohistochemistry, or by direct electron microscopy of intestinal contents or affected intestinal tissue.[61,62]

Parasitic Diseases

Protozoa

Cryptosporidiosis *Cryptosporidium* is an apicomplexan protist that is found mostly on the epithelium of the gastrointestinal, biliary, and respiratory tracts of mammals, birds, reptiles, and fish.[8] *Cryptosporidium parvum* is responsible for cryptosporidiosis in immunologically normal and immunosuppressed foals between 5 days and 6 weeks of age.[7,63,64] Clinically, cryptosporidiosis is characterized by self-limiting diarrhea, which is mainly caused by malabsorption, villus atrophy, and a predominance of immature enterocytes. The covering of a significant part of the surface area of absorptive cells by the organisms is probably a contributory factor for the diarrhea. Mortality is rare.[8,65]

Grossly, there is liquid content throughout the small intestine and, sometimes, the colon.[7,8] Diagnosis is confirmed by microscopic demonstration of oocysts in smears of feces or intestinal content stained with Giemsa, modified Ziehl-Neelsen, or auramine O, or with the fluorescent antibody technique. An ELISA technique is also available for detection of oocysts in feces and intestinal content. Histology of the intestine is also diagnostic. However, these techniques allow only identification at the genus level; identification of the species involved requires molecular methods, including PCR and loop-mediated isothermal DNA amplification.[66]

Ciliated protozoa Ciliated protozoa (*Balantidium* spp) and coccidia (*Eimeria leuckarti*) are occasionally seen on the colonic mucosa of healthy and sick horses, including animals with enteric and nonenteric problems. Although a role for pathogenicity has been suspected for these organisms, definitive evidence of their pathogenicity is missing. For practical purposes, these ciliated protozoa are considered normal inhabitants of the intestine.[8]

Nematodes

Strongyloides

Equine strongylosis is produced by members of the subfamilies Strongylidae (large strongyles) and Cyathostominae (small strongyles), including several genera in each subfamily.

Large strongyles *Strongylus vulgaris* is the most important of the large strongyles and is a common parasite of horses, although the development and use of improved anthelminthics has reduced the prevalence significantly

Horses of any age may be affected. The classic lesion produced by *S vulgaris* larvae is endoarteritis, most commonly involving the cranial mesenteric artery and its main branches, which in young horses may lead to arterial infarction of the colon. This condition manifests clinically as colic. Enlargement of the cranial mesenteric artery can be detected on rectal palpation and/or ultrasonography when the lesion is severe.[7,8] The adult forms of *S vulgaris* found in the intestine are responsible for anemia and ill thrift. An acute syndrome characterized by fever, anorexia, depression, weight loss, diarrhea or constipation, colic, and infarction of the intestine occurs in foals infected with large numbers of larvae for the first time, whereas this syndrome is uncommon in animals previously exposed to infection.[8]

The gross and histologic lesions of the larval form of the disease consist mostly of proliferative arteritis with thrombus formation and, when emboli are released from the large thrombi, they can obliterate smaller mesenteric arteries, arterioles, and capillaries, resulting in clearly demarcated areas of infarction in the colon. Gross lesions produced by adult large strongyles consist of encapsulated nodules in the subserosa of the cecum and colon.[8]

Diagnosis of *S vulgaris*–associated disease is based on clinical signs coupled with large numbers of strongyle eggs in feces and hyperbetaglobulinemia. The differentiation between large and small strongyle eggs cannot be achieved by microscopic examination alone and larval culture is required.[7,67]

Small strongyles (cyathostomes) This group includes more than 50 species, of which the larvae, and not the adult forms, are considered pathogenic.[68] Cyathostomiasis is more prevalent in horses up to approximately 1 year old, although the disease can occur in horses of any age. Clinical cyathostomiasis is the consequence of simultaneous emergence of large numbers of inhibited third-stage larvae from the cecal and colonic mucosa in the late winter, spring, and early summer in temperate climates. Encysted third-stage larvae may undergo hypobiosis, persisting in nodules in the colonic wall for as long as 2 years.[68] Over the past few years, cyathostomins have developed significant anthelmintic resistance.[69–71] Clinical signs of cyathostomiasis are nonspecific and include diarrhea, anorexia, weight loss, and edema of ventral parts.[8,68]

Gross findings include the presence of nodules of a few millimeters in diameter in the cecal and colonic mucosa. These nodules are formed by encysted larvae and are red or black and slightly elevated. The mucosa of the affected intestinal segments shows diffuse edema and congestion (**Fig. 10**).[8]

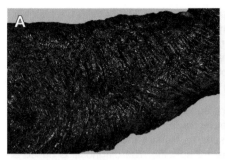 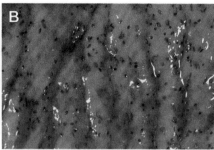

Fig. 10. Cyathostomiasis (small strongyles) in horses. (A) The large colon of a horse with diffusely reddened and edematous mucosa. (B) A close-up of the mucosal surface of a large colon with hundreds of coiled, red to brown, third-stage larvae encysted in the mucosa. (*Courtesy of* [A] Mark Anderson, DVM, PhD, DACVP, University of California Davis, Davis, CA; and [B] the Anatomic Pathology Service, School of Veterinary Medicine, UC Davis.)

Diagnosis of cyathostomiasis is based on clinical signs combined with increased strongyle egg counts in feces, anemia, and hyperbetaglobulinemia. Adult nematodes can occasionally be seen in feces. As explained earlier, larval culture is required to differentiate between large and small strongyle eggs.[7,67] A high fecal egg count is a useful diagnostic criterion and gives an idea of the number of adult parasites in the intestinal tract. However, the egg count is not representative of the encysted larval stage, for which the disease induced by the emergence of these larvae cannot be ruled out based on low egg count in feces. No diagnostic techniques are currently available for prepatent stages of *Strongylus* spp.[7]

Noninfectious or Parasitic Conditions

Inflammatory enteric disease in horses may be produced by intestinal displacements, and intoxication by nonsteroidal antiinflammatory drugs and other substances.

Intestinal displacements

Intestinal displacements that produce ischemic mucosal lesions but that are corrected with consequent reflow may cause chronic diarrhea and possibly cachexia. Because these lesions are initially noninflammatory, they are not discussed here.

Toxic enteric disease

Nonsteroidal antiinflammatory drugs These drugs are universally used to treat multiple ailments of horses and they have been associated with ulcerative colitis and typhlitis.

The pathogenesis of the syndrome is related to ischemia caused by reduced perfusion, which is a consequence of inhibition of synthesis of prostaglandin by inhibition of the cyclooxygenase enzyme.[72] Clinically, intoxication by NSAIDs is characterized by colic and diarrhea, and other signs associated with ulceration of the upper and lower alimentary system.[72] The most consistent clinicopathologic findings are hypoproteinemia and hypoalbuminemia.[72]

At necropsy, multifocal to coalescing widespread ulceration of the colonic and cecal mucosa is observed. Although the lesions tend to be most severe on the right dorsal colon (hence the name right dorsal colitis), the lesions can be found anywhere in the dorsal colon and occasionally in the ventral colon as well (Uzal and Diab, unpublished observation, 2015). Ulcers can also be seen in other locations, including the mouth, esophagus, and stomach. Renal papillary necrosis in the kidneys is a typical lesion but is not always present.[8,72,73]

No specific tests are available for the diagnosis of NSAID intoxication. A history of administration of NSAIDs coupled with hypoproteinemia and hypoalbuminemia is highly suggestive of intoxication by these drugs.[72] At necropsy, ulcerative lesions in the alimentary tract, mainly in the right dorsal colon, and the presence of necrotizing lesions in the renal papilla are suggestive of intoxication by NSAIDs, especially when other common causes of colitis have been ruled out.[8,72]

Other toxic causes of enteric disease Several substances[8,73] have an irritant effect on the alimentary tract of horses. Among these are cantharidin (the principal toxin of blister beetle),[74,75] *Nerium oleander*[76] and arsenic.[77] Neither the clinical signs nor the postmortem changes of these intoxications are specific. The diagnosis is based on the presence of compatible lesions (within the alimentary tract or other organs) and detection of these substances in intestinal contents or tissues of affected horses.

REFERENCES

1. Weese JS, Baird JD, Poppe C. Emergence of *Salmonella typhimurium* definitive type 104 (DT104) as an important cause of salmonellosis in horses in Ontario. Can Vet J 2001;42:788–92.
2. Feary DJ, Hassel DM. Enteritis and colitis in horses. Vet Clin Equine 2006;22: 437–79.
3. Diab SS, Kinde H, Moore J, et al. Pathology of *Clostridium perfringens* type C enterotoxemia in horses. Vet Pathol 2012;49:255–63.
4. Diab SS, Songer G, Uzal FA. *Clostridium difficile* infection in horses: a review. Vet Microbiol 2013;167:42–9.
5. Diab SS, Rodriguez-Bertos A, Uzal FA. Pathology and diagnostic criteria of *Clostridium difficile* enteric infection in horses. Vet Pathol 2013;50:1028–36.
6. Diab S, Giannitti F, Mete A, et al. Ulcerative enterocolitis and typhlocolitis associated with *Actinobacillus equuli* and *Streptococcus equi* in horses. Annual Meeting Proceedings. San Diego (CA): AAVLD; September 17–23, 2013.
7. van der Kolk JH, Veldhuis Kroeze EJ. Infectious diseases of the horse. London: Manson Publishing; 2013. p. 336.
8. Uzal FA, Plattner BL, Hostetter JM. Alimentary system. In: Maxie MG, editor. Jubb, Kennedy, and Palmer's pathology of domestic animals. 6th edition. St Louis (MO): Elsevier; 2015. p. 1–257.
9. Murray MJ. Gastric ulceration. In: Smith BP, editor. Large animal internal medicine. St Louis (MO): Mosby Elsevier; 2009. p. 695–702.
10. Andrews F, Bernard W, Byars D, et al. Recommendations for the diagnosis and treatment of equine gastric ulcer syndrome (EGUS): the Equine Gastric Ulcer Council. Equine Vet Educ 1999;11:262–72.
11. Murray MJ, Eichorn ES. Effects of intermittent feed deprivation, intermittent feed deprivation with ranitidine administration, and stall confinement with *ad libitum* access to hay on gastric ulceration in horses. Am J Vet Res 1996; 57:1599–603.
12. Johnson JH, Vatistas N, Castro L, et al. Field survey of the prevalence of gastric ulcers in thoroughbred racehorses and on response to treatment of affected horses with omeprazole paste. Equine Vet Educ 2001;13:221–4.
13. Ferrucci F, Zucca E, Di Fabio V, et al. Gastroscopic findings in 63 standardbred horses in training. Vet Res Com 2003;27:759–62.
14. Al-Mokaddem AK, Ahmed KA, Doghaim RE. Pathology of gastric lesions in donkeys: a preliminary study. Equine Vet J 2014. http://dx.doi.org/10.1111/evj.12336.

15. Dart AJ, Hutchins DR, Begg AP. Suppurative splenitis and peritonitis in a horse after gastric ulceration caused by larvae of *Gasterophilus intestinalis*. Aust Vet J 1987;64:155–8.
16. van der Kolk JH, Sloet van Oldruitenborgh-Oosterbaan MM, Gruys E. Bilateral pleuritic fistula in a horse as a complication of a *Gasterophilus* infection. Tijdschr Diergeneeskd 1989;114:769–74.
17. Sánchez-Andrade R, Cortiñas FJ, Francisco I, et al. A novel second instar *Gasterophilus* excretory/secretory antigen-based ELISA for the diagnosis of gasterophilosis in grazing horses. Vet Parasitol 2010;171:314–20.
18. Songer JG, Trinh HT, Dial SM, et al. Equine colitis X associated with infection by *Clostridium difficile* NAP1/027. J Vet Diagn Invest 2009;21:377–80.
19. Hazlett MJ, Kircanski J, Slavic D, et al. Beta 2 toxigenic *Clostridium perfringens* type A colitis in a three-day-old foal. J Vet Diagn Invest 2011;23:373–6.
20. Bacciarini LN, Boerlin P, Straub R, et al. Immunohistochemical localization of *Clostridium perfringens* beta2-toxin in the gastrointestinal tract of horses. Vet Pathol 2003;40:376–81.
21. Schoster A, Arroyo LG, Staempfli HR, et al. Presence and molecular characterization of *Clostridium difficile* and *Clostridium perfringens* in intestinal compartments of healthy horses. BMC Vet Res 2012;8:94.
22. Macias Rioseco M, Beingesser J, Uzal FA. Freezing or adding trypsin inhibitor to equine intestinal contents extends the lifespan of *Clostridium perfringens* beta toxin for diagnostic purposes. Anaerobe 2012;18:357–60.
23. McClane BA, Uzal FA, Fernandez Miyakawa ME, et al. The enterotoxic clostridia. In: Dworkin S, Falkow S, Rosenberg E, et al, editors. The prokaryotes, vol. 4, 3rd edition. New York: Springer-Verlag; 2006. p. 698–752.
24. Sayeed S, Uzal FA, Fisher DJ, et al. Beta toxin is essential for the intestinal virulence of *Clostridium perfringens* type C disease isolate CN3685 in a rabbit ileal loop model. Mol Microbiol 2008;67:15–30.
25. Lawrence GW. The pathogenesis of enteritis necroticans. In: Rood JI, McClane BA, Songer JG, et al, editors. The clostridia: molecular biology and pathogenesis. San Diego (CA): Academic Press; 1997. p. 197–207.
26. Drolet R, Higgins R, Cécyre A. Necrohemorrhagic enterocolitis caused by *Clostridium perfringens* type C in a foal. Can Vet J 1990;31:449–50.
27. Songer JG, Uzal FA. Clostridial enteric infections in pigs. J Vet Diagn Invest 2005;17:528–36.
28. Uzal FA, Diab SS, Blanchard P, et al. *Clostridium perfringens* type C and *Clostridium difficile* co-infection in foals. Vet Microbiol 2012;156:395–402.
29. Keel MK, Songer JG. The comparative pathology of *Clostridium difficile*-associated disease. Vet Pathol 2006;43:225–40.
30. Songer JG. Clostridia as agents of zoonotic disease. Vet Microbiol 2010;140:399–404.
31. Kuehne SA, Cartman ST, Heap JT, et al. The role of toxin A and toxin B in *Clostridium difficile* infection. Nature 2010;467:711–3.
32. Kuehne SA, Cartman ST, Minton NP. Both, toxin A and toxin B, are important in *Clostridium difficile* infection. Gut Microbes 2011;2:252–5.
33. Swerczek TW. Tyzzer's disease in foals: retrospective studies from 1969 to 2010. Can Vet J 2013;54:876–80.
34. Ganaway JR, Allem AM, Moore TD. Tyzzer's disease. In: Symposium on Diseases of Laboratory Animals Complicating Biomedical Research. 55th Annual Meeting of the Federation of American Societies for Experimental Biology. Chicago, October 5–6, 1971.

35. Borchers A, Magdesian KG, Halland S, et al. Successful treatment and polymerase chain reaction (PCR) confirmation of Tyzzer's disease in a foal and clinical and pathologic characteristics of 6 additional foals (1986–2005). J Vet Intern Med 2006;20:1212–8.

36. Alinovi CA, Ward MP, Couëtil LL, et al. Risk factors for fecal shedding of *Salmonella* from horses in a veterinary teaching hospital. Prev Vet Med 2003;60: 307–17.

37. Ernst NS, Hernandez JA, MacKay RJ, et al. Risk factors associated with fecal *Salmonella* shedding among hospitalized horses with signs of gastrointestinal tract disease. J Am Vet Med Assoc 2004;225:275–81.

38. McCain CS, Powell KC. Asymptomatic salmonellosis in healthy adult horses. J Vet Diagn Invest 1990;2:236–7.

39. Cheng CM, Lin W, Van KT, et al. Rapid detection of *Salmonella* in foods using real-time PCR. J Food Prot 2008;71:2436–41.

40. Giguère S, Cohen ND, Chaffin MK, et al. *Rhodococcus equi*: clinical manifestations, virulence, and immunity. J Vet Intern Med 2011;25:1221–30.

41. Reuss SM, Chaffin MK, Cohen ND. Extrapulmonary disorders associated with *Rhodococcus equi* infection in foals: 150 cases (1987–2007). J Am Vet Med Assoc 2009;235:855–63.

42. Tripathi NV, Harding WC, Willingham-Lane JM, et al. Conjugal transfer of a virulence plasmid in the opportunistic intracellular actinomycete *Rhodococcus equi*. J Bacteriol 2012;194:6790–801.

43. Palmer JE, Whitlock RH, Benson CE. Equine ehrlichial colitis (Potomac horse fever): recognition of the disease in Pennsylvania, New Jersey, New York, Ohio, Idaho, and Connecticut. J Am Vet Med Assoc 1986;189:197–9.

44. Dutra F, Schuch LF, Delucchi E, et al. Equine monocytic ehrlichiosis (Potomac horse fever) in horses in Uruguay and southern Brazil. J Vet Diagn Invest 2001; 13:433–7.

45. Bertin FR, Reising A, Slovis NM, et al. Clinical and clinicopathological factors associated with survival in 44 horses with equine neorickettsiosis (Potomac horse fever). Vet Intern Med 2013;27:977–81.

46. Gebhart CJ, Guedes RM. Lawsonia intracellularis. In: Gyles CL, Prescott JF, Songer JG, et al, editors. Pathogenesis of bacterial infections in animals. 3rd edition. Ames (IA): Blackwell; 2004. p. 363–72.

47. Pusterla N. Equine proliferative enteropathy caused by *Lawsonia intracellularis*. Equine Vet Educ 2009;21:415–9.

48. Pusterla N, Gebhart CJ. Equine proliferative enteropathy-a review of recent developments. Equine Vet J 2013;45:403–9.

49. Lavoie JP, Drolet R, Parsons D, et al. Equine proliferative enteropathy: a cause of weight loss, colic, diarrhoea and hypoproteinaemia in foals on three breeding farms in Canada. Equine Vet J 2000;32:418–25.

50. Cooper DM, Swanson DL, Gebhart CJ. Diagnosis of proliferative enteritis in frozen and formalin-fixed, paraffin-embedded tissues from a hamster, horse, deer and ostrich using a *Lawsonia intracellularis*-specific PCR assay. Vet Microbiol 1997;54:47–62.

51. Jordan DM, Knittel JP, Roof MB, et al. Detection of *Lawsonia intracellularis* in swine using polymerase chain reaction methodology. J Vet Diagn Invest 1999; 11:45–9.

52. Jordan DM, Knittel JP, Schwartz KJ, et al. A *Lawsonia intracellularis* transmission study using a pure culture inoculated seeder-pig sentinel model. Vet Microbiol 2004;104:83–90.

53. Holland RE, Grimes SD, Walker RD, et al. Experimental inoculation of foals and pigs with an enterotoxigenic *E. coli* isolated from a foal. Vet Microbiol 1996;52: 249–57.

54. Nunes J, Mackie JT, Kiupel M. Equine histoplasmosis presenting as a tumor in the abdominal cavity. J Vet Diagn Invest 2006;18:508–10.

55. Nemeth NM, Blas-Machado U, Hopkins BA, et al. Granulomatous typhlocolitis, lymphangitis, and lymphadenitis in a horse infected with *Listeria monocytogenes*, *Salmonella typhimurium*, and cyathostomes. Vet Pathol 2013;50:252–5.

56. Warner SL, Boggs J, Lee JK, et al. Clinical, pathological, and genetic character-ization of *Listeria monocytogenes* causing sepsis and necrotizing typhlocolitis and hepatitis in a foal. J Vet Diagn Invest 2012;24:581–6.

57. Papp H, Matthijnssens J, Martella V, et al. Global distribution of group A rotavirus strains in horses: a systematic review. Vaccine 2013;31:5627–33.

58. Elschner M, Prudlo J, Hotsel H, et al. Nested reverse transcriptase-polymerase chain reaction for the detection of group A rotaviruses. J Vet Med B Infect Dis Vet Public Health 2002;49:77–81.

59. Frederick J, Giguere S, Sanchez LC. Infectious agents detected in the faeces of diarrheic foals: a retrospective study of 233 cases (2003–2008). J Vet Intern Med 2009;23:1254–60.

60. Nemoto M, Imagawa H, Tsujimura K, et al. Detection of equine rotavirus by reverse transcription loop-mediated isothermal amplification (RT-LAMP). J Vet Med Sci 2010;72:823–6.

61. Fielding CL, Higgins JK, Higgins JC, et al. Disease associated with equine coro-navirus infection and high case fatality rate. J Vet Intern Med 2015;29(1):307–10.

62. Giannitti F, Diab SS, Mete A, et al. Necrotizing enteritis and hyperammonemic en-cephalopathy associated with equine coronavirus infection in equids. Vet Pathol 2015. [Epub ahead of print].

63. Chalmers RM, Grinberg A. Significance of *Cryptosporidium parvum* in horses. Vet Rec 2005;156:688.

64. Chalmers RM, Thomas AL, Butler BA, et al. Identification of *Cryptosporidium par-vum* genotype 2 in domestic horses. Vet Rec 2005;156:49–50.

65. De Souza PN, Bomfim TC, Huber F, et al. Natural infection by *Cryptosporidium* sp., *Giardia* sp. and *Eimeria leuckarti* in three groups of equines with different handlings in Rio de Janeiro, Brazil. Vet Parasitol 2009;160:327–33.

66. Bakheit MA, Torra D, Palomino LA, et al. Sensitive and specific detection of *Cryp-tosporidium* species in PCR-negative samples by loop-mediated isothermal DNA amplification and confirmation of generated LAMP products by sequencing. Vet Parasitol 2008;158:11–2.

67. Chapman MR, Hutchinson GW, Cenac MJ, et al. *In vitro* culture of equine Strong-ylidae to the fourth larval stage in a cell-free medium. J Parasitol 1994;80:225–31.

68. Love S, Murphy D, Mellor D. Pathogenicity of cyathostome infection. Vet Parasitol 1999;85:113–21.

69. Traversa D. The little-known scenario of anthelmintic resistance in equine cya-thostomes in Italy. Ann N Y Acad Sci 2008;1149:167–9.

70. Traversa D, Iorio R, Otranto D, et al. Species-specific identification of equine cy-athostomes resistant to fenbendazole and susceptible to oxibendazole and mox-idectin by macroarray probing. Exp Parasitol 2009;121:92–5.

71. Slocombe JO, Coté JF, de Gannes RV. The persistence of benzimidazole-resistant cyathostomes on horse farms in Ontario over 10 years and the effective-ness of ivermectin and moxidectin against these resistant strains. Can Vet J 2008; 49:56–60.

72. Jones SL. Nonsteroidal anti-inflammatory drug toxicity. In: Smith BP, editor. Large animal internal medicine. St Louis (MO): Mosby Elsevier; 2009. p. 754–7.
73. Jones SL. Medical disorders of the large intestine. In: Smith BP, editor. Large animal internal medicine. St Louis (MO): Mosby Elsevier; 2009. p. 742–50.
74. Helman RG, Edwards WC. Clinical features of blister beetle poisoning in equids: 70 cases (1983–1996. J Am Vet Med Assoc 1997;211:1018–21.
75. Schmitz DG. Cantharidin toxicosis in horses. J Vet Intern Med 1989;3:208–15 [Review].
76. Renier AC, Kass PH, Magdesian KG, et al. Oleander toxicosis in equids: 30 cases (1995–2010). J Am Vet Med Assoc 2013;242:540–9.
77. Casteel SW. Metal toxicosis in horses. Vet Clin North Am Equine Pract 2001;17: 517–27.

Skin Diseases in Horses

Bruce K. Wobeser, DVM, MVetSC, PhD

KEYWORDS

- Equine • Skin • Dermatitis • Alopecia • Biopsy

KEY POINTS

- Many skin lesions may require biopsy to definitively diagnose.
- Many skin lesions of horses are characterized by the formation of dermal nodular masses.
- Despite the frequency with which sarcoids are diagnosed, understanding of the development of sarcoids remains incomplete.

INTRODUCTION

Skin disease in horses is a common and potentially challenging clinical problem. Information pertaining to skin disease is lacking in horses when compared with that in other companion animal species. Certainly, both horse-specific and location-specific patterns are present, but these can often be confounded by other factors. There are many possible ways in which to organize skin disease; in this article, they are organized based loosely on their most common clinical feature (**Table 1**). Space limits the number of conditions that can be described here, and those chosen were seen relatively frequently in a multiinstitutional study of equine biopsies.[1,2]

USEFUL DIAGNOSTIC TECHNIQUES
Skin Scrapings

Skin scrapings, although common in smaller companion animals, are often less useful in horses. Superficial scrapings may have limited results, whereas deeper skin scrapings may be useful for *Demodex equi* and *Rhabditis strongyloides*. Deep skin scrapings are done by squeezing the skin between the fingers, adding a drop of oil to the skin, and then using a scalpel to scrape across the skin. The collected material can then be examined on a microscopic slide. Scraping of the skin until capillary bleeding occurs increases the sensitivity of the test.

Acetate Tape Impressions

Given the relatively low sensitivity of superficial skin scrapings, a simple alternative is the use of acetate tape. Clear tape when pressed to the skin of horses can collect

Department of Veterinary Pathology, Western College of Veterinary Medicine, University of Saskatchewan, 52 Campus Drive, Saskatoon, Saskatchewan, S7N 5B4, Canada
E-mail address: Bruce.wobeser@usask.ca

Vet Clin Equine 31 (2015) 359–376
http://dx.doi.org/10.1016/j.cveq.2015.04.007
0749-0739/15/$ – see front matter © 2015 Elsevier Inc. All rights reserved.

Table 1
Classification of skin disease based on common clinical features

Nodular	Ulcerative	Alopecic	Scaling
Sarcoid	Squamous cell carcinoma	Atopy	Dermatophytosis
Eosinophilic granuloma	Exuberant granulation tissue	Alopecia areata	Pemphigus foliaceus
Fungal Granulomas	Habronemiasis	Anagen/telogen effluvium	Dermatophilus
Cutaneous lymphoma	—	MEED	—
Mast cell tumors	—	—	—

surface debris and crusts. Clipping the skin is often useful for increasing material collection. Examples of pathogens detectable by this method are *Chorioptes bovis, Dermanyssus gallinae, Trombicula* (chigger mites), *Oxyuris equi,* and dermatophytes.

Hair Plucking

Useful information can be attained by microscopic examination of plucked hairs. Examination of the root of the hair can determine whether hairs are in the anagen or telogen stage of growth. Anagen hair bulbs are smooth and rounded, whereas telogen hair bulbs are rough and more pointed or irregular. Typically, hairs plucked should be a mixture of telogen and anagen.

Examination of the hair shaft can likewise be useful. Twisted or misshapen and irregular hair shafts suggest an underlying nutritional disorder. Fractured or clearly split hair shafts imply excessive grooming or self-trauma and are a good indicator of pruritus.

Fine-Needle Aspiration

Unlike dogs and cats, fine-needle aspiration (FNA) is sparingly used in equine skin lesions. The usefulness of this technique seems to be primarily in the diagnosis of nodular skin lesions. Some masses such as sarcoids may exfoliate poorly, whereas the presence of neutrophils and eosinophils may be helpful in diagnosing inflammatory lesions. FNA can be quite useful in the diagnosis of mast cell tumors.

Biopsy

Many skin lesions may require biopsy to definitively diagnose. Hints to improve biopsy success are included in **Box 1**. Biopsy should be performed if neoplasia is suspected, ulceration is persistent, treatment is unsuccessful, and lesions are spreading rapidly or the lesion is impairing the use of the animal.

Sampling the center of a skin lesion is important as biopsies from transitional zones between normal and affected skin may miss the lesion when sectioned for histologic processing. Inclusion of scale and crusts from lesion is vital because important diagnostic clues are present within the crusts in many lesions. As such, minimal sample site preparation is important so as not to disturb these superficial changes.

NODULAR SKIN DISEASES

Many skin lesions of horses are characterized by the formation of dermal nodular masses. The nature of these masses may vary from condition to condition, but

Box 1
Helpful hints to biopsy of skin lesions

Treat superficial bacterial skin infections before biopsy

Avoid the use of glucocorticoids before biopsy

Minimize preparation of the sample site before biopsy, and avoid clipping as much as possible

Use the largest biopsy punch possible; incisional biopsy with a scalpel may be useful in large lesions

Sample the center of the lesion or multiple areas if the lesion varies in morphology

Include the crust or scales of skin lesions

Fix samples immediately in 10% neutral buffered formalin

Clearly label samples; do not include normal skin samples in the same container as lesion samples

If shipping samples in freezing weather, after fixation for 24 hours transfer sample to 70% alcohol to ship

The more biopsy samples submitted, the greater is the likelihood of a diagnosis

many of these may appear clinically similar. Because of this similarity, nodular masses often require biopsy for definitive diagnosis. The following group of diseases includes the most common ones seen at veterinary diagnostic referral centers, but is by no means an exhaustive list of all possible lesions.[1,2]

Equine Sarcoids

Equine sarcoids are by a large margin the most common tumor of horses[1,3] and are locally invasive and potentially disfiguring tumors of fibroblasts. Equine sarcoids are notorious for becoming more aggressive after treatment or diagnostic attempts. However, this behavior is unpredictable and a subset of sarcoids may actually resolve spontaneously. The diagnosis of sarcoids can be clinically challenging because they can mimic many other conditions.

Microbiology
The development of sarcoids is associated with infection with one of 3 different bovine papillomaviruses (BPVs), namely, BPV-1, BPV-2, and BPV-13.[4,5] The relative frequencies of these papillomaviruses vary by the geographic region. No clinical differences between sarcoids caused by these papillomaviruses have been identified. The presence of a BPV in equine sarcoids is interesting because papillomaviruses are typically species specific, but there is some recent evidence to suggest that BPV-1 has only been present in horses for a relatively short period.[6]

Epidemiology
Horses of almost any age and breed can develop sarcoids, and sarcoids have been identified in horses worldwide. Simple infection with BPV alone is not sufficient for the development of sarcoids. Individual horse factors must be involved, but particular factors have not been identified and there are no tests available to determine if a particular horse is predisposed to the development of sarcoids.

Clinical presentation
A total of 5 different clinical types of sarcoids have been described, ranging from occult sarcoids, which may appear as an area of scaly skin with some alopecia, to

fibroblastic sarcoids, which can be very large proliferative ulcerated masses.[7] Given the wide range of clinical presentations, almost any persistent skin lesion in a horse has at least the possibility of being a sarcoid. Sarcoids are more commonly reported as being on the head or trunk of horses than in other locations.[1,8]

Pathogenesis

Despite the frequency with which sarcoids are diagnosed, an understanding of the development of sarcoids remains incomplete. Simple infection with appropriate papillomaviruses is not sufficient to create sarcoids, and re-creating sarcoids in horses under laboratory conditions has not been successful. Although contact with cattle is not required for the development of sarcoids, direct contact or contact with fomites carrying infectious material between sarcoid-affected and uninfected horses and stable flies have been suggested as possible routes of transmission.[9,10] It is worth noting that horses that develop one sarcoid seem to be predisposed to the development of other sarcoids and multiple sarcoids being present on a horse at one time seems to be relatively common.[8]

Specimen collection

It is difficult to give general information on collection of specimen for the diagnosis of sarcoids. The behavior of any particular sarcoid is impossible to predict. Some sarcoids resolve spontaneously, whereas others are markedly more aggressive. Given that biopsy may be the only way to diagnose sarcoid, excisional biopsy where possible is likely the best method to try to both diagnose and resolve the lesion. Biopsy of ulcerated areas increases the difficulty of making the diagnosis because typical epidermal changes seen in sarcoids will not be present in ulcerated samples.

Diagnosis

Histopathology is the gold standard of diagnosis. Sarcoids tend to exfoliate poorly, and so FNA tends to be unrewarding. The identification of neoplastic fibroblasts is required for the diagnosis of sarcoids. Ulceration and particularly the presence of granulation tissue complicates the diagnosis of sarcoid. Differentiating between exuberant granulation tissue (EGT) and an ulcerated sarcoid can be very difficult. As it currently stands, there are no secondary diagnostic tests to diagnose sarcoids. The level of papillomavirus antigen present in tissue is below the detection limit of immunohistochemistry. Polymerase chain reaction for papillomavirus in biopsies is unrewarding because BPV can be found in skin biopsies from horses without sarcoids.[11]

Treatment

Multiple treatment protocols have been developed to deal with sarcoids. None of these are effective in all cases. Generally speaking, complete removal of the lesion and surrounding skin seems to be the most effective common treatment. Successful use of several topical or subcutaneously administered products has been reported.[12–14] The number of horses in these trials is relatively small, and practicality and cost-effectiveness of these products is not clear.

Differential diagnoses

The various clinical types of sarcoids can mimic other skin conditions of horses. Dermatophytosis can resemble occult sarcoids. Papillomas can resemble verrucous sarcoids. Various types of granulomas can resemble nodular sarcoids. Squamous cell carcinomas and EGT can resemble fibroblastic sarcoids.

Eosinophilic Granulomas

Epidemiology
Eosinophilic granulomas are relatively common nonneoplastic skin lesions of horses. These granulomas represent between 3.5% and 12% of submissions to diagnostic laboratories.[2,15] Eosinophilic granulomas are most commonly reported as occurring in the spring or summer but are diagnosed at all times of year.[2,15,16] No age, breed, or sex predilections have been identified.

Clinical presentation
Lesions commonly occur in the saddle region and neck. Typically, they are raised, nonpainful, well-circumscribed nodules with normal overlying skin. The nodules can widely range in size from less than 1 cm in diameter to over 10 cm. Rarely, horses may have very large numbers of lesions spread across the body.

Pathogenesis
The pathogenesis is unclear. The presence of large numbers of eosinophils suggests an allergic or hypersensitivity-type reaction, but it does not appear that any single antigen is implicated in the development of this lesion. Given the location in the area of the saddle, trauma has also been suggested as a possible cause.[16,17] Silicone-coated needles have also been reported as a cause of eosinophilic granulomas.[18]

Diagnosis
FNA may be helpful in making the diagnosis. The presence of eosinophils, macrophages, lymphocytes, and plasma cells is consistent with eosinophilic granulomas. Histopathologic features vary somewhat depending on the age of the lesion. Lesions contain areas of eosinophilic and histiocytic inflammation in the dermis and occasionally extending deeper into the panniculus. Collagen coated with eosinophil granules (flame figures) are common. In older lesions, dystrophic mineralization may be a more common feature. The presence of large amounts of dystrophic mineralization may impart a gritty nature to the lesion on biopsy.

Treatment
Surgical removal of individual lesions or mineralized lesions is typically curative. Glucocorticoids administered sublesionally in the case of smaller numbers of lesions or orally in horses with large numbers of lesions have been reported to be effective.[16]

Fungal Granulomas

Microbiology
A variety of fungal species have been identified in fungal granulomas, and both pigmented and nonpigmented fungi have been found.

Epidemiology
The frequency with which equine fungal granulomas are reported seems to vary geographically from being relatively rare[16] to a more common nodular biopsy finding.[2,19] The occurrence seems to be year round but with more frequency in the warmer months of the year.[2,19]

Clinical presentation
Granulomas can be single or multiple and seem to occur more frequently on the head and neck. Fungal granulomas tend to be smaller than eosinophilic granulomas, often less than 1 cm in diameter.[19] However, there is a single case report of much larger lesions (10 cm diameter).[20] The skin overlying these lesions tends to be intact, and draining tracts are not a feature of these lesions.

Pathogenesis

These granulomas are thought to be caused by the introduction of the fungi via penetrating wounds.[21] The immune system has difficulty removing the fungal organisms, and this results in granuloma formation.

Diagnosis

FNA often only reveals inflammation. If fungal elements are found on aspiration, the diagnosis is made. However, fungal elements are often fairly rare and biopsy is frequently needed to make a definitive diagnosis.[20] The nature of the inflammation on histopathology seems to vary from primarily lymphoplasmacytic[19] to pyogranulomatous.[2]

Fungal culture is also a possible means for diagnosis. If this technique is performed, sampling from the deepest portion of the lesion may increase diagnostic sensitivity.

Treatments

Surgical excision of the granuloma seems to be the most effective treatment.[16] Treatment with antifungals is possible, and fluconazole has been reported to be effective.[20,22]

Cutaneous Lymphomas

Epidemiology

Cutaneous lymphoma is relatively uncommon,[1] and it seems that there may be a sex predilection for mares.[23–25] Horses of a variety of ages can be affected. There is no established breed predilection, but one study found thoroughbreds to be overrepresented.[1]

Clinical presentation

The most common clinical presentation seems to be multiple subcutaneous nodular masses that may be present for months to years. Occasionally, these nodules may become alopecic or ulcerated[26] and their size may wax and wane over time.[27]

Pathogenesis

Like many tumors, the underlying cause of these lesions is unknown. Many of these tumors are reported to be of B-cell origin with large numbers of nonneoplastic T cells, the so-called T-cell-rich B-cell lymphomas. However, a recent study of cutaneous lymphomas in a group of horses found them to be more constituent with T-cell origin.[25]

Diagnosis

Diagnosis is made based on biopsy results. The result of FNA is difficult to interpret because the neoplastic lymphocytes can resemble inflammatory lesions on FNA,[28] although flow cytometry may be useful.[25] Despite the long-term course of the disease in these horses, elevated numbers of lymphocytes are not present and complete blood cell count and serum biochemistries are often not useful in diagnosis.

Treatment

The prognosis for treatment is unknown. Anecdotally, there has been a report of remission after administration of synthetic progestin.[27] A multidrug chemotherapeutic regime has been suggested as well.[29]

Mast Cell Tumors

Epidemiology

Mast cell tumors are typically benign tumors that tend to affect horses of any age. There are no reported breed predilections; male horses may be overrepresented.[30]

Mast cell tumors have also been referred to as cutaneous mastocytosis, suggesting more of a dysregulated immune response rather than a true neoplasm, but no particular underlying antigen has been identified.

Clinical presentation
Tumors are commonly found on the head, trunk, and limbs.[16] On the head and trunk they may be fluctuant, and the overlying skin can range in appearance from normal through alopecia to ulcerated. Masses on the limbs are often found near joints and are firm and nonmovable.[16] On occasion, caseous material may be exuded by the masses. Mast cell tumors are typically slow to grow, but there has been a report of a slowly growing mass suddenly growing.[31]

Diagnosis
Diagnosis can often be made using FNA. Mast cells retrieved are typically well granulated and well differentiated. Older lesions can have abundant dystrophic mineralization, significant eosinophilic inflammation, and relatively lower numbers of mast cells.[16] Histopathology of biopsy samples can be helpful in this event to identify the mast cells.

Treatment
The prognosis for mast cell tumors in horses is generally very good and rarely, the lesions resolve spontaneously. Surgical excision of tumors is typically curative, and even masses that have been incompletely excised may undergo remission.[16]

ULCERATIVE LESIONS
Squamous Cell Carcinoma

Squamous cell carcinomas are a very frequently diagnosed cancer in the skin of horses.[1,3] Clinically, these tend to be locally destructive lesions, and the majority of owner concerns are because of local disease. However, it is worth noting that in one study approximately 17% of penile squamous cell carcinomas had metastasized to the local lymph node at the time of diagnosis.[32]

Microbiology
Traditionally, squamous cell carcinomas have been attributed to UV light exposure, with smaller numbers associated with areas of chronic inflammation.[16] Although this may still hold true for lesions of the eyelid and poorly pigmented or haired skin, there is increasing evidence that squamous cell carcinomas, particularly those on the penis, are associated with papillomavirus infections with equine papillomavirus 2.[33,34]

Epidemiology
Squamous cell carcinoma can occur in horses of a wide range of ages but most commonly affects horses aged between 12 and 16 years.[1,16] Appaloosas and American Paint horses seem to be predisposed to the development of the lesion, and males also seem to be at a slightly increased risk.[1] Most of these tumors occur in or around the eyelid, penis, and perianal region.[1,16]

Clinical presentation
The typical early appearance of these tumors is that of a solitary, ulcerating, proliferative nonhealing wound. As the disease progresses, the amount of necrosis and tissue destruction increases and foul smelling discharge is relatively common.

Pathogenesis
UV light exposure is thought to be involved with the development of tumors on the eyelid and in poorly pigmented skin, and early solar changes to the skin can be

seen in these areas. As previously mentioned, papillomavirus infections seem to be associated with the development of penile squamous cell carcinomas. Areas of chronic inflammation such as burn wounds or other poorly healing wounds are also possible sites for tumor development.

Diagnosis

FNA revealing dysplastic keratinocytes can be helpful, but marked epithelial dysplasia can also be seen with inflammatory conditions. So this finding is not unique. Histopathology is the most common diagnostic method. Invasive and irregular islands of neoplastic keratinocytes are typically found.

In horses with penile tumors, sedation may be required to better examine the extent of the lesions. Ultrasonography has been suggested to define the extent of the tumor. Rectal palpation and ultrasonography of inguinal and iliac lymph nodes to assess the presence of metastasis may be useful.[35]

Treatment

A standardized approach to the assessment and treatment of penile tumors has been suggested.[36] This approach is based on evaluation of the primary tumor site with histopathology and ultrasonography and evaluation for possible metastatic disease. Complete surgical excision of the tumor should be curative in the absence of metastatic disease. However, complete removal may not be feasible depending on the size and location of the tumor.[35] Cryotherapy has been used to treat smaller tumors.[37] With widespread metastasis, euthanasia may be the only viable option.

Exuberant Granulation Tissue

Wounds in horses often involve loss of a considerable amount of tissue, and primary closure is frequently not possible. Repair via secondary intention through the formation of granulation tissue can lead to the production of EGT (proud flesh).

Epidemiology

EGT is an unusual change in veterinary species apart from equids and can occur after wounds in any age, breed, or sex of horses.

Clinical presentation

EGT occurs almost always along wounds on the limbs and presents as raised ulcerated fleshy masses that grow along the edges and bulge into the center of the wounds.

Pathogenesis

The pathogenesis of EGT in horses is complex, and numerous observations have been made describing abnormalities in these lesions. Wounds on the limb, particularly when bandaged, have a tendency to heal via contraction and produce large amounts of granulation tissue, which can bulge and extend over the wound margins.[38] Myofibroblasts within this granulation tissue are reported to be haphazardly oriented and may have poor contractile activity.[39] In addition, mutant p53 has been found in limb wounds of horses, suggesting a possible abnormality in apoptosis.[40] Changes in the microvasculature of healing wounds has also been suggested as a possible factor in these lesions.[41]

Diagnosis

Diagnosis is based on the location of the lesion and its clinical appearance. Differentiating EGT from fibroblastic sarcoids can be difficult both clinically and histopathologically. Biopsy of suspect tissue should be performed if there is question as to its nature. FNA is unlikely to be useful in differentiating these 2 lesions because both can show similar changes.

Treatment
Prevention of EGT is likely the most important consideration. Limb wounds should be kept clean, foreign material should be removed, and necrotic tissue should be debrided. The issue of bandaging of wounds is complex. Bandaging of wounds after formation of a granulation tissue bed may enhance formation of EGT, but it also reduces wound contamination and desiccation.[42] Application of silicone gel dressings after granulation has been shown to reduce the likelihood of EGT formation.[43] Treatment of EGT consists largely of surgical excision of the excess tissue removing nonviable tissue and inflammation.

Habronemiasis

Microbiology
Habronemiasis within the skin is caused by third-stage larvae of 3 different gastric nematodes, *Habronema muscae, Habronema majus, and Draschia megastoma.* The adult worms live within the stomach, and skin lesions are caused by aberrant migration of larvae.[44] The larvae themselves are transmitted by flies.

Epidemiology
There are no age or sex predilections, and the disease has been reported worldwide.[16] Arabian and gray horses were overrepresented in a survey of habronemiasis in North America.[45]

Clinical presentation
Lesions are seen most commonly on the limbs, ventral abdomen, external genitalia, and ventral canthus of the eyes. Single or multiple lesions may be seen. Lesions appear as ulcerated masses that may bleed easily. These lesions can appear similar to EGT.

Diagnosis
Diagnosis can be made based on clinical appearance, cytology, and biopsy. Cytology of smears taken from the lesion can contain small (<1 mm) yellow granules, which may contain larvae. Biopsy samples show eosinophilic inflammation with areas of coagulation necrosis. Larvae may be seen within these areas of necrosis, but larva are often not seen in biopsy, although the disease is still suspected.[2]

Treatment
Surgical debulking of masses along with topical use of antiinflammatories has been used with success. Addition of macrocyclic lactones may improve treatment results.[46] Fly control to prevent infection of horses is an important preventive measure.

ALOPECIC DERMATOSES
Atopy

Atopy is the term for hypersensitivity to a variety of environmental stimuli. Atopy in horses is somewhat different from that in other veterinary species in that the amount of pruritus is variable.[47]

Epidemiology
Atopy in horses may initially present as a seasonal allergy, but often becomes nonseasonal. However, depending on the antigen involved, atopy may also present as

nonseasonal initially.[16] Horses of a wide range of ages have been diagnosed with atopy.[48] No study has found any breed, age or sex predilections.

Clinical presentation
Clinical presentation can be variable. Urticaria, both pruritic and nonpruritic, is a reported common clinical sign.[47,48] Alopecia, self-trauma, and pitting edema are also relatively common. Lesions are most common on the face, pinnae, trunk, and distal part of the legs.

Pathogenesis
Allergens involved can be quite variable and include insects, food hypersensitivity, pollen, dust, and mites.[49]

Diagnosis
Diagnosis is based largely on clinical suspicion. Intradermal skin testing has some scientific support, but serum allergy testing does not.[49]

Treatment
Allergen-specific immunotherapy has had reportedly good results with a response rate of 84%.[48] Treatment with antihistamines and glucocorticoids are commonly used to control symptoms.

Alopecia Areata

Epidemiology
There are no reported age, breed, or sex predilections for alopecia areata (AA). Lesions are often reported to worsen during spring and summer, but no reason for this seasonality has been proven.[50]

Clinical presentation
AA presents as patches of nonsymmetrical alopecia of the head, body, mane, and tail.[16,50] Skin within these areas can appear normal or have mild scaling. Alopecic areas can range in size from 2 cm to up to 80% of the body, mane, and tail.[50]

Pathogenesis
The underlying cause of AA is thought to be an autoimmune reaction to the hair follicles. T cells targeting anagen hair follicles cause destruction of these follicles leaving behind fibrosis and telogen hair follicles.

Diagnosis
Diagnosis is made based on clinical appearance and biopsy results. The typical histopathologic findings are peribulbar inflammation or the presence of fibrosis surrounding hair follicles.

Treatment
At present, no effective treatment of the condition has been found. Partial hair regrowth after initial presentation was present in most horses.[50]

Anagen/Telogen Effluvium

Epidemiology
Anagen effluvium (AE) and telogen effluvium (TE) are nonspecific alterations to the hair coat. AE and TE occur after some stressful change including fever, pregnancy, surgery, and anesthesia. AE alopecia usually takes place within a few days of the insult.[51] In TE, at 1 to 4 months after this change there is sudden marked alopecia.[52] There are no sex, breed, or age predispositions.

Clinical presentation
Clinical presentation is of a rapid alopecic hair loss that is typically roughly bilaterally symmetric. The amount of hair loss can vary from a focal area to most of the hair on the horse. Skin in the alopecic areas is typically normal in appearance. In AE, the skin may have a slightly stubbled feel to it.[16]

Pathogenesis
Hair follicles go through a cycle of growth with an anagen or growth phase followed by a transitional catagen phase and finally a telogen resting phase. Telogen hairs are typically displaced from below by the newly emerging anagen hair. In TE, there is disruption of this normal hair cycle and large groups of hair follicles in the anagen phase suddenly stop growth. This process leads to synchronization of these large number of follicles, and when new hair growth occurs later, all the synchronized telogen hairs fall out at the same time leading to alopecia.

AE is similar, but rather than the hairs entering telogen, they restart growth. This interruption in growth leads to abnormalities in the hair shaft, which result in weakening of the shaft at that point. Breakage of the shaft leads to the alopecia seen, and the remaining portions of the shaft within the skin account for the stubbled feeling.

Diagnosis
Diagnosis is based on clinical examination, history, and hair examination. Abnormalities in the hair shaft may be seen microscopically in anagen defluxion, but in the case of already broken hairs, no changes may be noted. Biopsy is typically unrewarding; in the case of TE, large numbers of anagen-phase hair bulbs are noted.[16]

Treatment
If the initial inciting cause is removed, no treatment is required and regrowth of new hair soon fills in the alopecic areas.

SCALY DERMATOSES
Dermatophytosis

Dermatophytosis or ringworm, as it is more commonly called, is potentially a concern for both its veterinary and zoonotic potential.

Microbiology
In horses, most infections are caused by the fungi *Trichophyton equinum* or *Microsporum canis* (*Microsporum equinum* is an equine-adapted *M canis*), although other fungi are occasionally found. Both these fungi grow worldwide, although they are more common in warmer and humid environments.

Epidemiology
Dermatophytes are relatively widespread, present on 9% of riding horses in one study.[53] Once introduced into an environment, dermatophytes spread easily from one animal to another through environmental contamination or fomites.[54] In endemic infections, younger animals are affected and animals seldom have recurrent infections.[55]

Clinical presentation
Most lesions occur in the saddle area or other locations in contact with tack. Initially, they commonly present as areas of raised hair that progress to alopecia with scaling, erythema and crusting. Often these lesions are circular with an area of erythema in the center. Single lesions are common, but lesions can coalesce and occasionally animals can have widespread lesions.

Occasionally, animals develop a military dermatitis with exudation. This lesion is more commonly associated with infection with *Trichophyton mentagrophytes*.[55]

Pathogenesis
Infections are superficial with colonization of hair shafts and the superficial layers of the skin.

Diagnosis
Diagnosis can be performed in many ways. Some strains of *M canis* fluoresce under UV light. Arthroconidia can sometimes be seen microscopically using plucked hairs or skin scrapings. Skin scrapings are most useful when taken from the margins of the lesion, and digestion with 10% to 20% potassium hydroxide removes debris and makes visualization of the fungi easier. Acetate tape is another method of rapidly collecting and viewing samples. Fungal culture can also be performed on these samples, or a new toothbrush can be used to brush the area and collect the sample. Biopsy can be useful when lesions are less superficial.

Treatment
The disease is self-limiting in most animals, but given the concerns for transmission and the zoonotic potential, treatment should be considered. Topical therapy is useful to speed resolution. The area should be clipped to provide better access. Any tools used when treating or cleaning the area need to be disinfected to prevent their acting as fomites. A variety of antifungal shampoos are available and effective. Given that there is likely contamination of the hair coat beyond the lesion, the entire coat should be treated.[56] Systemic treatment with oral antifungals can be attempted, but efficacy studies in horses are largely lacking. Given the costs of this treatment and the potential side effects (teratogenesis with griseofulvin), systemic treatment may not be useful.

Disinfection of the property can be undertaken when practical. A dilute solution of bleach (1:10) kills dermatophyte arthroconidia.[57] All grooming equipment, stalls, and trailers could be washed using this solution.

Pemphigus Foliaceus

Pemphigus foliaceus (PF) is the most common autoimmune disease of horses.[2,16,58]

Epidemiology
PF has been identified in animals ranging in age from 2.5 months to over 20 years.[59] There is no breed or sex predilection. Cases are more likely to be diagnosed during the cooler months of the year.[59]

Clinical presentation
PF presents initially as vesicles on the face or limbs, which may then spread to other areas of the body. These vesicles are short lived, however, and alopecic, scaling, or crusting lesions are more commonly seen. The degree of pruritus, pain, and edema can be variable,[58] but limb edema has been reported in more than half of the cases.[16]

Pathogenesis
PF is caused by the production of autoantibodies to intraepidermal adhesion proteins. Binding of these antibodies causes dissolution of the intercellular bonds between keratinocytes and production of acantholytic cells and clefts or pustules within the skin. Rupture of these clefts leads to the scaling and crusting seen clinically.

Diagnosis

Diagnosis can be made cytologically via identification of individual or rafts of acantholytic cells within vesicles. These vesicles are often short lived, however, and biopsy of the crusted sites is a good second choice. Because of the importance of the identification of these acantholytic cells and intraepidermal clefts, surgical preparation before biopsy is contraindicated because these delicate structures may be lost. Immunohistochemical identification of immunoglobulin deposition helps to confirm the diagnosis.

Treatment

Treatment is usually via glucocorticoid administration, although other substances have also been tried. Treatment is likely to be prolonged, for weeks to months, although a small proportion of horses undergo spontaneous remission.

Dermatophilosis

Microbiology

Dermatophilus congolensis is an anaerobic non-acid-fast gram-positive bacterium with worldwide distribution, and it can infect a wide variety of species including horses, sheep, and cattle.

Clinical presentation

Both acute and chronic forms of dermatophilosis have been identified in horses. The acute form appears as thick scabs of matted hair with viscous yellow purulent discharge that are firmly attached to the skin surface and when removed cover ulcerated skin. In chronic forms of the disease, these crusts become progressively drier and the ulceration beneath them begins to heal.[60] Lesions are usually present on the back, sides, and hind legs.

Pathogenesis

Dermatophilus are opportunistic bacteria that affect horses with an impaired skin barrier or immune function. Although the disease itself is relatively common, risk factors have not been formally identified.[56] Excessive skin moisture whether from environmental conditions or because of an excessive hair coat caused by other conditions are commonly seen.

The bacteria can be found on the skin of clinically normal horses, and these may represent carrier animals. However, if these are important in the disease is unknown.[56]

Diagnosis

The presence of these distinctive crusts, particularly with a history of being in a wet environment or thick hair coats, is highly suggestive of *Dermatophilus*. Impression smears of the crusts can demonstrate the classical laminated appearance of the bacteria. The bacteria can be cultured from the crusts, or the disease can be diagnosed via histopathology.[56] The diagnosis of dermatophilosis in animals with no history of being wet should trigger an investigation for other underlying conditions.

Treatment

As an important adjunct to specific treatment, improving environmental conditions such as getting the animals dry speeds healing of the lesions. Soaking crusts with a dilute chlorhexidine solution (4%) facilitates removal. Vigorous scrubbing should be avoided because this tends to delay healing. Similar dilute chlorhexidine solutions can be applied as a shampoo for generalized cases or as a spray for more focal lesions. The solution should be allowed to sit on the affected tissue for 10 to 15 minutes before rinsing.[56] Antibiotic treatment is rarely required.

Equine Multisystemic Eosinophilic Epitheliotropic Disease

Equine multisystemic eosinophilic epitheliotropic disease (MEED) is a relatively rare chronic progressive disease associated with exfoliative dermatitis and infiltrations of eosinophils and lymphocytes in various organs.[2,61,62]

Epidemiology

Clinical reports are relatively limited, but there appears to be a breed predisposition for the development of MEED in standardbreds.[62] Affected animals are typically young, but animals as old as 19 years have been reported.

Clinical presentation

Most animals have generalized dermatitis characterized by alopecia and a poor hair coat. Pruritus, although reported, is not typical of most cases. Lesions typically progress slowly, but rapid progression was seen in 1 case.[62] Other signs seen in MEED include weight loss and diarrhea, with epistaxis and other respiratory signs rarely reported.[63] Skin lesions most commonly begin on the distal part of the limbs and spread, in 1 case report becoming generalized.[61] Changes to the proximal gastrointestinal tract are commonly seen, and these include hyperkeratosis of the esophagus and nonglandular stomach. The intestine may also become thickened in a nodular or diffuse pattern.[61,62] Similarly, thickening of the bile duct and fibrosis within the pancreas are reported.

Pathogenesis

The underlying cause of MEED remains unknown. Eosinophilic inflammation is a relatively common reaction pattern in the horse and can be associated with parasitism, hypersensitivity, and other causes. The systemic nature of the eosinophilic infiltrates has been possibly related to migrating parasites,[61] but due to a seasonal reaction pattern seen in some reports an allergen or toxin may also be a possibility.[64]

Diagnosis

Diagnosis can be challenging and depends on clinical findings, history, and ultimately biopsy of affected tissues. Surprisingly, considering the widespread eosinophilic inflammation, eosinophilia is only seen in a small proportion of cases. Other blood chemistry changes are nonspecific such as hypoproteinemia and hypoalbuminemia or are associated with biliary or pancreatic disease (elevated levels of alkaline phosphatase and Gamma-glutamyl transpeptidase).

The gross changes to the gastrointestinal tract with concurrent skin disease are highly suggestive of MEED.

Treatment

Treatment is likely to be unrewarding. Of the nearly 50 cases in the literature, only 4 horses survived past 8 months[63,65,66]; all others were euthanized. These 4 horses were treated with dexamethasone at varying doses. A similar condition in humans also relied on corticosteroid treatment, but newer medications that target eosinophils within the blood are now used. Whether these would work in horses is unknown.

SUMMARY

In summary, skin disease in horses is relatively common and can occur for a wide variety of different reasons. Many of these lesions appear similar clinically and frequently further diagnostic work is required. Dermatopathology in horses can be complex and developing a good relationship with an experienced dermatopathologist can be very valuable. Like disease in any other body system, good observational skills, good history taking and wise selection of biopsy material can aid in making the diagnosis more quickly and efficiently.

REFERENCES

1. Schaffer PA, Wobeser B, Martin LE, et al. Cutaneous neoplastic lesions of equids in the central United States and Canada: 3,351 biopsy specimens from 3,272 equids (2000-2010). J Am Vet Med Assoc 2013;242(1):99–104.
2. Schaffer PA, Wobeser B, Dennis MM, et al. Non-neoplastic lesions of equine skin in the central United States and Canada: a retrospective study. Can Vet J 2013; 54(3):262–6.
3. Valentine BA. Survey of equine cutaneous neoplasia in the Pacific Northwest. J Vet Diagn Invest 2006;18(1):123–6.
4. Lunardi M, de Alcântara BK, Otonel RA, et al. Bovine papillomavirus type 13 DNA in equine sarcoids. J Clin Microbiol 2013;51(7):2167–71.
5. Teifke JP. Morphologic and molecular biologic studies of the etiology of equine sarcoid. Tierarztl Prax 1994;22(4):368–76 [in German].
6. Trewby H, Ayele G, Borzacchiello G, et al. Analysis of the long control region of bovine papillomavirus type 1 associated with sarcoids in equine hosts indicates multiple cross-species transmission events and phylogeographical structure. J Gen Virol 2014;95(Pt 12):2748–56.
7. Knottenbelt DC. A suggested clinical classification for the equine sarcoid. Clin Tech Equine Pract 2005;4:278–95.
8. Wobeser BK, Davies JL, Hill JE, et al. Epidemiology of equine sarcoids in horses in western Canada. Can Vet J 2010;51(10):1103–8.
9. Nasir L, Campo MS. Bovine papillomaviruses: their role in the aetiology of cutaneous tumours of bovids and equids. Vet Dermatol 2008;19(5):243–54.
10. Finlay M, Yuan Z, Burden F, et al. The detection of Bovine Papillomavirus type 1 DNA in flies. Virus Res 2009;144(1–2):315–7.
11. Wobeser BK, Hill JE, Jackson ML, et al. Localization of Bovine Papillomavirus in equine sarcoids and inflammatory skin conditions of horses using laser microdissection and two forms of DNA amplification. J Vet Diagn Invest 2012;24(1):32–41.
12. Stadler S, Kainzbauer C, Haralambus R, et al. Successful treatment of equine sarcoids by topical aciclovir application. Vet Rec 2011;168(7):187.
13. Christen-Clottu O, Klocke P, Burger D, et al. Treatment of clinically diagnosed equine sarcoid with a mistletoe extract (Viscum album austriacus). J Vet Intern Med 2010;24(6):1483–9.
14. Scagliarini A, Bettini G, Savini F, et al. Treatment of equine sarcoids. Vet Rec 2012;171(13):330.
15. Valentine BA. Equine cutaneous non-neoplastic nodular and proliferative lesions in the Pacific Northwest. Vet Dermatol 2005;16(6):425–8.
16. Scott D, Miller W. Equine dermatology. 2nd edition. Maryland Heights (MO): Saunders; 2011.
17. Mathison P. Eosinophilic nodular dermatoses. Vet Clin North Am Equine Pract 1995;11:75–89.
18. Slovis NM, Watson JL, Affolter VK, et al. Injection site eosinophilic granulomas and collagenolysis in 3 horses. J Vet Intern Med 1999;13(6):606–12.
19. Valentine BA, Taylor GH, Stone JK, et al. Equine cutaneous fungal granuloma: a study of 44 lesions from 34 horses. Vet Dermatol 2006;17(4):266–72.
20. Schwarz B, Burford J, Knottenbelt D. Cutaneous fungal granuloma in a horse. Vet Dermatol 2009;20(2):131–4.

21. Blackford J. Superficial and deep mycoses in horses. Vet Clin North Am Large Anim Pract 1984;6:47–58.
22. Latimer FG, Colitz CM, Campbell NB, et al. Pharmacokinetics of fluconazole following intravenous and oral administration and body fluid concentrations of fluconazole following repeated oral dosing in horses. Am J Vet Res 2001;62(10): 1606–11.
23. Gerard MP, Healy LN, Bowman KF, et al. Cutaneous lymphoma with extensive periarticular involvement in a horse. J Am Vet Med Assoc 1998;213(3):391–3.
24. Hermeyer K, Seehusen F, Gehlen H, et al. Cutaneous T-cell-rich B-cell lymphoma in a horse. Berl Munch Tierarztl Wochenschr 2010;123(9–10):422–4.
25. de Bruijn CM, Veenman JN, Rutten VP, et al. Clinical, histopathological and immunophenotypical findings in five horses with cutaneous malignant lymphoma. Res Vet Sci 2007;83(1):63–72.
26. Taintor J, Schleis S. Equine lymphoma. Equine Vet Educ 2011;23(4):205–13.
27. Henson KL, Alleman AR, Cutler TJ, et al. Regression of subcutaneous lymphoma following removal of an ovarian granulosa-theca cell tumor in a horse. J Am Vet Med Assoc 1998;212(9):1419–22.
28. Adams R, Calderwood-Mays MB, Peyton LC. Malignant lymphoma in three horses with ulcerative pharyngitis. J Am Vet Med Assoc 1988;193(6):674–6.
29. Burns T, Couto C. Systemic chemotherapy for oncologic diseases. In: Robinson N, editor. Current therapy in equine medicine. St Louis (MO): Saunders; 2009. p. 15–8.
30. Mair TS, Krudewig C. Mast cell tumours (mastocytosis) in the horse: a review of the literature and report of 11 cases. Equine Vet Educ 2008;20(4):177–82.
31. Mcentee MF. Equine cutaneous mastocytoma - morphology, biological behavior and evolution of the lesion. J Comp Pathol 1991;104(2):171–8.
32. van den Top JG, de Heer N, Klein WR, et al. Penile and preputial tumours in the horse: a retrospective study of 114 affected horses. Equine Vet J 2008;40(6):528–32.
33. Lange CE, Tobler K, Lehner A, et al. EcPV2 DNA in Equine Papillomas and in situ and invasive squamous cell carcinomas supports papillomavirus etiology. Vet Pathol 2013;50(4):686–92.
34. Knight CG, Munday JS, Peters J, et al. Equine penile squamous cell carcinomas are associated with the presence of equine papillomavirus type 2 DNA sequences. Vet Pathol 2011;48(6):1190–4.
35. Van den Top JG, Ensink JM, Barneveld A, et al. Penile and preputial squamous cell carcinoma in the horse and proposal of a classification system. Equine Vet Educ 2011;23(12):636–48.
36. Van Den Top JG, Ensink JM, Gröne A, et al. Penile and preputial tumours in the horse: literature review and proposal of a standardised approach. Equine Vet J 2010;42(8):746–57.
37. Stick J. Cryosurgery. In: Auer JA, Stick JA, editors. Equine surgery. 3rd edition. St Louis (MO): Elsevier; 2006. p. 172–6.
38. Theoret CL, Barber SM, Moyana TN, et al. Preliminary observations on expression of transforming growth factors beta1 and beta3 in equine full-thickness skin wounds healing normally or with exuberant granulation tissue. Vet Surg 2002; 31(3):266–73.
39. Theoret CL, Olutoye OO, Parnell LK, et al. Equine exuberant granulation tissue and human keloids: a comparative histopathologic study. Vet Surg 2013;42(7):783–9.
40. Lepault E, Céleste C, Doré M, et al. Comparative study on microvascular occlusion and apoptosis in body and limb wounds in the horse. Wound Repair Regen 2005;13(5):520–9.

41. Theoret CL, Wilmink JM. Aberrant wound healing in the horse: naturally occurring conditions reminiscent of those observed in man. Wound Repair Regen 2013; 21(3):365–71.

42. Woollen N, DeBowes RM, Liepold HW, et al. A comparison of four types of therapy for the treatment of full-thickness skin wounds of the horse. In: Proceedings of the annual convention of the American Association of Equine Practitioners (USA). 1988. p. 569–76.

43. Hackett R. How to prevent and treat exuberant granulation tissue. In: Proceedings of the Annual Convention of the American Association of Equine Practitioners. San Antonio (TX): Blackwell; 2011. p. 367–73.

44. Fadok VA. Parasitic skin diseases of large animals. Vet Clin North Am Large Anim Pract 1984;6(1):3–26.

45. Pusterla N, Watson JL, Wilson WD, et al. Cutaneous and ocular habronemiasis in horses: 63 cases (1988-2002). J Am Vet Med Assoc 2003;222(7):978–82.

46. Pugh DG, Hu XP, Blagburn B. Habronemiasis: biology, signs, and diagnosis, and treatment and prevention of the nematodes and vector flies. J Equine Vet Sci 2014;34(2):241–8.

47. Rosenkrantz W, White S. Clinical aspects of equine atopic disease, in veterinary allergy. Chichester (West Sussex): John Wiley & Sons, Ltd; 2013. p. 334–7.

48. Stepnik CT, Outerbridge CA, White SD, et al. Equine atopic skin disease and response to allergen-specific immunotherapy: a retrospective study at the University of California-Davis (1991-2008). Vet Dermatol 2012;23(1):29–35 e7.

49. Fadok VA. Update on equine allergies. Vet Clin North Am Equine Pract 2013; 29(3):541–50.

50. Hoolahan DE, White SD, Outerbridge CA, et al. Equine alopecia areata: a retrospective clinical descriptive study at the University of California, Davis (1980-2011). Vet Dermatol 2013;24(2):282-e64.

51. Rosychuk RA. Noninflammatory, nonpruritic alopecia of horses. Vet Clin North Am Equine Pract 2013;29(3):629–41.

52. Jubb TF, Graydon RJ. Telogen defluxion associated with hypersensitivity causing alopecia in a horse. Aust Vet J 2007;85(1–2):56–8.

53. Moretti A, Boncio L, Pasquali P, et al. Epidemiological aspects of dermatophyte infections in horses and cattle. Zentralbl Veterinarmed B 1998;45(4):205–8.

54. Lund A, Deboer DJ. Immunoprophylaxis of dermatophytosis in animals. Mycopathologia 2008;166(5–6):407–24.

55. Chermette R, Ferreiro L, Guillot J. Dermatophytoses in animals. Mycopathologia 2008;166(5–6):385–405.

56. Weese JS, Yu AA. Infectious folliculitis and dermatophytosis. Vet Clin North Am Equine Pract 2013;29(3):559–75.

57. Rycroft AN, McLay C. Disinfectants in the control of small animal ringworm due to Microsporum canis. Vet Rec 1991;129(11):239–41.

58. Rosenkrantz W. Immune-mediated dermatoses. Vet Clin North Am Equine Pract 2013;29(3):607–13.

59. Vandenabeele SI, White SD, Affolter VK, et al. Pemphigus foliaceus in the horse: a retrospective study of 20 cases. Vet Dermatol 2004;15(6):381–8.

60. Awad W, Nadra-Elwgoud M, El-Sayed A. Diagnosis and treatment of bovine, ovine and equine dermatophilosis. J Appl Sci Res 2008;4(4):367–74.

61. Pucheu-Haston CM, Del Piero F. Equine multi-systemic eosinophilic epitheliotropic disease. Equine Vet Educ 2013;25(12):614–7.

62. Bosseler L, Verryken K, Bauwens C, et al. Equine multisystemic eosinophilic epitheliotropic disease: a case report and review of literature. N Z Vet J 2013;61(3):177–82.

63. Carmalt J. Multisystemic eosinophilic disease in a quarter horse. Equine Vet Educ 2004;16(5):231–4.
64. Nimmo Wilkie JS, Yager JA, Nation PN, et al. Chronic eosinophilic dermatitis: a manifestation of a multisystemic, eosinophilic, epitheliotropic disease in five horses. Vet Pathol 1985;22(4):297–305.
65. McCue ME, Davis EG, Rush BR, et al. Dexamethasone for treatment of multisystemic eosinophilic epitheliotropic disease in a horse. J Am Vet Med Assoc 2003; 223(9):1320–3, 1281.
66. Gibson KT, Alders RG. Eosinophilic enterocolitis and dermatitis in two horses. Equine Vet J 1987;19(3):247–52.

Diseases of the Equine Urinary System

Shannon McLeland, DVM

KEYWORDS

- Equine • Glomerulonephritis • Interstitial nephritis • Renal • Tubular necrosis
- Urinary

KEY POINTS

- Diseases of the equine urinary system have multiple potential etiologies, including infectious agents, toxins, developmental abnormalities, and neoplasia.
- A minimum diagnostic database is essential for diagnosis of urinary diseases and should include a complete blood count, serum biochemistry, and urinalysis, in addition to a thorough physical examination and medical history.
- Renal and urinary bladder biopsies are valuable tools in determining a definitive diagnosis in cases of equine urinary diseases.

INTRODUCTION

Urinary diseases of equines encompass many disease entities at various locations within the urinary tract and can be an indicator of systemic health. The urinary system can be divided into an upper, or renal, and a lower urinary tract, which consists of ureters, bladder, and urethra. Although perhaps not common, renal disease can be caused by a variety of infectious, immune-mediated, developmental, and toxic insults, which if not identified and addressed may result in a poor outcome for the animal. As a clinician, quickly and definitively identifying an etiology for renal disease may be impeded by vague, nonspecific clinical presentations and potentially by the lack of sensitive, accessible diagnostic parameters as an indicator of renal impairment. Because of these limitations, the clinician should be well equipped with the knowledge of equine urinary pathology and various etiologies that will produce lesions in the urinary tract, which is the focus of this review.

A minimum database that includes a thorough history, physical examination, complete blood count, serum biochemistry, and urinalysis is essential for identification of urinary disease. Glomerular disease is distinguished by the presence of persistent

Department of Microbiology, Immunology and Pathology, College of Veterinary Medicine and Biomedical Sciences, Colorado State University, 1619 Campus Delivery, Fort Collins, CO 80523, USA
E-mail address: Shannon.mcleland@colostate.edu

Vet Clin Equine 31 (2015) 377–387
http://dx.doi.org/10.1016/j.cveq.2015.04.005
0749-0739/15/$ – see front matter Published by Elsevier Inc.

vetequine.theclinics.com

proteinuria with or without azotemia.[1,2] This can be differentiated from tubulointersti-tial disease, which frequently lacks significant proteinuria, but alterations in baseline serum creatinine and urine-concentrating abilities should be evident.[1] Lower urinary tract diseases can present with variable clinical symptoms and clinicopathologic ab-normalities. Urinary bladder distention, dysuria, or pollakiuria can be the result of an obstruction from urolithiasis or neoplasia. Urinary incontinence may be indicative of a developmental anomaly such as ectopic ureter.

Additional diagnostic modalities can further help localize disease, tailor treatment, and have prognostic relevance. A few of these include renal biopsy, imaging such as ultrasound, cystoscopy, and microbiologic, molecular, and serologic assays. **Fig. 1** outlines the major categories of equine urinary diseases discussed here for an easy, quick reference to this review.

UPPER URINARY TRACT DISEASES
Glomerular Diseases

Glomerular injury can be mediated by immunologic and nonimmunologic pro-cesses.[3,4] Antibodies directed at glomerular antigens or soluble immune complexes that deposit within glomeruli are the 2 major routes of immunologic injury to glomeruli of domestic animals.[5] Although glomerular disease is not commonly clinically apparent, immune-complex glomerulonephritis occurs with some frequency in horses.[5–8] Equine infectious anemia and *Streptococcus equi* have been implicated in immune-complex membranous and membranoproliferative glomerulonephritis of

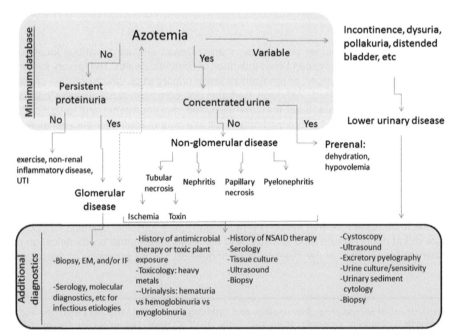

Fig. 1. Flow chart of equine urinary diseases discussed in this review. Solid lines represent clinicopathologic derangements associated with general categories of urinary diseases. Dashed line indicates that persistent proteinuria is typical of glomerular disease although concurrent azotemia may or may not be present. EM, electron microscopy; IF, immunofluorescence.

horses.[6,7,9,10] Idiopathic immune-mediated and non–immune-mediated glomerulone-phritides have been sporadically reported as well.[11–13] Glomerular amyloidosis in horses is unusual.[3,14]

Clinically, horses presenting with glomerular disease suffer from symptoms that could include anorexia, weight loss, depression, or dependent edema. Clinicopatho-logic derangements include persistent proteinuria with or without hematuria.[2,3] Azotemia, electrolyte abnormalities, metabolic acidosis, and decreased urine specific gravity are variable depending on the severity of disease and involvement of the tubu-lointerstitium. Hypoproteinemia and hypoalbuminemia may be present as a result of injury to the glomerular filtration barrier, which may manifest clinically as edema; how-ever, protein-losing nephropathy is infrequently reported in horses.[15] Clinicians should be cautious in diagnosing glomerular disease based solely on the presence of protein on urinary reagent strip tests. Proteinuria can be the result of lower urinary tract dis-ease such as cystitis, physiologic due to nonrenal inflammatory diseases, or transient proteinuria after heavy exercise.[3,15,16] Persistent, proteinuria confirmed with a com-plete urinalysis with sediment cytology and urine protein-to-creatinine ratio is strongly encouraged, along with an initial thorough physical examination and minimum diag-nostic database (ie, complete blood count, serum biochemistry, and urine specific gravity and reagent strip test).

Renal biopsy is an effective and relatively safe diagnostic tool to aid in the diagnosis of renal disease such as glomerulonephritis.[17] Histologically, glomeruli should have evidence of basement membrane thickening, remodeling depending on the course of disease, or increased cellularity. The addition of special histochemical stains, such as periodic-acid Schiff reaction, Jones methenamine silver, Masson trichrome, and Congo red, aid in identification of these features. Electron-dense deposits, fibrils, and remodeling of glomerular basement membranes are confirmed by electron micro-scopy with identification of immune complexes by immunofluorescence. Infectious agents should be ruled out by serologic, molecular, and microbiologic assays. Gross abnormalities, observed on postmortem examination, of the kidneys may be absent or subtle with evidence of acute renal injury, such as swelling and bulging of the cortex on cut surface. With progressive disease, whole nephron units could be affected with scarring, which on gross examination the kidneys could be shrunken, pale, and firm.

Tubulointerstitial Diseases

Renal tubular and interstitial compartments are structurally and functionally interre-lated and, therefore, insults and disease processes that affect tubules invariably involve the interstitial compartment and are referred to collectively as tubulointerstitial diseases.[1] Acute tubular degeneration and necrosis is in general the consequence of either ischemia or toxin exposure, whereas interstitial inflammation and subsequent tubular injury (interstitial nephritis) is the result of hematogenous or urogenous dissem-ination (pyelonephritis) of infectious agents.[1,18] Acute tubular necrosis may be severe enough to result in acute kidney failure or with time and sustained injury lead to chronic kidney disease.[3] Histologically, tubulointerstitial diseases are characterized by vari-able degrees of tubular degeneration, atrophy, interstitial inflammation, edema, and fibrosis.[1] Clinically, diseases affecting the tubulointerstitium can be identified by azotemia, a decrease in urine concentration (ie, isosthenuria), and an inability to prop-erly process electrolytes or maintain acid-base hemostasis.[1,3]

Numerous nephrotoxins originating from plants, medications, or heavy metals have been implicated as causative etiologies for tubular necrosis in equines.[19] Ingestion of oak (*Quercus* spp.) flowers, leaf buds, or acorns with toxic gallotannins results in tubular necrosis and characteristic intratubular hemorrhagic casts.[19–21]

Clinicopathologic abnormalities are typical of tubular injury as stated previously. Oxalate-containing plants have been reported in other species to cause precipitation of calcium oxalate crystals in tubular lumina and tubular necrosis; however, horses appear to be resistant to tubular injury.[3,19,22,23] Diagnosis of oxalate nephrosis is supported by the presence of calcium oxalate crystalluria. Red maple (*Acer rubrum*) leaves if ingested will cause hemolysis, pigmentary nephrosis, and ischemic tubular necrosis.[19] Toxicants in red maple are metabolized by ileal microbes into pyrogallol, an oxidizing agent that is responsible for methoglobinemia and hemolysis.[24] Evidence of oxidative damage to erythrocytes should be evident on complete blood count in addition to biochemical derangements of acute kidney disease.

Several antimicrobials and vitamins have the potential to be nephrotoxic with associated tubular injury in equines. Tubular degeneration and necrosis culminating in acute renal failure can occur with aminoglycosides, sulfonamides, oxytetracylines, and amphotericin B.[1,19] The toxic potential of aminoglycosides, like other medications, is potentiated by other factors, such as concurrent nephrotoxic therapy, hypovolemia, or dehydration.[19] The aminoglycoside with intermediate nephrotoxicity, gentamicin, is concentrated in proximal tubules, which leads to loss of brush border integrity and cell viability in horses.[25] Gamma-glutamyl transferase, a leakage enzyme in tubular epithelial cells, can be elevated in the urine early in the course of disease.[19,25] In addition, imidocarb dipropionate and menadione sodium bisulfite (vitamin K_3) have been documented to produce tubular necrosis in horses.[19] Overzealous supplementation with vitamin D will result in dystrophic mineralization of the soft tissues, such as the kidney, tendons, ligaments, heart, and vasculature.[19]

Ingestion of inorganic mercury or arsenic can result in acute tubular necrosis in the horse.[19] Mercury is concentrated in proximal tubules, binding with metallothionein in the endoplasmic reticulum and slowly released over weeks.[19,26] Arsenic primarily affects the gastrointestinal tract, but will cause acute tubular necrosis in horses.[19,27,28] Definitive diagnosis of either metal can be made with toxicologic evaluation of metal concentrations in urine or kidney tissue.[19,27] Rarely, cadmium has been reported in horses to cause nephrocalcinosis and chronic renal failure.[19,27]

Myoglobulinuria and hemoglobinuria, a consequence of myonecrosis and hemolysis, respectively, can cause acute tubular necrosis due to the release and filtration of heme proteins.[29,30] Mechanisms of injury by heme proteins are attributable to renal ischemia via vasoconstriction, tubular stasis via obstructive casts, and direct cytotoxicity by ischemic and oxidative damage.[29,30] Differentials for myonecrosis in horses include infectious (*Clostridia* spp and *S. equi*), nutritional (vitamin E/selenium deficiency), toxic plants and drugs (eg, ionophores), genetic (polysaccharide storage myopathy), and exertional rhabdomyolysis.[31] Intravascular hemolysis with subsequent hemoglobinuria is caused by infectious agents (eg, equine infectious anemia, piroplasmosis, or ehrlichiosis), toxic plants (eg, red maple), and immune-mediated diseases.[29,32]

Macroscopic hematuria and pigmenturia may be obvious when urine is collected, by a red to red-brown discoloration, and confirmed by a positive reagent test. Centrifugation of urine will distinguish between pigmenturia and hematuria; urine will remain discolored with pigmenturia.[29] Red discoloration of serum in conjunction with pigmenturia is supportive of hemolysis, whereas the serum should remain clear in cases of myonecrosis.[29] Hematuria may be the result of numerous upper or lower urinary tract diseases, including glomerulonephritis, pyelonephritis, idiopathic hematuria, cantharidin toxicosis, and neoplasia, to name a few.[29,33–36] Last, renal lipofuscin has been reported as an incidental finding in a horse with diffuse black pigmentation to the renal cortices.[37]

Infectious causes of equine nephritis include viral, bacterial, and parasitic etiologies. Renal tubular necrosis and tubulointerstitial nephritis similar to that seen in human kidney transplant recipients with BK polyomavirus has been reported in horses with confirmed equine polyomavirus infection.[38,39] In domestic animals, leptospirosis is frequently associated with reproductive loss and acute disease, such as septicemia, hepatitis, and nephritis.[1] Leptospirosis in horses, however, is more often subclinical or manifests as chronic disease, such as uveitis and reproductive failure.[3,40–42] Horses are only rarely affected by leptospirosis nephritis.[1,42,43] Morphologic changes consist of tubular degeneration, pigment casts, interstitial edema, and chronically with interstitial fibrosis.[42] *Leptospira interrogans* serovar *pomona* is the most prominent serovar in the US equine population.[42] Tissue culture can be unrewarding, whereas Warthin-Starry histochemical stain of tissues and serology is a reliable diagnostic tool.[42] Septicemia from *Actinobacillus* species in adult horses and foals will disseminate and shower the kidney, resulting in embolic nephritis.[1,44] Emboli histologically consist of multiple cortical abscesses that grossly appear as pinpoint, slightly raised, tan-gray foci.[1] *Actinobacillus equuli* subspecies *equuli* is most commonly encountered with equine septicemia, embolic pneumonia, and nephritis due to Actinobacillosis.[44]

Sporozoan *Klossiella equi* is typically nonpathogenic in horses, but with high parasitic load, tubular degeneration and interstitial nephritis have been reported.[1,45] The life cycle involves glomerular endothelial cells, proximal convoluted tubules, and the loop of Henle before release of sporocysts into the urine.[1] Sporocysts can be identified with sugar flotation of urine in infected horses or by renal histopathology.[1,45,46] Granulomas in multiple organs, including the kidneys, are associated with the rhabditiform nematode *Halicephalobus gingivalis* infection in equids.[29,47–51] The presence of parasites in close proximity to blood vessels and associated inflammation supports the pathogenesis of a hematogenous dissemination to multiple organs, including the kidney, by this parasite in equids.[50] Nematodes can be identified by histologic examination of the kidneys within regions of granulomatous inflammation or free within the urine.[48,50]

Renal Pelvis

Nonsteroidal anti-inflammatory drugs (NSAIDs) are a common therapy to ameliorate pain and inflammation associated with acute and chronic diseases in veterinary medicine. Most NSAIDs are capable of reversibly inhibiting the conversion of arachidonic acid to prostaglandins by cyclooxygenase.[52] Prostaglandins are widely expressed throughout the kidney and affect renal blood flow and glomerular filtration rate primarily by their vasodilatory effects.[52] Inhibition of prostaglandin synthesis has no deleterious consequences in healthy animals. However, horses with concurrent dehydration, hypovolemia, or other conditions that may diminish renal function are at risk for renal medullary ischemia and necrosis if treated with NSAIDs.[19,52] Additionally, NSAIDs are known to have direct toxic effects on renal medullary cells, which may account for the localization of necrosis within the renal papilla.[1,53,54] Phenylbutazone has the greatest nephrotoxicity potential of NSAIDs in the horse in addition to colonic ulceration.[55] Hypoproteinemia and hypoalbuminemia due to enteric loss with azotemia, increased phosphorus, and mild decrease in serum calcium may be present.[19] Inability to concentrate urine is a potential sequela to medullary necrosis from NSAID toxicity.[1] Loss of medullary architecture is evident on ultrasonography, which corresponds grossly with a well-demarcated region of necrosis outlined by a rim of hyperemia or hemorrhage.[1,19]

Pyelonephritis is most frequently attributable to an ascending infection of the lower urinary tract into the renal pelvis, resulting in inflammation and necrosis of the tubulointerstitium.[1] Clinically, horses can present with hematuria and variable clinicopathologic abnormalities indicative of renal disease, such as azotemia, electrolyte imbalance, and inadequate urine concentration.[33,56,57] Urine culture and antimicrobial sensitivity are indicated with hematuria and/or suspected cases of pyelonephritis.[29] Urinary stasis, cystitis, urolithiasis, and other causes of urinary obstruction are all predisposing factors for pyelonephritis.[29] Grossly acute pyelonephritis results in hyperemia and hemorrhage of the papilla that can radiate into the outer medulla and cortex with variable pyelectasia, ulceration, and suppurative exudation.[1] Chronic pyelonephritis can appear as wedge-shaped scars extending from cortex to medulla with irregular pitting and adhesions of the cortex to the renal capsule.[1] Ultrasonography is a helpful diagnostic tool for the diagnosis of pyelonephritis. Typical changes observed with ultrasound include increased parenchymal echogenicity, loss of corticomedullary distinction, pyelectasia, and pelvic debris.[29,33]

Other

Congenital anomalies of the horse kidney include renal dysplasia, hypoplasia, polycystic kidney disease, and horseshoe kidney. Renal dysplasia is the result of abnormal nephrogenesis of one or both kidneys.[1,58,59] Hypoplastic kidneys can be confused with dysplastic kidney based on gross appearance.[1] Dysplastic kidneys are typically small and misshapen with poor corticomedullary distinction.[60] In contrast, renal hypoplasia is defined as a reduction in normal parenchyma.[1,59] Histologically, dysplastic kidneys contain immature glomeruli, primitive mesenchyme and anomalous renal components.[1,60] Chronic kidney disease, azotemia, and electrolyte abnormalities are often the consequence of renal dysplasia, whereas concurrent congenital anomalies are frequently encountered complicating clinical manifestations of urinary disease.[61–64] Congenital polycystic kidney disease (PKD) with no known heritable trait has been reported in horses.[65,66] Grossly, kidneys are often enlarged due to multiple, variably sized fluid-filled cysts throughout the renal parenchyma.[1] Horses with PKD may eventually develop chronic kidney disease with typical clinical symptoms of weight loss, anorexia, depression, and lethargy.[65,66] Horseshoe kidneys are fused at either pole, which occurs during migration and renal development with little to no adverse consequences to renal function.[1,67]

Primary renal neoplasia is rare in horses with an incidence of approximately 0.11% of necropsied horses.[68,69] Renal carcinoma is the most common primary renal neoplasia in horses with reports of renal adenomas, sarcomas, and less frequently transitional and squamous cell carcinomas.[69] Tumors are typically unilateral, originating from either the cranial or caudal pole, and can be well-demarcated expansile masses or diffusely obliterating the normal parenchyma with necrosis and hemorrhage.[69,70] Renal carcinoma tumors are locally aggressive with metastasis to the lung and liver.[71] Clinically, horses present for nonspecific symptoms of weight loss, anorexia, and colic.[71] Clinicopathologic abnormalities are inconsistent among horses with renal carcinoma; however, hematuria is most frequently reported.[71] Renal ultrasound and biopsy are helpful diagnostic tools for a definitive diagnosis of renal neoplasia.[69]

LOWER URINARY TRACT DISEASES

Horses with congenital anomalies of the lower urinary tract frequently present with variable weight loss, depression, dysuria, hematuria, and mild colic.[59] The most common congenital anomaly in horses is ectopic ureters, with greater prevalence in females than males.[72] Ectopia is the result of abnormal embryologic development of the metanephric bud with termination of either unilateral or bilateral ureters caudal to the bladder.[59,72,73] Urinary incontinence from a young age is the most consistent clinical presentation, with variable incidence of urinary tract infections, hydronephrosis, or functional impairment of the kidneys.[59,72,74] Diagnosis can be made by cystoscopy, ultrasound, or excretory urography.[59,75–78]

Uroliths are composed mostly of inorganic crystalloid components with a smaller proportion of organic matrix.[79] In horses, the crystalloid component is most commonly calcium carbonate with a mucoprotein organic matrix.[79–81] Urolithiasis is more prevalent in male horses.[82] Uroliths will cause clinical symptoms in horses if located within the bladder and urethra due to urine outflow obstruction.[82,83] Clinical symptoms can include dysuria, tenesmus, and colic.[80,82,84] Clinicopathologic abnormalities include proteinuria, microscopic hematuria, and pyuria on urinalysis, with biochemical evidence of renal dysfunction.[80,82,84,85]

Bacterial or idiopathic cystitis is rare in horses.[29] Urolithiasis, neoplasia, or other causes of urine retention will predispose some horses to cystitis.[19,29,69] Ingestion of cyanogenic grasses of the *Sorghum* species will cause axonal degeneration and demyelination of lumbar and sacral nerve fibers with possible urinary bladder atony, urine retention, and secondary cystitis.[19,86,87]

Squamous cell carcinoma is the most frequently encountered neoplasm of the urinary bladder in horses, with reports of lymphosarcoma, transitional cell carcinoma, and fibromatous polyps.[69,88–90] Clinical presentation of horses with bladder neoplasia includes pollakiuria and hematuria similar to that seen in cases of urolithiasis.[89,90] Cystitis and pyelonephritis are reported sequelae of bladder neoplasia.[89] Diagnosis can be made by rectal palpation, ultrasound, or cystoscopy with biopsy.[69]

SUMMARY

Diseases of the urinary system in horses are uncommon. However, infectious, immune-mediated, developmental, toxic, and neoplastic etiologies are capable of affecting the equine urinary tract. Early in renal disease, glomerular and tubulointerstitial diseases may be differentiated. In general, moderate to marked loss of protein through the glomerulus occurs with glomerular diseases versus retention of metabolic waste by-products and loss of urine concentration, which predominates in tubulointerstitial diseases. However, there is typically overlap in these disease processes with progression, and therefore a definitive distinction between the 2 entities based on clinicopathologic derangements can be difficult. Clinical presentation, in conjunction with baseline clinicopathologic diagnostics, can guide the practitioner in localizing urinary tract diseases. Additional diagnostics are often warranted, such as renal biopsy or imaging, in addition to ancillary molecular, serologic, and microbiologic assays.

ACKNOWLEDGMENTS

The author acknowledges Dr Jessica Quimby for her time and consideration in reviewing this article.

REFERENCES

1. Maxie M, Newman S. Urinary system. In: Maxie M, editor. Pathology of domestic animals, vol. 2, 5th edition. Philadelphia: Elsevier Saunders; 2007. p. 425–522.
2. van Biervliet J, Divers T, Porter B, et al. Glomerulonephritis in horses. Compend Contin Educ Vet 2002;24:892–902.

3. Schott HC. Chronic renal failure in horses. Vet Clin North Am Equine Pract 2007; 23:593–612.

4. Osborne CA, Hammer RF, Stevens JB, et al. The glomerulus in health and disease: a comparative review of domestic animals and man. Adv Vet Sci Comp Med 1977;21:207–85.

5. Slauson DO, Lewis RM. Comparative pathology of glomerulonephritis in animals. Vet Pathol 1979;16:135–64.

6. Banks KL, Henson JB, McGuire TC. Immunologically mediated glomerulitis of horses. I. Pathogenesis in persistent infection by equine infectious anemia virus. Lab Invest 1972;26:701–7.

7. Banks KL, Henson JB. Immunologically mediated glomerulitis of horses. II. Antiglomerular basement membrane antibody and other mechanisms in spontaneous disease. Lab Invest 1972;26:708–15.

8. Sabnis SG, Gunson DE, Antonovych TT. Some unusual features of mesangioproliferative glomerulonephritis in horses. Vet Pathol 1984;21:574–81.

9. Roberts MC, Kelly WR. Renal dysfunction in a case of purpura haemorrhagica in a horse. Vet Rec 1982;110:144–6.

10. Divers TJ, Timoney JF, Lewis RM, et al. Equine glomerulonephritis and renal failure associated with complexes of group-C streptococcal antigen and IgG antibody. Vet Immunol Immunopathol 1992;32:93–102.

11. Mcsloy A, Poulsen K, Fisher PJ, et al. Diagnosis and treatment of a selective immunoglobulin M glomerulonephropathy in a quarter horse gelding. J Vet Intern Med 2007;21:874–7.

12. Wilkinson JE, Smith CA, Castleman WL, et al. Fibrillary deposits in glomerulonephritis in a horse. Vet Pathol 1985;22:647–9.

13. Linke RP, Geisel O, Mann K. Equine cutaneous amyloidosis derived from an immunoglobulin lambda-light chain. Immunohistochemical, immunochemical and chemical results. Biol Chem Hoppe Seyler 1991;372:835–43.

14. Jakob W. Spontaneous amyloidosis of mammals. Vet Pathol 1971;8:292–306.

15. Savage CJ. Urinary clinical pathologic findings and glomerular filtration rate in the horse. Vet Clin North Am Equine Pract 2008;24:387–404.

16. Mills PC, Auer DE, Kramer H, et al. Effects of inflammation-associated acute-phase response on hepatic and renal indices in the horse. Aust Vet J 1998;76:187–94.

17. Tyner GA, Nolen-Walston RD, Hall T, et al. A multicenter retrospective study of 151 renal biopsies in horses. J Vet Intern Med 2011;25:532–9.

18. Geor RJ. Acute renal failure in horses. Vet Clin North Am Equine Pract 2007;23: 577–91.

19. Schmitz DG. Toxins affecting the urinary system. Vet Clin North Am Equine Pract 2007;23:677–90.

20. Smith S, Naylor RJ, Knowles EJ, et al. Suspected acorn toxicity in nine horses. Equine Vet J 2014. [Epub ahead of print].

21. Anderson GA, Mount ME, Vrins AA, et al. Fatal acorn poisoning in a horse: pathologic findings and diagnostic considerations. J Am Vet Med Assoc 1983;182: 1105–10.

22. Walthall JC, McKenzie RA. Osteodystrophia fibrosa in horses at pasture in Queensland: field and laboratory observations. Aust Vet J 1976;52:11–6.

23. Collier M, Brown C, Stick J. Renal disease and oxalosis in horses. Mod Vet Pract 1985;66:641–4, 735–739.

24. Agrawal K, Ebel JG, Altier C, et al. Identification of protoxins and a microbial basis for red maple (*Acer rubrum*) toxicosis in equines. J Vet Diagn Invest 2013;25: 112–9.

25. van der Harst MR, Bull S, Laffont CM, et al. Gentamicin nephrotoxicity—a comparison of in vitro findings with in vivo experiments in equines. Vet Res Commun 2005;29:247–61.
26. Schuh JC, Ross C, Meschter C. Concurrent mercuric blister and dimethyl sulphoxide (DMSO) application as a cause of mercury toxicity in two horses. Equine Vet J 1988;20:68–71.
27. Casteel SW. Metal toxicosis in horses. Vet Clin North Am Equine Pract 2001;17: 517–27.
28. Pace LW, Turnquist SE, Casteel SW, et al. Acute arsenic toxicosis in five horses. Vet Pathol 1997;34:160–4.
29. Schumacher J. Hematuria and pigmenturia of horses. Vet Clin North Am Equine Pract 2007;23:655–75.
30. Zager RA. Rhabdomyolysis and myohemoglobinuric acute renal failure. Kidney Int 1996;49:314–26.
31. Quist EM, Dougherty JJ, Chaffin MK, et al. Equine rhabdomyolysis. Vet Pathol 2011;48:E52–8.
32. Morris D. Review of anemia in horses, part II: pathophysiologic mechanisms, specific diseases and treatment. Equine Pract 1989;2:34–46.
33. Kisthardt KK, Schumacher J, Finn-Bodner ST, et al. Severe renal hemorrhage caused by pyelonephritis in 7 horses: clinical and ultrasonographic evaluation. Can Vet J 1999;40:571–6.
34. Schumacher J, Varner DD, Schmitz DG, et al. Urethral defects in geldings with hematuria and stallions with hemospermia. Vet Surg 1995;24:250–4.
35. Schott HC, Hines MT. Severe urinary tract hemorrhage in two horses. J Am Vet Med Assoc 1994;204:1320.
36. Helman RG, Edwards WC. Clinical features of blister beetle poisoning in equids: 70 cases (1983–1996). J Am Vet Med Assoc 1997;211:1018–21.
37. Marcato PS, Simoni P. Pigmentation of renal cortical tubules in horses. Vet Pathol 1982;19:572–3.
38. Bohl DL, Brennan DC. BK virus nephropathy and kidney transplantation. Clin J Am Soc Nephrol 2007;2(Suppl 1):S36–46.
39. Jennings SH, Wise AG, Nickeleit V, et al. Polyomavirus-associated nephritis in 2 horses. Vet Pathol 2013;50:769–74.
40. Hogan PM, Bernard WV, Kazakevicius PA, et al. Acute renal disease due to *Leptospira interrogans* in a weanling. Equine Vet J 1996;28:331–3.
41. Morter RL, Williams RD, Bolte H, et al. Equine leptospirosis. J Am Vet Med Assoc 1969;155:436–42.
42. Hodgin EC, Miller DA, Lozano F, et al. Leptospira abortion in horses. J Vet Diagn Invest 1989;1:283–7.
43. Divers TJ, Byars TD, Shin SJ. Renal dysfunction associated with infection of *Leptospira interrogans* in a horse. J Am Vet Med Assoc 1992;201:1391–2.
44. Layman QD, Rezabek GB, Ramachandran A, et al. A retrospective study of equine actinobacillosis cases: 1999–2011. J Vet Diagn Invest 2014;26:365–75.
45. Ballweber LR, Dailey D, Landolt G. *Klossiella equi* infection in an immunosuppressed horse: evidence of long-term infection. Case Rep Vet Med 2012;2012:1–4.
46. Reppas GP, Collins GH. *Klossiella equi* infection in horses; sporocyst stage identified in urine. Aust Vet J 1995;72:316–8.
47. Ruggles AJ, Beech J, Gillette DM, et al. Disseminated *Halicephalobus deletrix* infection in a horse. J Am Vet Med Assoc 1993;203:550–2.
48. Kinde H, Mathews M, Ash L, et al. *Halicephalobus gingivalis* (*H. deletrix*) infection in two horses in southern California. J Vet Diagn Invest 2000;12:162–5.

49. Isaza R, Schiller CA, Stover J, et al. *Halicephalobus gingivalis* (Nematoda) infection in a Grevy's zebra (*Equus grevyi*). J Zoo Wildl Med 2000;31:77–81.

50. Henneke C, Jespersen A, Jacobsen S, et al. The distribution pattern of *Halicephalobus gingivalis* in a horse is suggestive of a haematogenous spread of the nematode. Acta Vet Scand 2014;56:56.

51. Akagami M, Shibahara T, Yoshiga T, et al. Granulomatous nephritis and meningoencephalomyelitis caused by *Halicephalobus gingivalis* in a pony gelding. J Vet Med Sci 2007;69:1187–90.

52. Black HE. Renal toxicity of non-steroidal anti-inflammatory drugs. Toxicol Pathol 1986;14:83–90.

53. Rocha GM, Michea LF, Peters EM, et al. Direct toxicity of nonsteroidal antiinflammatory drugs for renal medullary cells. Proc Natl Acad Sci U S A 2001;98: 5317–22.

54. Khan KN, Venturini CM, Bunch RT, et al. Interspecies differences in renal localization of cyclooxygenase isoforms: implications in nonsteroidal antiinflammatory drug-related nephrotoxicity. Toxicol Pathol 1998;26:612–20.

55. MacAllister CG, Morgan SJ, Borne AT, et al. Comparison of adverse effects of phenylbutazone, flunixin meglumine, and ketoprofen in horses. J Am Vet Med Assoc 1993;202:71–7.

56. Held JP, Wright B, Henton JE. Pyelonephritis associated with renal failure in a horse. J Am Vet Med Assoc 1986;189:688–9.

57. Hamlen H. Pyelonephritis in a mature gelding with an unusual urinary bladder foreign body: a case report. J Equine Vet Sci 1993;13:4.

58. Zicker SC, Marty GD, Carlson GP, et al. Bilateral renal dysplasia with nephron hypoplasia in a foal. J Am Vet Med Assoc 1990;196:2001–5.

59. Chaney KP. Congenital anomalies of the equine urinary tract. Vet Clin North Am Equine Pract 2007;23:691–6.

60. Anderson WI, Picut CA, King JM, et al. Renal dysplasia in a standardbred colt. Vet Pathol 1988;25:179–80.

61. Gull T, Schmitz DG, Bahr A, et al. Renal hypoplasia and dysplasia in an American miniature foal. Vet Rec 2001;149:199–203.

62. Ronen N, van Amstel SR, Nesbit JW, et al. Renal dysplasia in two adult horses: clinical and pathological aspects. Vet Rec 1993;132:269–70.

63. Jones SL, Langer DL, Sterner-Kock A, et al. Renal dysplasia and benign ureteropelvic polyps associated with hydronephrosis in a foal. J Am Vet Med Assoc 1994;204:1230–4.

64. Brown CM, Parks AH, Mullaney TP, et al. Bilateral renal dysplasia and hypoplasia in a foal with an imperforate anus. Vet Rec 1988;122:91–2.

65. Aguilera-Tejero E, Estepa JC, López I, et al. Polycystic kidneys as a cause of chronic renal failure and secondary hypoparathyroidism in a horse. Equine Vet J 2000;32:167–9.

66. Rhind S, Keen J. Polycystic kidney disease in a mature horse: report and review of previously reported cases. Equine Vet Educ 2004;16:178–83.

67. Shojaei B, Kheirandish R, Azizi S. Morphological observation of a horseshoe (fused) kidney and its vascular pattern in a horse. Anat Histol Embryol 2012;41:388–91.

68. Haschek WM, King JM, Tennant BC. Primary renal cell carcinoma in two horses. J Am Vet Med Assoc 1981;179:992–4.

69. Traub-Dargatz J. Urinary tract neoplasia. Vet Clin North Am Equine Pract 1998; 14:495–504.

70. Brown PJ, Holt PE. Primary renal cell carcinoma in four horses. Equine Vet J 1985; 17:473–7.

71. Wise LN, Bryan JN, Sellon DC, et al. A retrospective analysis of renal carcinoma in the horse. J Vet Intern Med 2009;23:913–8.
72. Pringle JK, Ducharme NG, Baird JD. Ectopic ureter in the horse: three cases and a review of the literature. Can Vet J 1990;31:26–30.
73. Owen RR. Canine ureteral ectopia—a review. 1. Embryology and aetiology. J Small Anim Pract 1973;14:407–17.
74. Houlton JE, Wright IM, Matic S, et al. University incontinence in a shire foal due to ureteral ectopia. Equine Vet J 1987;19:244–7.
75. MacAllister CG, Perdue BD. Endoscopic diagnosis of unilateral ectopic ureter in a yearling filly. J Am Vet Med Assoc 1990;197:617–8.
76. Blikslager A, Green E, MacFadden K, et al. Excretory urography and ultrasonography in the diagnosis of bilateral ectopic ureters in a foal. Vet Radiol Ultrasound 1992;33:41–7.
77. Coleman M, Chaffin M, Arnold C, et al. The use of computed tomography in the diagnosis of an ectopic ureter in a Quarter horse filly. Equine Vet Educ 2011;23: 597–602.
78. Tomlinson JE, Farnsworth K, Sage AM, et al. Percutaneous ultrasound-guided pyelography aided diagnosis of ectopic ureter and hydronephrosis in a 3-week-old filly. Vet Radiol Ultrasound 2001;42(4):349–51.
79. Osborne CA, Clinton CW. Urolithiasis. Terms and concepts. Vet Clin North Am Small Anim Pract 1986;16:3–17.
80. Duesterdieck-Zellmer KF. Equine urolithiasis. Vet Clin North Am Equine Pract 2007;23:613–29.
81. Diaz-Espineira M, Escolar E, Bellanato J, et al. Structure and composition of equine uroliths. J Equine Vet Sci 1995;15:27–34.
82. Laverty S, Pascoe JR, Ling GV, et al. Urolithiasis in 68 horses. Vet Surg 1992;21: 56–62.
83. Holt PE, Mair TS. Ten cases of bladder paralysis associated with sabulous urolithiasis in horses. Vet Rec 1990;127:108–10.
84. Laing JA, Raisis AL, Rawlinson RJ, et al. Chronic renal failure and urolithiasis in a 2-year-old colt. Aust Vet J 1992;69:199–200.
85. Ehnen SJ, Divers TJ, Gillette D, et al. Obstructive nephrolithiasis and ureterolithiasis associated with chronic renal failure in horses: eight cases (1981–1987). J Am Vet Med Assoc 1990;197:249–53.
86. Cheeke PR. Endogenous toxins and mycotoxins in forage grasses and their effects on livestock. J Anim Sci 1995;73:909–18.
87. Knight PR. Equine cystitis and ataxia associated with grazing of pastures dominated by sorghum species. Aust Vet J 1968;44:257.
88. Patterson-Kane JC, Tramontin RR, Giles RC, et al. Transitional cell carcinoma of the urinary bladder in a thoroughbred, with intra-abdominal dissemination. Vet Pathol 2000;37:692–5.
89. Fischer AT, Spier S, Carlson GP, et al. Neoplasia of the equine urinary bladder as a cause of hematuria. J Am Vet Med Assoc 1985;186:1294–6.
90. Sweeney RW, Hamir AN, Fisher RR. Lymphosarcoma with urinary bladder infiltration in a horse. J Am Vet Med Assoc 1991;199:1177–8.

Reproductive Disorders in Horses

Timothy A. Snider, DVM, PhD

KEYWORDS

- Horse • Theriogenology • Reproduction • Male • Female • Ovary • Testicle
- Abortion

KEY POINTS

- Reproductive disease is relatively common in the horse, resulting in a variable, yet significant, economic impact on individual horsemen as well as the entire industry.
- Diverse expertise from the veterinary community ensures and improves individual and population health of the horse.
- Communication between veterinarian, diagnostic pathologist, and owner provides best environment to provide accurate diagnoses.

INTRODUCTION

Reproductive disorders are common in the horse and can represent a significant proportion of the caseload to the equine practitioner. The diagnostic approach to reproductive disorders of the horse could be quite variable, inclusive of physical examination, ultrasonography,[1] rectal palpation, clinical endocrinology,[2] molecular genetics,[3] cytogenetics,[4] surgical pathology, and necropsy, among many approaches. Owing to the scope and title of this article, it focuses on pathology and diagnostic approaches to equine reproductive disorders. This focus necessitates exclusion of comprehensive or incidental coverage of other important aspects of equine reproduction, including mammary pathology.

The construction of this review is further limited, by pragmatism and principle, largely to discussions of reproductive disorders described from gross observations. Histopathologic techniques, although important and usually more specific and refining of morphologic observations, are not commonly pursued in intact equine breeding animals, with the necessary exception of the endometrial biopsy discussed later. Therefore, this review focuses more heavily on gross lesions and salient gross observations.

This review is divided into 2 main parts beginning with consideration of pathology and diagnostics of the female horse with reproductive disorders and ending with consideration of pathology and diagnostics of the male horse with reproductive

Department of Pathobiology, 250 McElroy Hall, Oklahoma State University, Stillwater, OK 74078, USA
E-mail address: tim.snider@okstate.edu

Vet Clin Equine 31 (2015) 389–405
http://dx.doi.org/10.1016/j.cveq.2015.04.011
0749-0739/15/$ – see front matter © 2015 Elsevier Inc. All rights reserved.

disorders. Intersex conditions are important in the horse, occurring with modest frequency, and have been recently reviewed.[5]

REPRODUCTIVE DISORDERS OF THE FEMALE
ABORTION AND STILLBIRTH

Abortion and stillbirth conditions cause significant economic impact on individual equine enthusiasts and the industry as a whole. Although the causes of equine abortion range from the toxic to the infectious, practical epidemiology and other realities limit the scope of discussion to the infectious causes, with 1 exception, the mare reproductive loss syndrome (MRLS), covered last. The delineation between an abortion and a stillbirth is often arbitrary and does not significantly alter the following discussion. However, a stillbirth is generally distinguished from an abortion in that the stillborn equine fetus is born dead in a late term time frame where it otherwise could have been expected to live.

Equine Arteritis Virus

Equine arteritis virus, an RNA virus in the *Arterivirus* genus, is an important cause of reproductive loss in horses. There can be remarkable strain differences in virulence, and acute infection of adult horses ranges from very mild signs to severe fevers and manifestations of edema.[6] The virus can be transmitted via respiratory secretions between horses having close contact. Importantly, stallions, usually carriers of the virus, can transmit the virus to susceptible mares via breeding.[6]

Infection of the pregnant mare with equine arteritis virus usually results in abortion or stillbirth, usually a few weeks after the acute febrile episode. Fetal lesions are usually nonexistent or very nonspecific. Term foals born alive often die within a few days and display widespread histologic inflammatory lesions, often focusing on vessels.[6,7]

Diagnosing equine arteritis can be accomplished by virus isolation and/or polymerase chain reaction (PCR) from nasopharyngeal or conjunctival swabs or from semen. Serologic tests are also available, and immunohistochemical staining techniques can be used on histologic specimens.[6,7]

Equine Herpesvirus 1

Equine herpesvirus 1 (EHV-1) is a DNA virus causing 3 presentations of equine illness. Abortion is a major presentation and is thus included here, but EHV-1 also causes a mild, transient upper respiratory tract infection and a severe, sporadic equine herpes myeloencephalopathy.[7]

EHV-1 is contagious, and transmission is readily completed via respiratory pathway. It is thought that most horses are affected before they are yearlings, and the virus can enter a period and locale of latency. Immunity to the virus is usually considered fairly low, and immunization regimens are recommended for pregnant mares.[7]

EHV-1 abortion is almost always a third trimester abortion, and yet the infectious event and timing is often not known, either ranging from recrudescence of a latent infection or mare exposure to another infected horse on the premises. Also, the incubation period could range from days to months, yet infection of mares before the fifth month of gestation usually does not incite abortion.[7,8]

The virus infects the vasculature of the placenta, and expelled fetuses exhibit an array of changes ranging from quite modest to more-specific changes. Fetuses are usually edematous and have some meconium staining. There may be variable to significant multifocal necrosis of the lungs and the liver. Within the liver, these foci may be grossly detectable as disseminated white foci (**Fig. 1**). Lungs may display significant

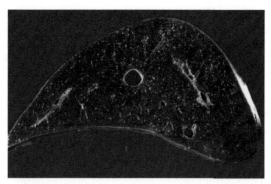

Fig. 1. Cross section of equine fetal liver. Note disseminated white foci of necrosis on section; EHV-1 abortion. (*Courtesy of* Oklahoma State CVHS Pathobiology Teaching File, Stillwater, OK; with permission.)

pulmonary edema. Diagnostic considerations range from the intranuclear inclusion bodies detected by pathologists to fluorescent antibody and PCR testing on placenta or fetal tissues.[7,8]

Nocardioform

The nocardioform equine abortions are less common but notable for some unique features of disease and gross lesions. The etiologic agent is any of several actinomycetes (gram-positive filamentous bacteria) with *Crossiella equi* being frequently mentioned in the literature. This etiologic agent is increasingly detected in equine abortions of central Kentucky. Usually causative of late-term abortions, the placentitis it causes is unique in that it affects the chorionic surface at the cranial uterine body, distant from the cervical star. The fetus is not infected.[7,9]

Leptospira

Leptospires are a minor cause of equine abortion, but this may be an underdiagnosis explained by lack of specific diagnostic pursuits.[9] No specific trends in involved serovars are apparent, yet confirmed leptospiral equine abortions are reported. This fact emphasizes the importance of fetal and maternal serology in abortion diagnostics. Submissions of fixed kidney may provide the pathologist a suitable sample for diagnostics as well.[7,10–12]

Miscellaneous Bacterial Agents

The following bacterial agents are discussed as miscellaneous, not because of any perceived lack of importance, but because of the generalities of pathogenesis and clinical signs they induce. The bacteria under consideration may frequently cause equine abortion, and they include various β-hemolytic *streptococci, Escherichia coli, Staphylococcus aureus, Klebsiella pneumoniae*, and *Actinobacillus equuli*. Regardless of the agent, these often infect the chorionic surface of the placenta via a patent cervix, but could also be of blood-borne origin. Because of the transcervical pathogenesis of infection, exudative changes are often seen at the placental region adjacent to the internal cervical os, the cervical star. Culture of fresh placenta is indicated, if available.[7]

Miscellaneous Protozoa and Fungi

Additional miscellaneous infectious pathogens are included here for the sake of completeness. Dimorphic fungal agent *Histoplasma capsulatum* can induce second or third trimester abortions.[13] Fungi such as *Aspergillus fumigatus* can opportunistically infect the placenta in a transcervical ascending manner.[14] Finally, *Encephalitozoon cuniculi* is a microsporidian protozoan parasite that can cause equine abortion, resulting in a viscous chorionic exudate and swollen joints of the foal in a single case report. Histology of fixed chorion was diagnostic, and PCR testing was confirmatory.[7,15]

Mare Reproductive Loss Syndrome

MRLS emerged in Kentucky in 2001 and resulted in significant economic impacts to the racing industry of that state. MRLS occurred in adjacent states as well, but the major geographic focus was Kentucky. MRLS led to 3 equine reproductive pathologies—early embryonic death, late-term abortions, and red bag deliveries—but the etiology remained elusive for months while research projects were begun. Eventually, portions of the exoskeleton of the eastern tent caterpillar were circumstantially, and then experimentally, shown to induce the abortion syndrome. Aborted fetuses and conceptuses usually had significant bacterial isolates recovered from them, including *Streptococcus* spp and *Actinobacillus* spp, and fetal bacteremia was thought to significantly contribute to the syndrome.[7,16]

General Considerations

Although the article by Frank and colleagues elsewhere in this issue provides recommendations on field necropsies, specific recommendations germane to abortion investigations are included here. If proximity or courier services permit, the best diagnostic sample to submit for an equine abortion investigation is the entire fetus and accompanying placenta. In most situations, this is not possible. After field necropsy of the equine fetus, a complete battery of tissues should be collected in duplicate, one set collected fresh and the additional set immersion fixed in 10% buffered neutral formalin. Essential organs include lung, spleen, liver, heart, kidney, and brain. Eyelid in formalin is increasingly recommended and often reveals infectious and inflammatory processes. In addition, aspiration of stomach contents should be pursued with contents submitted for bacteriology. Clotted or liquid blood from the heart or great vessel should be collected for fetal serology.[7]

Submission of the placenta greatly increases diagnostic yield because infectious agents can often be more readily recovered.[7] Two practical issues provide limitations on the goal. First, if the mare is foaling under field conditions, the placenta is often not recovered because of ingestion or scavenging. Second, again under field conditions, the placental culture steps may yield an array of contaminating bacteria bearing no significance on the case.

Maternal sera should be submitted simultaneously with the fetus to test maternal sera within a panel of various equine abortifacient infectious agents.[7]

ENDOMETRIAL AND UTERINE PATHOLOGY
Endometrium

Perhaps the most important aspect of equine female reproductive disorders and their associated pathology and diagnostics is a thorough understanding of endometrial pathology, its impact on indices of fertility, and use and interpretation of the endometrial biopsy procedure.

Within the clinical investigation of any mare failing to conceive and carry a foal to term, once the stallion has been evaluated and has successfully passed a breeding soundness examination, attention turns to the mare for evaluation. Much of that attention is placed on the endometrium because it represents the interface of endometrial luminal epithelium and placental trophoblast cells once pregnancy is established.[17,18]

The major pathologic lesion of the endometrium is inflammation, termed endometritis. Gross changes, observed via endoscopy or necropsy, could include hyperemia, edema, and exudates ranging from purulent to mucoid to rarely fibrinous. The changes are characterized more definitively via histopathology after endometrial biopsy, and these changes include various inflammatory infiltrates ranging from purulent to lymphoplasmacytic to rarely granulomatous. A second pathologic lesion, detected by endometrial biopsy, is fibrosis. Fibrosis, the long-term scarring occurring in reparative processes, is irreversible and encircles glands and the branching points, leading to loss of glandular functions. Other histologic lesions encountered frequently include eosinophilic infiltrates, lymphatic cysts, and detection of some infectious agents.[17,18]

Aspects of endometritis and the endometrial biopsy have been thoroughly reviewed recently[17,18] after early work published by Kenney[19,20] along with Doig.[21] Salient procedural and interpretive points are summarized here, but the reader is directed to the primary literature and recent reviews for more comprehensive coverage.

Clinical indications for the endometrial biopsy include barren mares or repeat breeders, mares in which genital tract pathology is palpable, mares enrolled in embryo transfer programs or research projects in which offspring are critical, unexplained anestrus during breeding seasons, or mares with grossly observed pyometra or mucometra.[18] The procedure is relatively straightforward, but guidance from an experienced mentor is recommended in lieu of this brief summary. The mare is appropriately restrained, sometimes with supplemental chemical sedation as needed; the tail is wrapped and diverted from the external genitalia; and the genitalia are appropriately cleansed. The biopsy instrument (Jackson equine uterine biopsy forcep, Jorgensen Laboratories, Loveland, CO) is advanced with closed jaws within the caudal reproductive tract, traversing the external and internal cervical os, until the closed jaws are near the junction between 1 uterine horn and the uterine body. The operator's other arm, via rectal palpation, guides and brings into close contact the dorsal endometrial surface to the instrument and the jaws are opened and then closed to procure the biopsy.[18] Some evidence indicates that a single biopsy is considered representative of the entirety of the endometrial surface, yet there is additional evidence indicating that additional sites may exhibit milder or more severe changes.

Once procured, biopsy materials are placed into 10% buffered neutral formalin or Bouin solution and forwarded to a veterinary diagnostic laboratory.[18] Tissues are then routinely processed and hematoxylin-eosin–stained slides are prepared for interpretation by a pathologist or theriogenologist.[17,18]

Pathologic observations on the endometrial biopsy are focused on 2 principal changes, inflammation (endometritis) and fibrosis, and a subjective-objective observational rubric can be used to assign the biopsy a grade, eponymously named the Kenney-Doig grading system.[21] In addition to the Kenney-Doig biopsy grade, the pathologist should render a morphologic diagnosis and comment that provides additional context for the case. This additional information might further integrate the history and biopsy observations or might be a record of additional changes that are not scored within the Kenney-Doig rubric.[7,17,18]

The 4 endometrial biopsy grades—1, 2A, 2B, and 3—range from essentially normal tissue or minimal changes (grade 1) to additive, marked endometritis and fibrosis (grade 3).[17,18,21] The comprehensive assessment tool is described or comprehensively summarized elsewhere,[17,18,22] but is briefly summarized, along with predictions of likelihood of the mare carrying a foal to term, in **Table 1**. The construction of this grading system and associated percentages is focused not on conception rates,

Table 1
Summary of Kenney-Doig endometrial biopsy grades

Grade	Typical Findings	Foaling Rate Prediction (%)
1	Essentially normal tissue; minimal inflammation or fibrosis sparsely scattered	80–90
2A	Mild, multifocal inflammation; mild fibrosis	50–80
2B	Moderate, scattered inflammation; moderate fibrosis	10–50
3	Severe, irreversible fibrosis; severe inflammation	<10

Mares barren for greater than 2 years increases the grade assigned.
Qualifying lesions are considered additive in nature.

which may be predictably higher, but on rates of carrying the foal to term gestation.[17,18,21]

Other Uterine Pathology

Other equine uterine pathologic conditions, exclusive of abortion and endometritis, are summarized briefly.

Endometrial hyperplasia rarely occurs in the mare and is a more common lesion of the dog.[23] Endometrial maldifferentiation, an emerging observational goal of the biopsy technique, is a research focus of Schoon and colleagues,[24] who describe variants of the condition with various morphologies.

Pyometra is the accumulation of purulent exudate in the uterine lumen; its occurrence in the mare is usually postpartum, and the usual infectious agents are *Streptococcus equi* subspecies *zooepidemicus, E coli, Pasteurella*, and others.[7,25] Hydrometra, the intrauterine accumulation of watery fluid, and mucometra, the intrauterine accumulation of mucinous fluid, are reported in the horse, but uncommonly.[7]

Uterine torsions and uterine prolapses occur with some frequency in the equine species. Circulatory embarrassment and trauma and associated changes are the major pathologic findings of note; usually clinical obstetric emergencies, they are not often the subject of requested diagnostic assistance and are not further discussed.[7] Rupture of the middle uterine artery can occur during a dystocia event. Mares often die of exsanguination and hypovolemic shock. Diagnostic assistance via necropsy is often required to confirm and demonstrate this lesion and diagnosis.[7]

Contagious Equine Metritis

Contagious equine metritis is a venereal disease of horses caused by *Taylorella equigenitalis*, a gram-negative coccobacillus.[7,26] A disease of regulatory importance and a bacterial threat of financial significance to the equine industry, the agent emerged in the 1970s in the United Kingdom and has been detected around the world since. Sporadic reports occur in the United States, with the most recent cases in 2013.[27]

The disease causes temporary infertility in mares, and it can take months to clear the agent. Gross hallmarks of the disease in mares include a mucopurulent discharge in the uterine lumen. The disease can present clinically as a cervicitis; a salpingitis can also occur. Histologically, mild to moderate endometrial inflammation and edema are recognized, persisting for 2 to 3 weeks.[28] Although clinically recovered, mares represent a reservoir of infection, especially with localization of the bacteria within clitoral crypts and fossae. Stallions can also serve as a reservoir of infection and pass it onto susceptible mares, but stallions do not exhibit disease.[7,26,27]

Diagnostic approaches of contagious equine metritis are of regulatory importance on an import and export basis. Bacterial culture is the main diagnostic approach. Because of the regulatory landscape, sampling should be conducted by veterinarians accredited by the US Department of Agriculture and samples should only be submitted to approved laboratories, with state government diagnostic laboratories usually having the capability. The genitalia of mares and stallions is usually swabbed for culture processes, and 3 samples are usually acquired. The swabs require special handling, and it is recommended that the laboratory receive the sample within 48 hours. Serology testing via the complement fixation test is available for mare; it is not available for stallions because they do not demonstrate an immune response. Finally, test breeding of an infected stallion should be done to at least 2 naive mares.[26,27] Infection with *T equigenitalis* can be reliably eliminated with a lengthy antibiotic regimen.[27]

SELECTED PATHOLOGY OF THE OVARY AND OVIDUCT

The practitioner or the pathologist must have an understanding of the range of normal cyclic changes that can occur in the ovary in order to recognize many lesions. Moreover, some ovarian changes are lesions of no clinical significance, yet must be defined and identified to prevent diagnostic confusion leading to inappropriate therapies. Some normal cyclic changes range from maturing and tertiary follicles to corpora hemorrhagica and corpora lutea, as well as ovulation tags.[7]

Paraovarian cysts are lesions of little clinical significance, although their size and position can be diagnostically confusing to the inexperienced ultrasonographer. Derived from mesonephric tubules, they are positioned next to the ovary on the cranial surface (most common) or the caudal surface. These cysts are thin walled and freely movable and are histologically lined by epithelium; they can be seen in mares of any age.[7]

Germinal inclusion cysts are somewhat common in the mare. Also known as fossa cysts, they are initiated at ovulation when small pieces of peritoneum are entrapped in the ovulation fossa. They are seldom clinically significant, but they can occasionally become large enough to interfere with ovulation.[7]

Oviductal pathology is extremely uncommon. Salpingitis is usually an extension of an endometritis and often resolves with the endometritis resolution.[7] Oviductal blockage and concerns about patency are increasingly studied as potential causes of mare infertility.[29]

SELECTED PATHOLOGY OF CERVIX, VAGINA, AND VULVA

There are few notable pathologies of the caudal reproductive tract of the mare. Of those, neoplasia is discussed in the following section. Traumatic lesions of this portion of the tract are worth highlighting and can result from artificial or natural breeding and from parturition, assisted or otherwise. Usually, the diagnosis of these conditions is straightforward via observation. Lesions range from focal hemorrhages to lacerations to secondary infections.[7]

Equine coital exanthema is a venereal disease of horses caused by EHV-3. In mares, after a short incubation period, multiple raised papules of the vaginal and vulvar mucosa and perineal skin can arise (**Fig. 2**). These papules then progress to a vesicular and a pustular stage before ulcerating and eventually healing. The virus is contagious, but the disease is relatively mild and heals within a few weeks.[7,30]

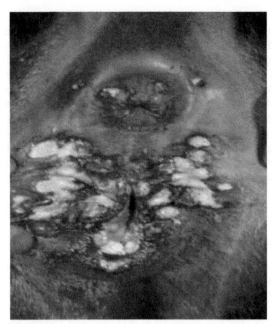

Fig. 2. External genitalia and perineal skin of grade mare. Note multifocal, large, healing depigmented foci of vulva and perineum; EHV-3. (*Courtesy of* Oklahoma State CVHS Pathobiology Teaching File, Stillwater, OK; with permission.)

FEMALE REPRODUCTIVE TRACT NEOPLASIA

Most female horses spend their lives sexually intact, so one might expect that equine female reproductive tract neoplasia occurs with some frequency. However, although numerous tumors are described, their overall occurrence rate is qualitatively low. This brief summation addresses the potential neoplasms from a cranial to caudal anatomic standpoint. Undoubtedly, from a comparative basis, almost any neoplasm reported in other species could affect the equine similarly. For example, mesenchymal neoplasia such as fibromas, leiomyomas (**Fig. 3**), and leiomyosarcomas could be expected

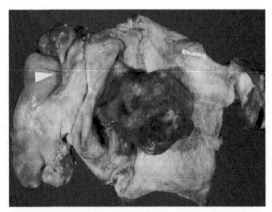

Fig. 3. Uterus of an aged mare. Note intraluminal, red to tan mass arising in the body of the uterus. Smaller pedunculated serosal leiomyoma (*arrowhead*). (*Courtesy of* Oklahoma State CVHS Pathobiology Teaching File, Stillwater, OK; with permission.)

within the cervix, vagina, and vulva, yet they are infrequently reported. Thus, the neoplasms selected for inclusion in this section represent those that occur with some degree of frequency. Before beginning, lymphosarcoma of the horse is well described, and it could be detected in any portion of the equine female tract; hence, it should remain on a list of differential diagnoses.

The granulosa-theca cell tumor is perhaps the most frequently occurring tumor of all tumors included for discussion; it is a gonadal stromal tumor that is usually unilateral and benign. There are defined clinical behavioral syndromes associated with these tumors and their functional products. These syndromes include stallion-like behavior, persistent estrus behavior, and persistent anestrus. These tumors can reach great sizes before being detected.[7]

The granulosa-theca cell tumor is composed of granulosa cells with fewer theca cells. Granulosa cells normally produce and secrete the steroid hormone inhibin, and elevated inhibin concentrations can be detected in tumor-bearing mares. Grossly, the surface of the tumor is usually smooth. On section, these tumors are white to yellow, having solid to cystic foci, and may have regions of hemorrhage and rarely, necrosis (**Fig. 4**). Histologically, they are benign sheets of duplicative granulosa cells, sometimes forming a characteristic rosette known as a Call-Exner body. The contralateral ovary is often atrophic.[7,31]

The dysgerminoma is an ovarian germ cell tumor; it is the female counterpart of the male seminoma.[7] McEntee[32] summarizes the case of 2 mares affected by ovarian dysgerminomas. Both the mares were reported to have hypertrophic osteopathy.

The teratoma is another ovarian germ cell tumor, distinguished from a dysgerminoma in that tissues from multiple germ cell lines are within the tumor. Uniformly, these are incidental neoplasms detected usually in the context of breeding soundness examinations or other routine procedures. Teratomas are usually large, multilobulated, and can be cystic; they are gross and histologic curiosities, having cartilage, respiratory epithelium, hair, sebaceous glands, and other tissues (**Fig. 5**). No age or breed susceptibilities are identified, yet some recent cases were reported in younger mares.[7,33,34]

Primary uterine neoplasia is infrequently reported in mares. An endometrial carcinoma was reported in a mare; it metastasized to lung.[35] Melanomas can affect the perineum and external genitalia of aged gray mares and can extend into the caudal reproductive tract; they are easily grossly detectable as black to gray masses, usually

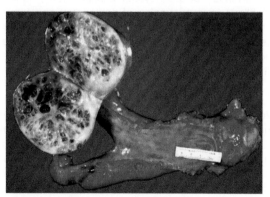

Fig. 4. Uterus and ovary of an aged mare. Granulosa-theca cell tumor. Note smooth surface. On section, the tumor has many cavities and cysts. Tumor is tan to red. (*Courtesy of* Oklahoma State CVHS Pathobiology Teaching File, Stillwater, OK; with permission.)

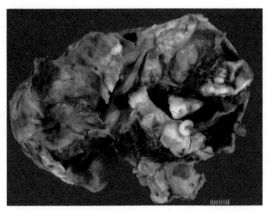

Fig. 5. Ovary of an aged mare. Ovarian teratoma. Note irregular surfaces and tissues. Bone, hair, glandular material, cartilage, and possible rudimentary teeth are visible. (*Courtesy of Oklahoma State CVHS Pathobiology Teaching File, Stillwater, OK; with permission.*)

raised and firm and often spherical. Growth patterns and behavior can be quite variable, and clinical observations are usually most informative. Many such tumors exist for years and only grow very slowly. Some melanomas grow slowly for a period of months and then increase their growth and spread rates remarkably.[7,36] Squamous cell carcinoma can affect the mare's vulva.[7]

REPRODUCTIVE DISORDERS OF THE MALE
Pathology of Scrotum and Tunica Vaginalis

In consideration of pathology of the scrotum and tunica vaginalis of the male horse, there are very few pathologic conditions and diagnostic issues of significance. Yet, the anatomy and terminologies are briefly reviewed and some lesions are described.

The scrotum is sparsely haired, relatively thin perineal skin that is lined by peritoneum and contains the testicles; it provides some functionality to temperature control of the testicles via contraction of the dartos muscle.[37] Some gross developmental anomalies of the scrotum can be seen in intersex conditions. Scrotal edema can be seen in equine viral arteritis[38] or other systemic inflammatory conditions.[37]

The tunica vaginalis is an outpouching of peritoneum and forms a cavity that is continuous with it. Hydrocele is accumulation of fluid within this cavity and can be seen in other edematous conditions, especially ascites.[37] Longstanding hydrocele can be associated with testicular degeneration. Hematocele is the accumulation of blood in this cavity, and it is usually associated with trauma.[37]

Pathology of the Testicle, Epididymis, and Spermatic Cord

Numerous pathologic conditions of the testicle, epididymis, and spermatic cord are documented in the intact equine male. This section begins with anomalies and disorders of growth and ends with inflammatory and circulatory diseases.

Cryptorchidism is defined as incomplete descent of one or both testicles. The embryology and endocrinology are reviewed more comprehensively elsewhere.[39] The equine testicles should completely descend before birth.[37]

Cryptorchidism is usually unilateral, with apparently no convincing trend regarding which side is more commonly affected. However, abdominal retention of the testicle is more commonly left sided, whereas inguinal retention is more common on the right side. Cryptorchid testicles are prone to the development of various testicular neoplasms (see below). A strong basis for heritability of cryptorchidism exists for the equine, but is not proven. Medical and surgical approaches to induce descent of a retained testicle exist, but are questionable and controversial because of the ethical concerns raised.[37,40]

A cryptorchid testicle is usually much smaller than the contralateral testicle; proper descent and location allow normal spermatogenesis to progress based on the temperature differential, and the active testicle is larger. Therefore, histologically, the cryptorchid testicle often shows lack of spermatogenesis, lack of spermatogonia, and a relative or absolute increase in interstitial cells. Diagnostic pathologists may be involved when their opinion is sought on the histologic identity of resected tissues from presumed cryptorchid stallions.[37]

Size differences in the equine testicle are summarized by testicular hypoplasia, testicular atrophy, and testicular hypertrophy. The former 2 are represented grossly by smaller than normal testicles and are difficult to differentiate and reconcile unless much clinical history is available; even then it is difficult. Testicular hypoplasia is seen in cryptorchidism and some intersex conditions. Testicular degeneration, usually recognized in descended testicles, can result from a broad array of potential insults, ranging from aging to vitamin deficiencies to toxins, as well as others. Testicular hypertrophy is the general response of a normal, descended testicle to a pathologic insult or hemicastration of the contralateral testicle. This condition is most recognizable in the boar; it may be recognized in the descended testicle of a cryptorchid stallion, but otherwise should be uncommon as hemicastration of stallions is rarely pursued.[37]

Orchitis and epididymitis are considered together, although they may occur independently. Orchitis, inflammation of the testicle, mainly occurs in the bull and is generally considered rare in males of other domestic species.[37] Although this is likely descriptive of clinical disease, subclinical orchitis is detected via histology in most stallions subjected to complete reproductive tract examinations at termination. The inflammation described is minimal to mild and likely not clinically significant.[41] With minimal or mild orchitis, the initiating stimulus may not be known. More defined instances of orchitis can be attributed to *Salmonella abortus equi*, various hemolytic streptococci, and migrating nematodes including *Strongylus edentatus* and *Halicephalobus gingivalis*. Viral pathogens equine infectious anemia virus and equine arteritis virus may also incite orchitis directly or via vascular insult.[37,38]

Epididymitis, inflammation of the epididymis, is usually infectious or parasitic, and the etiologic differentials, again, include equine arteritis virus[38] and various bacteria and parasitic nematodes mentioned above.[37]

Testicular torsion can occur in cryptorchid testicles in many species but occurs in the context of the descended testicle most notably in the stallion. Torsion occurs on the long axis of the spermatic cord, compressing thin-walled veins and compromising venous return. The result is usually a markedly congested testicle and eventual hemorrhagic infarction. This condition is reported clinically as colic-like pain and often results in complete loss of testicular function and spermatogenesis.[37] Other circulatory or vascular disorders of the testicular cord are related to viral insults such as equine arteritis virus[38] or migrating strongyles.[37]

Selected Pathology of Accessory Sex Glands

The accessory sex glands of the male horse include the bulbourethral glands, seminal vesicles, ampullae, and prostate. Lesions of these glands in the equine species are uncommon,[37] and diagnostic assistance is rarely requested.

Cystic dilation of seminal vesicular ducts can occur in the male horse. Inflammation of the accessory sex glands appears within the literature and textbooks as the most frequent pathologic disorder in the region.[37] Notably, equine arteritis virus causes inflammation of these glands, and the ampullae and bulbourethral glands are sites of predilection for recovery and long-term maintenance of the virus.[38] Seminal vesiculitis and ampullitis is reported in the stallion with recovery in pure culture of either *Pseudomonas aeruginosa* in one case or *Streptococcus equisimilis* in another case.[42]

Pathology of Penis and Prepuce

A survey of pathology of the equine penis and prepuce ranges from developmental to infectious and inflammatory causes. Neoplasia of these structures is discussed below.

Abnormalities of the penis (hypospadias) may occur with some intersex conditions. Traumatic insults have resulted in rupture of the penile corpus cavernosum. The stallion has well-developed penile periurethral veins and with age, these can dilate and become noticeable varices.[37] Trauma can also result in paraphimosis, an inability to retract the penis, in the stallion. Some tumors are also associated with the condition. Penile paralysis has also been described, occurring as a result of a focal neurologic insult, in chronically and severely debilitated stallions,[37,40] or in cases of tranquilization with phenothiazine derivatives.[40,43]

Penile inflammation is termed balanitis; preputial inflammation is termed posthitis. The co-occurrence, often encountered, is termed balanoposthitis. Inflammation of these anatomic structures is almost exclusively because of infectious agents or parasites.[37]

Equine coital exanthema, caused by EHV-3, is a venereal disease of horses. In the stallions, it initiates with large watery vesicles on the body of the penis typically, with foci on the prepuce or glans penis occurring less commonly. Over a period of days, these vesicles progress to yellow pustules and then ulcerate (**Fig. 6**), leaving behind a series of well-circumscribed unpigmented foci. Complete resolution usually requires approximately 3 weeks.[37]

Cutaneous habronemiasis is often associated with balanitis or balanoposthitis. The cause is usually *Habronema* spp, but *Draschia megastoma*, a related nematode, can be incriminated as well. In geographic regions where it is expected, lesions of the male genitalia are initiated by bites and larval deposition by carrier flies. The nematode is not thought to complete its life cycle in this aberrant diversion but instead is thought to incite a severe, localized hypersensitivity reaction to the larvae. These lesions are grossly recognized as nodular swellings, sometimes ulcerated; may hemorrhage; and may be somewhat fibrous depending on maturity (**Fig. 7**). Differential diagnoses include other minor causes of balanitis included below, or also squamous cell carcinoma. It is notable to mention that the literature suggests that the larvae often infect sites of squamous cell carcinoma. Thus, resection with histopathologic analysis is recommended.[37,44]

Rare to uncommon causes of balanitis or posthitis include *H gingivalis*, *Molluscum contagiosum virus*, *Pythium insidiosum*, and *Trypanosoma equiperdum*, the causal agent of dourine, a disease foreign to the United States.[37]

Male Reproductive Tract Neoplasia

Although the exceeding majority of male horses are castrated during young adult years, neoplasia of the male reproductive tract can still be encountered frequently with neoplasms of the external genitalia occurring commonly and neoplasms of the testicle of intact stallions occurring not uncommonly.[37] This section reviews equine male reproductive tract neoplasia from the scrotum and testicles distally to the external genitalia.

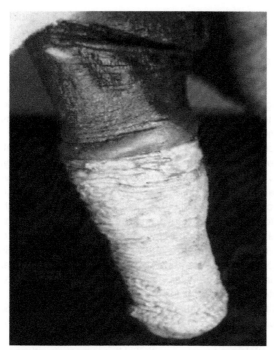

Fig. 6. Penis of a stallion. Note multifocal, circumscribed, slightly raised healing ulcers on the glans and body of the penis; EHV-3. (*Courtesy of* Oklahoma State CVHS Pathobiology Teaching File, Stillwater, OK; with permission.)

As briefly mentioned in the section on female horses, it is emphasized that lymphosarcoma as a multicentric neoplasm can affect the male reproductive tract.

Equine scrotal neoplasia is rare. Occasional single neoplasm reports of equine scrotal neoplasia exist but only serve to highlight that resident tissue components

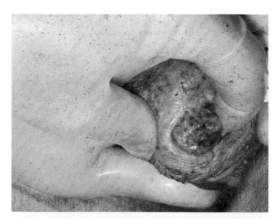

Fig. 7. Penis of a stallion. Note raised, fibrous, hyperemic nodule at the junction of the penile skin and penile urethral mucosa. Eosinophilic and granulomatous reaction to *Habronema* larvae. (*Courtesy of* Oklahoma State CVHS Pathobiology Teaching File, Stillwater, OK; with permission.)

can undergo neoplastic transformation as in other locales. An unpublished report of an equine mesothelioma of the tunica vaginalis is cited in one review.[40]

The seminoma is a germ cell tumor and represents the most common testicular tumor of the aged stallion. Usually unilateral, cryptorchidism is a known risk factor for development. These tumors can become quite large and usually are clinically detected via testicular enlargement and associated pain. On resection via castration, these tumors bulge on section, are white to gray-white, and occasionally are somewhat lobulated (**Fig. 8**). Although these tumors are often benign in most domestic species, they have the most malignant potential in the equine species.[37,45]

The interstitial cell tumor, or Leydig cell tumor, occurs in the horse at a frequency between those of seminomas and the rare Sertoli cell tumor. Again, cryptorchidism is a known risk factor. Following resection by castration, these tumors have efface regional architecture and are composed of slightly bulging lobules of orange to tan-orange, well-delineated parenchyma. Biological behavior of these tumors is usually benign.[37]

Testicular teratoma, sometimes involving the scrotum as well (scrotal teratoma), is uncommon in the horse, but when occurring, is almost exclusively diagnosed in the young horse, and is the most common tumor of the young stallion. This condition often arises in the cryptorchid testicle and is composed of tissues representing multiple germ cell layers, including bone, hair, glandular materials, and the like. Some of these tumors are reported as congenital lesions.[37,45–47]

Rare reports of the Sertoli cell tumor and a teratocarcinoma as testicular neoplasms exist in the horse.[37] Neoplasia of the testicular cord structures as well as accessory sex glands is extremely uncommon in the horse.[37]

Penile and preputial neoplasms of epithelial lineage occur with modest frequency in aged stallions and geldings. The reported tumors are benign squamous papilloma and squamous cell carcinoma. Smegma retention is a reported risk factor underpinning development of these tumors. The malignant squamous cell carcinoma can become invasive quite early in its progression, and early intervention is important. Papillomas and carcinomas can be presumptively distinguished from each other grossly based on discrete margins and minimal ulceration for the benign tumor versus ill-defined margins, scarring, and ulceration seen more commonly in the malignant tumor.[37,45] However, histology of resected lesions is required for definitive diagnosis. Miscellaneous

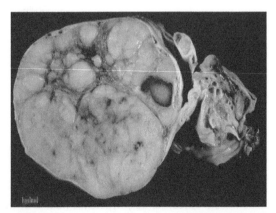

Fig. 8. Testicle of a stallion. Note multilobulated mass expanding and effacing normal testicular parenchyma. Lobules of neoplasia are white to tan. Testicular seminoma. (*Courtesy of* Oklahoma State CVHS Pathobiology Teaching File, Stillwater, OK; with permission.)

penile and preputial tumors reported in the horse include fibroma, sarcoid, melanoma, lipoma, and hemangioma.[48]

REFERENCES

1. Ginther OJ. How ultrasound technologies have expanded and revolutionized research in reproduction in large animals. Theriogenology 2014;81(1):112–25.
2. Ousey JC. Hormone profiles and treatments in the late pregnant mare. Vet Clin North Am Equine Pract 2006;22(3):727–47.
3. Chowdhary BP, Paria N, Raudsepp T. Potential applications of equine genomics in dissecting diseases and fertility. Anim Reprod Sci 2008;107(3–4):208–18.
4. Lear TL, Bailey E. Equine clinical cytogenetics: the past and future. Cytogenet Genome Res 2008;120(1–2):42–9.
5. Lear TL, McGee RB. Disorders of sexual development in the domestic horse, *Equus caballus*. Sex Dev 2012;6(1–3):61–71.
6. Del Piero F. Equine viral arteritis. Vet Pathol 2000;37(4):287–96.
7. Schlafer DH, Miller RB. Female genital system. In: Maxie MG, editor. Pathology of domestic animals, vol. 3, 5th edition. Philadelphia: Elseview; 2007. p. 429–564.
8. Lunn DP, Davis-Poynter N, Flaminio MJ, et al. Equine herpesvirus-1 consensus statement. J Vet Intern Med 2009;23(3):450–61.
9. Donahue JM, Williams NM. Emergent causes of placentitis and abortion. Vet Clin North Am Equine Pract 2000;16(3):443–56, viii.
10. Ellis WA, Bryson DG, O'Brien JJ, et al. Leptospiral infection in aborted equine foetuses. Equine Vet J 1983;15(4):321–4.
11. Ellis WA, O'Brien JJ, Cassells JA, et al. Leptospiral infection in horses in Northern Ireland: serological and microbiological findings. Equine Vet J 1983;15(4):317–20.
12. Pinna AE, Martins G, Hamond C, et al. Molecular diagnostics of leptospirosis in horses is becoming increasingly important. Vet Microbiol 2011;153(3–4):413.
13. Rezabek GB, Donahue JM, Giles RC, et al. Histoplasmosis in horses. J Comp Pathol 1993;109(1):47–55.
14. Monga DP, Tiwari SC, Prasad S. Mycotic abortions in equines. Mykosen 1983; 26(12):612–4.
15. Patterson-Kane JC, Caplazi P, Rurangirwa F, et al. *Encephalitozoon cuniculi placentitis* and abortion in a quarterhorse mare. J Vet Diagn Invest 2003;15(1):57–9.
16. Cohen ND, Carey VJ, Donahue JG, et al. Descriptive epidemiology of late-term abortions associated with the mare reproductive loss syndrome in central Kentucky. J Vet Diagn Invest 2003;15(3):295–7.
17. Schlafer DH. Equine endometrial biopsy: enhancement of clinical value by more extensive histopathology and application of new diagnostic techniques? Theriogenology 2007;68(3):413–22.
18. Snider TA, Sepoy C, Holyoak GR. Equine endometrial biopsy reviewed: observation, interpretation, and application of histopathologic data. Theriogenology 2011; 75(9):1567–81.
19. Kenney RM. Prognostic value of endometrial biopsy of the mare. J Reprod Fertil Suppl 1975;(23):347–8.
20. Kenney RM. Cyclic and pathologic changes of the mare endometrium as detected by biopsy, with a note on early embryonic death. J Am Vet Med Assoc 1978;172(3):241–62.
21. Kenney RM, Doig PA. Equine endometrial biopsy. current therapy in theriogenology 2. Philadelphia: WB Saunders; 1986. p. 723–9.

22. Van Camp SD. Endometrial biopsy of the mare - a review and update. Vet Clin N Am Equine Pract 1988;4(2):229–45.

23. McEntee K. The uterus: atrophic, metaplastic, and proliferative lesions. reproductive pathology of domestic mammals. San Diego (CA): Academic Press; 1990. p. 167–223.

24. Schoon HA, Wiegandt I, Schoon D, et al. Functional disturbances in the endometrium of barren mares: a histological and immunohistochemical study. J Reprod Fertil Suppl 2000;56:381–91.

25. Hughes JP, Stabenfeldt GH, Kindahl H, et al. Pyometra in the mare. J Reprod Fertil Suppl 1979;27:321–9.

26. Timoney PJ. Horse species symposium: contagious equine metritis: an insidious threat to the horse breeding industry in the United States. J Anim Sci 2011;89(5): 1552–60.

27. USDA. Contagious equine metritis. In: APHIS. USDA; 2014.

28. Acland HM, Kenney RM. Lesions of contagious equine metritis in mares. Vet Pathol 1983;20(3):330–41.

29. Arnold CE, Love CC. Laparoscopic evaluation of oviductal patency in the standing mare. Theriogenology 2013;79(6):905–10.

30. Barrandeguy M, Thiry E. Equine coital exanthema and its potential economic implications for the equine industry. Vet J 2012;191(1):35–40.

31. Bailey MT, Troedsson MH, Wheato JE. Inhibin concentrations in mares with granulosa cell tumors. Theriogenology 2002;57(7):1885–95.

32. McEntee K. Ovarian neoplasms. reproductive pathology of domestic mammals. San Diego (CA): Academic Press; 1990. p. 69–93.

33. Catone G, Marino G, Mancuso R, et al. Clinicopathological features of an equine ovarian teratoma. Reprod Domest Anim 2004;39(2):65–9.

34. Lefebvre R, Theoret C, Dore M, et al. Ovarian teratoma and endometritis in a mare. Can Vet J 2005;46(11):1029–33.

35. Gunson DE, Gillette DM, Beech J, et al. Endometrial adenocarcinoma in a mare. Vet Pathol 1980;17(6):776–80.

36. Smith SH, Goldschmidt MH, McManus PM. A comparative review of melanocytic neoplasms. Vet Pathol 2002;39(6):651–78.

37. Foster RA, Ladds PW. Male genital system. In: Maxie MG, editor. Pathology of domestic animals, vol. 3, 5th edition. Philadelphia: Elsevier; 2007. p. 565–620.

38. Holyoak GR, Little TV, McCollam WH, et al. Relationship between onset of puberty and establishment of persistent infection with equine arteritis virus in the experimentally infected colt. J Comp Pathol 1993;109(1):29–46.

39. Amann RP, Veeramachaneni DN. Cryptorchidism in common eutherian mammals. Reproduction 2007;133(3):541–61.

40. Edwards JF. Pathologic conditions of the stallion reproductive tract. Anim Reprod Sci 2008;107(3–4):197–207.

41. Birch SM. Survey of testicular lesions in stallions: veterinary biomedical sciences. Stillwater (OK): Oklahoma State University; 2008.

42. McEntee K. Bulbourethral, vesicular, and prostate glands. reproductive pathology of domestic mammals. San Diego (CA): Academic Press; 1990. p. 333–58.

43. Nie GJ, Pope KC. Persistent penile prolapse associated with acute blood loss and acepromazine maleate administration in a horse. J Am Vet Med Assoc 1997;211(5):587–9.

44. Pugh DG, Hu XP, Blagburn B. Habronemiasis: biology, signs, and diagnosis, and treatment and prevention of the nematodes and vector flies. J Equine Vet Sci 2014;34:241–8.

45. Brinsko SP. Neoplasia of the male reproductive tract. Vet Clin North Am Equine Pract 1998;14(3):517–33.
46. Misdorp W. Congenital tumours and tumour-like lesions in domestic animals. 3. Horses. A review. Vet Q 2003;25(2):61–71.
47. Stick JA. Teratoma and cyst formation of the equine cryptorchid testicle. J Am Vet Med Assoc 1980;176(3):211–4.
48. McEntee K. Penis and prepuce. Reproductive pathology of domestic mammals. San Diego (CA): Academic Press; 1990. p. 359–74.

Musculoskeletal Pathology

Frances J. Peat, BVSc, PGCertSc, Christopher E. Kawcak, DVM, PhD*

KEYWORDS

- Musculoskeletal • Orthopedic • Osteochondrosis • Osteoarthritis • Tendon
- Muscle • Infectious • Laminitis

KEY POINTS

- Juvenile osteochondral conditions (JOCC) in young, growing horses include lesions that occur as a direct result of osteochondrosis, as well as avulsion fractures of ossifying bones and physitis. Conformational deformities are discussed separately.
- It is now recognized that most exercise-induced pathology in the horse are consequences of cumulative microdamage caused by repetitive cyclic loading, rather than a single episode of high-energy trauma.
- Bacterial infection of synovial structures, bone, and soft tissue can have devastating long-term consequences for soundness in the horse and may be life threatening.
- Current knowledge of laminitis indicates that it should be regarded as a clinical syndrome with a variety of possible distinct mechanisms of structural failure, which originate from inflammatory, metabolic, traumatic, and vascular causes.

The current understanding of pathology as it relates to common diseases of the equine musculoskeletal system is reviewed in this article. Diseases have been organized according to the fundamental classifications of developmental, exercise-induced, infectious, and miscellaneous pathology.

DEVELOPMENTAL MUSCULOSKELETAL PATHOLOGY

A variety of specific growth-related musculoskeletal conditions occur in young horses, namely, osteochondral fragmentation, subchondral cystic lesions, physitis, incomplete cuboidal bone ossification, angular limb deformities, and flexural limb deformities. Traditionally, the term developmental orthopedic disease (DOD) has been used to encompasses all these conditions.[1] A new classification of equine JOCC has recently been proposed.[2] This classification encompasses lesions that occur as a direct result of osteochondrosis and also includes avulsion fractures of ossifying bones and physitis (**Fig. 1**).

Equine Orthopaedic Research Center, College of Veterinary Medicine and Biomedical Sciences, Colorado State University, 300 West Drake Rd, Fort Collins, CO 80523, USA
* Corresponding author.
E-mail address: Christopher.Kawcak@colostate.edu

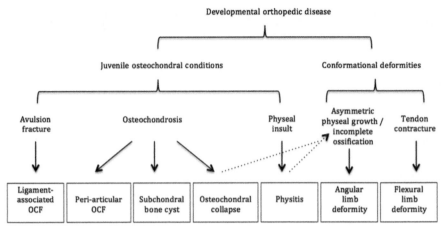

Fig. 1. Classification of developmental musculoskeletal pathology in the horse.

Epidemiology

Juvenile osteochondral conditions

The age range for JOCC is considered to be the first 2 years of life.[2] However, lesions that have developed within this time frame may not become clinically apparent until after a horse commences athletic training. Subchondral bone cysts that manifest clinically within the first 2 years of life are considered to be a result of osteochondrosis.[3] However, subchondral cystic lesions can also develop in older horses as a result of exercise-induced trauma.[4] A large-scale study following up Irish thoroughbred foals up to the age of 18 months found that 11% had some form of DOD that required treatment. In 73% of these foals, the specific condition requiring treatment was either angular limb deformity or physitis.[5] The incidence of physitis peaks between 4 and 8 months of age, but it can occur at any time before closure of the growth plate. In a separate study investigating radiographically evident lesions of osteochondrosis in over 9000 warmblood horses, the overall prevalence of such lesions was 14%.[6]

Conformational deformities

Angular and flexural limb deformities can be present congenitally or can be acquired postnatally. Their prevalence has been shown to decrease from birth to weaning in multiple breeds.[7] Prematurity or dysmaturity often results in angular deformities within the first 2 weeks of life, because of incomplete ossification of the cuboidal bones of the carpus or tarsus, or ligamentous laxity of the supporting periarticular soft tissues. Most angular deformities originate at the level of a distal growth plate, and the deviation is described with reference to the adjacent joint. Rarely, angular deviation can occur as a result of a bend within the metaphysis or diaphysis itself.[8] The most common angular limb deformities in neonates are carpal valgus, tarsal valgus, and fetlock valgus or varus.

Pathophysiology

Osteochondrosis

Osteochondrosis is a multifactorial disease process that involves focal failure of endochondral ossification within the articular epiphyseal growth cartilage or metaphyseal growth cartilage.[9] There is compelling evidence across multiple species of a polygenetic heritable component to the disease.[10] It is often assumed that the hereditary influence is linked to certain anatomic characteristics and a predisposition for higher growth rates. Current scientific evidence does not support a direct correlation with rapid growth rates or overnutrition, or mineral imbalances that have at times been implicated.[11,12]

Endochondral ossification occurs through a sequence of chondrocyte proliferation, extracellular matrix synthesis, cellular hypertrophy, vascular invasion, and matrix mineralization.[10] At the ossification front, there is an abrupt change in biomechanical strength, and the arterioles that traverse this zone are particularly vulnerable to insult.[13,14] In osteochondrosis, biomechanical loading is thought to result in focal microvascular changes that lead to ischemia, retention of cartilage cores, and subsequent chondronecrosis. Mechanical dissection of the lesion results in an osteochondral flap, which may detach and become a free-floating fragment within the joint.[3] Alternatively, continued biomechanical loading on retained chondronecrotic lesions can lead to the development of a juvenile subchondral bone cyst. Variations in biomechanical loading and pressure distribution at different anatomic sites could explain the occurrence of common distinct lesions of osteochondrosis.[2,3] These lesions are identified in **Table 1**.

Physitis

The clinical significance of asymptomatic growth plate enlargement is controversial, and recent research has suggested that there may be physiologic swelling associated with normal bone remodeling.[15] True pathology within an active physis is thought to result from persistent asymmetric loading that disrupts normal endochondral ossification. This condition can lead to asymmetric growth and subsequent angular deformity if not corrected. Common causes of unequally distributed, high-strain loading of physes in foals include excessive exercise combined with laxity of periarticular soft tissue structures, incomplete cuboidal bone ossification, incorrect foot trimming, contralateral limb lameness, and heavy body weight. The most commonly affected physes are those of the distal radius and distal third metacarpus or metatarsus.

Clinical Presentation

JOCC may remain clinically silent. Lesions that do become clinically apparent usually present with sudden-onset joint effusion and varying degrees of lameness because of debris or loose fragments causing synovitis within the joint.[3] Most commonly affected are the femoropatellar, tarsocrural, and metacarpophalangeal joints. Bilateral joint involvement was present in 26% of tarsocrural and 25% of femoropatellar cases in the study of over 9000 Hanoverian warmblood foals.[6] The scapulohumeral joint is less frequently involved. Overt lameness attributable to osteochondritis dissecans (OCD) is most common in the femoropatellar and scapulohumeral joints. Effusion without lameness is more common in OCD of the tarsocrural and metacarpophalangeal joints.[16]

The introduction of presale yearling radiograph systems has resulted in a significant increase in the diagnosis of clinically silent, but radiographically apparent lesions.[17] Prospective data relating to their potential clinical significance in future athletic careers are still needed for many of these minor lesions.

Diagnosis

Lesions of osteochondrosis are most frequently diagnosed via radiography. Ultrasonography can be useful in detecting lesions that only affect cartilage, although arthroscopy is often necessary for definitive diagnosis in such cases. Radiographic findings include the presence of an osteochondral flap or discrete fragment, articular surface irregularity or flattening, or lucencies within the subchondral bone and surrounding

Table 1
Juvenile osteochondral conditions

Type of JOCC	Lesion	Anatomic Region	Common Sites	Type of Biomechanical Overload
Osteochondrosis	Articular surface osteochondral fragment	Prominent articular ridge	Lateral trochlear ridge of the femur Sagittal ridge of metacarpal/tarsal condyle	Compression/shear
Osteochondrosis	Periarticular osteochondral fragment	Articular margin	Distal intermediate ridge of the tibial cochlea Dorsoproximal margin of proximal phalanx	Compression at end ranges of joint motion
Osteochondrosis	Subchondral bone cyst	Heavily loaded (convex) articular surface	Medial femoral condyle Distal aspect of proximal phalanx Metacarpal/tarsal condyle	Compression/shear
Avulsion Fracture	Extra-articular avulsed osteochondral fragment	Epiphyseal entheses	Palmar/plantar eminence of proximal phalanx at attachment of distal and oblique sesamoidean ligaments	Tension
Osteochondral Collapse	Physitis	Physeal cartilage	Distal radius, distal third metacarpus/tarsus	Pressure
Osteochondral Collapse	Deformation	Articular surface	Cuboidal bones of tarsus and carpus, proximal interphalangeal joint of hind limbs, scapulohumeral joint	Pressure

Adapted from Denoix JM, Jeffcott LB, McIlwraith CW, et al. A review of terminology for equine juvenile osteochondral conditions (JOCC) based on anatomical and functional considerations. Vet J 2013;197(1):29–35.

sclerosis.[18] Lesions that are not apparent radiographically are most common in the hock.[19] Radiographic changes of pathologic physitis are variable. The most common finding is paraphyseal bone production, often termed physeal lipping or metaphyseal flaring. Physeal radiolucency or widening is less commonly observed and can be difficult to interpret.

When the clinical presentation involves joint effusion accompanied by lameness, intra-articular anesthesia can be used to confirm the lameness that originates from the effused joint. Acute-onset joint effusion in foals also requires cytologic analysis of synovial fluid to rule out septic arthritis or hemarthrosis as the cause of lameness, which is important irrespective of radiographic findings, because radiographically evident osteochondrotic lesions can be clinically silent. OCD lesions are usually associated with synovial fluid total nucleated cell counts (TNCCs) of less than 1.0×10^9 cells/L.

Treatment

Osteochondrosis

Osteochondrosis is a dynamic process in horses younger than 12 months, and some lesions heal naturally.[20] For example, some tarsocrural lesions have been shown to resolve radiographically in foals aged up to 5 months. In the same study, resolution occurred with some femoropatellar lesions up to the age of 8 months, after which lesions tended to persist.[21] Lesions causing lameness or significant effusion are unlikely to heal without intervention, and in these cases, arthroscopic debridement is indicated.[22] Arthroscopy can be used simultaneously as a method of diagnosis and treatment when radiographic findings are inconclusive. A recent review of surgical versus conservative management of osteochondrosis discusses the topic in full detail.[23]

Surgical removal of palmar or plantar avulsion fragments of the proximal phalanx has been described,[24] but is of questionable necessity. Although previously associated with low-grade, high-speed lameness in racehorses,[25] a recent study showed no effect on the racing performance of standardbred trotters.[26]

Angular limb deformities

Management of angular deformities varies depending on the joint involved and the direction and severity of the deviation. Normal growth-related changes dictate that correct conformation for a skeletally mature horse does not equate to ideal conformation for a foal. A 2° to 5° carpal valgus deviation is normal through to weaning age and self-corrects during a period of rapid growth and chest widening at around 8 to 10 months of age. Conversely, fetlock varus deformities tend to worsen with age up to the age of 6 months.[27] Foals with incomplete cuboidal bone ossification require immediate restriction and splinting to facilitate even loading and increase the likelihood of normal ossification and long-term soundness.

Minor angular deviations are managed conservatively, and correct conformation is achieved via the Hueter-Volkmann law of mechanical modulation of epiphyseal growth.[28] Conservative treatment involves exercise restriction, modification of hoof conformation to minimize compressive forces on the affected physis, and weekly evaluation. Surgical intervention is indicated for deviations in excess of 10° to 15°, under which modeling does not result in self-correction.[29] The most reliable current surgical techniques are aimed at temporary unilateral physeal growth retardation, via transphyseal bridging in the form of staples, screws and wires, plating, or lag or positional screws across one side of physis.[30] Hemicircumferential transection and stripping of the periosteum was commonly used to accelerate growth on the concave aspect of the affected metaphysis but has been shown to be not more effective than stall confinement and hoof trimming alone.[31] With cessation of active physeal growth, the window for correction using the above methods closes. Subsequent correction is difficult and requires a surgical wedge ostectomy or step osteotomy.[32]

Prognosis

Osteochondrosis

The prognosis accompanying lesions of osteochondrosis depends on the extent of cartilage erosion and presence of degenerative changes identified within the joint at the time of arthroscopy.[19] Of the joints affected by OCD, the prognosis is typically least favorable in the shoulder. Subchondral bone cysts are associated with a poorer prognosis because they occur on central weight-bearing areas and surgical treatment is limited.[3]

Angular limb deformities

The prognosis for angular limb deformities depends on the severity of the deviation and subsequent degenerative change because of abnormal loading. Mild carpal valgus deformities have been shown to be protective for carpal injuries in racing thoroughbreds.[33] Conversely, fetlock varus deformities are more problematic and can predispose to lameness if uncorrected before physeal closure. Angular deviation resulting from physeal fracture or cuboidal bone collapse carries a poor prognosis.

EXERCISE-INDUCED MUSCULOSKELETAL PATHOLOGY

Exercise-induced injury to tissues of the musculoskeletal system is one of the most significant causes of pathology in the horse and is responsible for the shortened careers of many horses used in athletic disciplines. It is now recognized that most exercise-related injuries are a consequence of cumulative microdamage caused by repetitive cyclic loading, rather than a single episode of high-energy trauma.

Epidemiology

Bone injuries are common in horses exposed to high-intensity exercise, especially racehorses.[34] Horses working out long distances at high speeds, or that rapidly work out at a high speed within a short period of training, are more likely to develop fatal skeletal injuries than horses exercising at lower intensities.[35]

Soft tissue musculoskeletal injuries also occur most frequently in horses with a high level of cumulative biomechanical loading. The soft tissues of the palmar metacarpus and digits are those most commonly plagued by tendinous and ligamentous injury in the horse. Injury to a forelimb superficial digital flexor tendon reportedly accounts for 6% to 13% of all racing-related injuries.[36] The risk of tendon injury also increases with age.[37]

Muscular pathology that is exercise induced occasionally involves acute high-energy biomechanical trauma, but exertional rhabdomyolysis is more common. The 2 most-studied causes are recurrent exertional rhabdomyolysis (RER), which affects 5% to 10% of thoroughbreds in training, and polysaccharide storage myopathy (PSSM) in quarter horses.[38]

Pathophysiology

Bone

Exercise-induced bone injury occurs when biomechanical loading overwhelms the normal adaptive processes that function to replace pockets of weakened bone and strengthen areas subject to high strain, in accordance with Wolff law.[39] Repetitive cyclic overloading of bone results in focal microdamage, such as trabecular microfractures and focal breaks in the calcified cartilage layer identified in the metacarpal condyle of racehorses.[40] When cellular remodeling is activated to repair areas of weakened bone, osteoclasts exert their effect more rapidly than osteoblasts, resulting in a transient decrease in bone density. The potential exists for fracture propagation within the area of weakened bone if high cyclic loading continues.[41] Studies have identified the presence of such microdamage in sites of spontaneous fracture in racehorses, supporting the hypothesis that these are fatigue failure injuries.[42,43]

Adaptive cortical modeling is commonly seen in the third metacarpus of racehorses as increased dorsal cortical thickness and increased distal subchondral bone density.[44] Trabecular bone adaptation is evidenced by sclerosis within the radial facet of the third carpal bone and the palmar aspect of the metacarpal condyle.[45] Although this adaptive modeling affords increased strength to the areas sustaining high loads, excessive sclerosis alters the elastic deformation properties of the subchondral bone and is thought to result in stiffer, brittle bone that is predisposed to fracture.[46] When horses are rested from training, bone density in areas previously under high strain decreases, predisposing them to fracture on return to work if training is not resumed gradually.[47]

Joints

Osteoarthritis is a disorder of moveable joints characterized by degeneration and loss of articular cartilage.[48] Although previously believed to be the result of cartilage wear and tear, the pathophysiology is likely to involve complex mechanical and biochemical interactions between the synovium, cartilage, subchondral bone, periarticular bone, fibrous joint capsule, and periarticular soft tissue joint stabilizers.[49] Damage to one or more of these joint tissues may have the potential to initiate a perpetuating cycle of degenerative change within the joint as a whole, through release of inflammatory mediators, direct trauma, loss of joint stability, or loss of shock absorption.[48,50]

Synovitis, in particular, is now recognized as a critical feature in the development and progression of osteoarthritis.[49,50] The inflammatory nature of osteoarthritis and the role of soluble inflammatory mediators, such as cytokines and prostaglandins, has increasingly been the subject of osteoarthritis research. The activity of cytokines, such as interleukin-1 and tumor necrosis factor, and synovial macrophages in the presence of synovitis may play an important role in the activation of chondrocyte matrix-metalloproteinase–mediated cartilage degradation and osteophyte formation.[51]

Tendons

Exercise-induced tendon injuries are believed to be preceded by subclinical degeneration, which progressively weakens the resistive strength of the tendon. Repetitive loading during high-speed exercise induces isolated fibrillar microdamage and matrix degeneration. During loading, a greater strain is placed on the central tendon fibers and strain-induced lesions most frequently occur within the tendon core.[52] Proteolytic enzyme activity to remove necrotic collagen results in an increase in size of the lesion within the first 2 weeks postinjury.[53] Fibroblasts then synthesize scar tissue in the form of randomly arranged type III collagen that lacks elasticity. Subsequent remodeling causes conversion to type I collagen over a period of months. Controlled exercise is important during this period to align fibrils with the predominant loading forces, thereby improving the eventual strength of the tendon.

There is evidence to suggest that low- to moderate-intensity exercise induces adaptive hypertrophy within the superficial digital flexor tendon of foals, which may increase its ability to withstand biomechanical loading later in life.[54] In older horses, studies have shown a reduced crimp morphology of central tendon fibers, decreased sliding of tendon fascicles, and altered levels of proteins involved in matrix organization, which may be the result of age-related deterioration or an accumulation of exercise-related damage.

Muscle

Traumatic myopathy results from acute tearing of muscle fibers, often during extreme athletic maneuvers such as sliding stops, or when attempting to rise after a long period of recumbency. Specific reports include rupture of the gastrocnemius and gracilis muscles. Fibrotic myopathy is a separately recognized condition in which fibrosis tends to be chronic and progressive, with low-grade inflammation, muscle fiber atrophy, and replacement with fibrous tissue.[55] The semitendinosus muscle is usually involved, resulting in a characteristic gait with slapping of the foot at the end of a shortened cranial phase of stride.

RER in thoroughbreds is caused by an autosomal dominantly inherited abnormality in myocyte intracellular calcium regulation. PSSMs involve a deficiency of energy within muscle cells because of abnormal glycogen storage. A heritable defect in the glycogen synthase gene (GSY1) is responsible for a substantial proportion of PSSM in some breeds, including quarter horses. RER and PSSM both involve impaired myofilament relaxation, persistent painful contractures, and segmental myonecrosis.[56]

Regardless of the cause, macrophage infiltration occurs within 72 hours of muscle injury and regenerative myotubes form within 3 to 4 days. Within a month of injury, myofilaments are produced and aligned, forming new mature muscle fibers. If myofibers are damaged beyond their regenerative capacity by extensive trauma, prolonged compression, or ischemia, then fibrosis ensues.[56]

Clinical Presentation

The clinical presentation of exercise-induced pathology can range from acute, debilitating injury to insidious low-grade lameness that manifests as poor athletic performance. Pathology involving joints usually presents with effusion and pain on flexion. Injury involving the diaphsyses of long bones or the palmar metacarpal soft tissues presents with pain on palpation and varying degrees of surrounding edema. Muscular pathology manifests with focal, painful swelling, which in the case of exertional rhabdomyolysis may become extremely firm and is accompanied by a stiff gait, shifting lameness, or reluctance to move entirely. Severe myolysis causes sweating, tachypnea, elevated heart rate, coliclike signs, and variable myoglobinuria.

Diagnosis

Exercise-induced pathology is diagnosed by incorporating clinical and historical findings with variable use of diagnostic anesthesia, imaging, and arthroscopy. Increasing use of MRI and computed tomography, in addition to radiography, ultrasonography, and scintigraphy, has enhanced the diagnosis of some injuries, particularly those within the distal part of the limb. Current research into the identification of serum biomarkers suggests that these may become valuable indicators of pathology in the future and allow for detection of subclinical disease.[57–59]

In RER, suggestive clinical signs are associated with significantly elevated serum creatinine kinase (CK) enzyme activity 4 to 6 hours postexercise, indicating cell membrane damage because of myonecrosis.[56] Serum muscle enzyme activity does not always reflect the severity of clinical signs, but serial measurements can be used to determine the progression of injury.[56] Serum aspartate aminotransferase (AST) activity is not specific for myonecrosis and increases more slowly than CK activity. Serum AST activity peaks 12 to 24 hours after a muscle insult and has a half-life of approximately 7 to 8 days, in contrast to the 2-hour half-life of CK.[60] Therefore, elevated AST activity in the presence of normal or reducing CK activity indicates that muscle damage is no longer occurring. The gold standard for diagnosis of PSSMs involves genetic testing of a blood sample for the GYS1 mutation (Type 1 PSSM), followed by a semimembranosus muscle biopsy for histologic evidence of abnormal polysaccharide storage in horses that test negative for the mutation (Type 2 PSSM).

Prognosis

The prognosis for full return to athletic function depends on the severity of tissue damage and the extent to which it disrupts normal function. The presence of pathology is not always associated with a negative outcome.[61] However, the prognosis suffers greatly once disease is advanced, which can be because tissue repair is inherently not possible, as is currently thought to be the case with degradation of articular cartilage; it can also be because exercise conditions were not conducive to repair, as evidenced by the progression of bone stress-related injury to catastrophic fractures, or because the mechanical properties of the repaired tissue are inferior to those of the original. The latter is currently the case with many tendon injuries. Rates of return to racing after injury to the superficial digital flexor tendon currently range from 20% to 60%, with an injury recurrence rate of up to 80%.[62]

Improved prevention and management of exercise-related pathology requires early detection, which can be extremely difficult. Advances in diagnostic imaging and the development of biomarkers show promise in addressing this difficulty. Further research is required to better understand when certain normal adaptive change becomes pathologic.

INFECTIOUS MUSCULOSKELETAL PATHOLOGY

Musculoskeletal tissue can be infected by bacteria, fungi, viruses, and parasites. However, bacteria are by far the most common infectious agents. Bacterial infection of synovial structures, bone, and soft tissue can have devastating long-term consequences for soundness in the horse and may be life threatening.

Epidemiology

Musculoskeletal infection is estimated to cause death in approximately 5% of foals.[63] Neonatal foals with failure of passive transfer of immunity are at high risk of developing synovial and osseous infection. The most common cause of infectious arthritis in this age group is hematogenous spread of bacteria. *Rhodococcus equi* infection may also cause a reactive polysynovitis and does so in approximately 25% of affected foals.[64] In mature horses, traumatic wounds are reportedly responsible for 37% of joint infections and 55% of tendon sheath infections.[65] In the same study, intra-articular injection was responsible for 34% of joint infections and 22% of tendon sheath infections.

Pathophysiology

Synovial structures
Infection of joints, tendon sheaths, and bursae may result from wounds, intrasynovial injections, postoperative complications, hematogenous spread, or idiopathic causes. The most common pathogens in synovial sepsis of mature horses are coagulase-negative staphylococci and *Streptococcus equi* subsp *zooepidemicus*. Specifically, *Staphylococcus aureus* is the most common agent in postoperative and postinjection sepsis and *Escherichia coli* is the most common agent in septic arthritis of foals.[66]

Bone
Osteomyelitis is a process in which an infecting microorganism causes inflammation and destruction of bone.[67] Infection that does not involve bone marrow, such as in the distal phalanx, is termed osteitis. In foals, as with septic arthritis, the bacteria most commonly isolated from hematogenous osteomyelitis and physitis are enteric gram-negative organisms. Osteomyelitis in adult horses can be caused by a mixed infection involving staphylococci, Enterobacteriaceae, and streptococcal species.[68]

Muscle

Infection of skeletal muscles with clostridial species, most often *Clostridium perfringens* or *Clostridium septicum*, causes life-threatening clostridial myonecrosis or gas gangrene. Dormant spores have been detected in normal skeletal muscle, and the inciting cause of their germination may be a change in the muscle milieu via puncture wounds or intramuscular injection.[69] Irritating intramuscular solutions, especially those that have an alkaline pH or lower redox potential within muscle, are implicated.[55] The most commonly associated intramuscular injection is that of flunixin meglumine.[70] Clostridial toxins produce severe tissue necrosis, and animals may be found recumbent with painful muscle swellings or dead. Focal suppurative myositis can be caused by a range of bacteria including *Streptococcus* and *Staphylococcus* sp and, in some geographic regions of the United States, *Corynebacterium pseudotuberculosis*.[55]

Subcutaneous tissue

Cellulitis is an infection of the subcutaneous tissues, which in severe cases involves a deep suppurative process that dissects through soft tissue planes and causes extensive damage. Commonly identified exotoxin-producing cellulitis pathogens are coagulase-positive *Staphylococcus* sp, most commonly *S aureus* and *Staphylococcus intermedius*.[71]

Establishment of infection

Regardless of the tissue involved, bacterial colonization requires adhesion and subsequent permanent attachment of the bacteria to the substrata. Conditions that prevent effective elimination of transient bacterial contamination by host defense mechanisms include an overwhelming level of inoculum relative to the cellularity of the tissue, impaired host defense, trauma to tissue surfaces, or presence of a foreign body.[72] After bacterial colonization, leukocytes and various inflammatory factors contribute to necrosis of the infected tissue. In osteomyelitis, ischemic bone can become separated to form a sequestrum.[67] This isolated fragment of bone can continue to harbor bacteria and act as a persistent focus of infection. The smooth articular surfaces of cartilage and cortical bone are predisposed to bacterial colonization because they have low cellularity and lack a protective layer. Furthermore, the ability of pathogenic bacteria to form a biofilm slime layer from their extracapsular polysaccharides enhances adhesion, promotes survival of microcolonies on the surface of infected tissues, and affords resistance to antimicrobials.[73]

Clinical Presentation

Clinical signs of musculoskeletal infection vary according to the location, duration, and severity of infection. Synovial infection usually results in rapid development of a severe, minimally weight-bearing lameness.[66] Common differentials include subsolar abscessation and fracture. Lameness, focal swelling, effusion, pain, heat, and pyrexia are all variably associated with tissue infection, and rapid progression of disease is a key characteristic.

Diagnosis

Musculoskeletal infection is diagnosed on the basis of clinical and historical findings, combined with the results of hematology, serum biochemistry, and synovial fluid analysis and culture. Imaging may provide useful information in the later stages of disease. Radiographic findings are often unremarkable in the early stages bone and joint infection.[18] Infection must cause 50% to 70% demineralization of bone before lysis is detectable radiographically, and this can take up to 21 days.[74] Scintigraphy can identify areas of infection involving bone but lacks specificity, particularly in skeletally immature horses with active physes. Ultrasonography of septic synovial structures may reveal effusion with anechoic or echogenic fluid, synovial thickening, and fibrinous loculations; however, these findings vary depending on the time that has lapsed between the onset of clinical signs and veterinary examination.[75]

Hematology and serum biochemistry in the presence of bacterial musculoskeletal infection typically reveals leukocytosis, elevated serum amyloid A (SAA) levels, and later, hyperfibrinogenemia. Synovial fluid analysis is of prime importance in the diagnosis of synovial infections, unless compromised overlying tissue prevents an aseptic approach to the joint, sheath, or bursa. Increases in synovial fluid TNCC are seen within 8 hours of joint inoculation and reach significant levels within 12 to 24 hours. Diagnostic criteria for sepsis usually include a synovial fluid protein concentration greater than 40 g/L; TNCC greater than 30×10^9 cells/L, with a differential count of at least 80% neutrophils; or a positive result of bacterial culture. However, some cases of septic arthritis have lower values.[76] The total protein concentration and TNCC may vary depending on the duration of sepsis and the virulence of the bacteria. Transient increases have also been demonstrated in response to repeated synoviocentesis and injection with amikacin.[77] SAA concentrations in serum and synovial fluid have been shown to be greater than 1000 mg/L in the presence of septic arthritis.[78] This acute-phase inflammatory protein may be synthesized locally by chondrocytes, in addition to its systemic production by the liver, and evidence suggests that synovial fluid SAA concentration is a useful marker of local infection.[79]

Bacteria may sequester in the synovial membrane, and conventional methods of bacterial culture from synovial fluid are often unrewarding. However, the use of blood culture medium enrichment has shown a culture rate of up to 79% of infected joints and allows for fast isolation of bacteria and susceptibility testing.[80] Polymerase chain reaction analysis of bacterial DNA in synovial fluid may also become clinically available in the future.[76]

Prognosis

The factor considered by most to have the greatest influence on outcome of a septic synovial structure is the time between the onset of clinical signs and presentation for treatment.[81] A delay of greater than 24 hours has been shown to reduce the likelihood of survival to discharge.[82] Separate research has shown only evidence of bone or tendon involvement to negatively affect survival and athletic function.[83] Both these studies reported a rate of return to athletic function of approximately 50% after synovial sepsis.[82,83] Synovial total protein concentrations greater than 55 to 60 g/L preoperatively, and moderate to severe synovial inflammation at surgery, have been negatively associated with odds of survival to hospital discharge.[84] Synovial fluid analysis at 4 to 6 days after initiation of treatment has useful prognostic value.[83] Culture identification of antimicrobial-resistant bacteria carries a grave prognosis.[85]

MISCELLANEOUS MUSCULOSKELETAL PATHOLOGY
Laminitis

Laminitis is a debilitating disease of the equine foot that involves separation of the dermal and epidermal laminae. Progressive failure of the lamellar interdigitations can result in rotation of the distal phalanx away from the dorsal hoof wall or complete distal displacement away from the middle phalanx.

Epidemiology

Estimated rates of naturally occurring laminitis range from 1.5% to 34%, and a recent large-scale study in Great Britain indicates that active laminitis is the reason for 1 in every 200 cases seen by equine veterinarians.[86] In a hospital setting, laminitic subsets of particular concern include supporting limb laminitis and sepsis-related laminitis. Clinical signs of endotoxemia have been shown to be significantly associated with the development of acute laminitis during hospitalization.[87] Supporting limb laminitis develops after an average of 2 weeks postinjury and reportedly occurs in 0.02% of hospitalized horses.[88]

Pathophysiology

Current knowledge indicates that laminitis should be regarded as a clinical syndrome in which there are several distinct possible mechanisms of structural failure. Inflammatory, metabolic, traumatic, and vascular causes have been proposed.[89] A comprehensive review of the following models used to produce and study laminitis was recently published.[90]

Systemic inflammatory response syndrome laminitis

Laminitis that occurs in association with carbohydrate overload, exposure to black walnut extract, intestinal compromise, endometritis, or other causes of sepsis is thought to have a common link via initiation of a systemic inflammatory response syndrome (SIRS) that triggers lamellar dermal inflammation. A similar inflammatory response is seen in both forelimb and hind limb laminae, suggesting that mechanical factors are important in the progression to clinical laminitis in the forelimbs.[91]

Endocrinopathic laminitis

Endocrinopathic laminitis is most commonly seen in horses and ponies affected by equine metabolic syndrome or pituitary pars intermedia dysfunction and may be associated with hyperinsulinemia. Lamellar failure is thought to be triggered by insulin-mediated changes in the metabolism and structure of the basal epidermal cells, rather than being a primary inflammatory condition.[92] Contrary to historical and widely held beliefs, there is no strong scientific evidence that intra-articular administration of normal doses of exogenous corticosteroids increases the risk of laminitis in systemically healthy horses.[93–95]

Supporting limb laminitis

Supporting limb laminitis occurs in the contralateral limb because of a separate musculoskeletal condition that has resulted in persistent, unilateral lameness with minimal weight bearing. Loss of a normal cyclic pattern of loading, rather than merely an increase in load, is thought to cause hypoperfusion, hypoxia, and energy failure within the lamellar dermis of the weight-bearing foot.[96] Inflammatory events seem to be secondary in this form of laminitis as well.[97]

Traumatic laminitis

A distinct presentation of laminitis is hypothesized to occur because of repetitive hoof trauma or concussion and appears with some frequency in feral horse populations. The description is similar to that of road founder, a long-accepted cause of foot pain in heavy working horses.[89] This form of laminitis seems to be unrelated to body condition or carbohydrate overload, but the contribution of pony breeds to the genetic makeup of some feral horses diagnosed with chronic traumatic laminitis has been noted.[98]

Regardless of the primary cause that triggers laminitis, a threshold is reached at which there is sufficient loss of adhesion between the epidermal and dermal laminae that the remaining intact interdigitations fail to withstand the forces of weight bearing. Thus, tearing of the remaining laminae and rotation or distal displacement of the distal phalanx results. A temporary radiolucent area is seen adjacent to the dorsal margin of the distal phalanx on radiographs when this occurs. Proliferation of epithelial germinal cells leads to filling of this space by a wedge of disorganized epithelial tissue, which can make realignment of the distal phalanx within the hoof capsule difficult.

Clinical Presentation

The 3 recognized stages of laminitis are the prodromal stage before the onset of clinical signs, the acute stage in which there are clinical signs but no radiographic change, followed by the chronic stage, which is defined by the presence of radiographic change. The most common clinical signs associated with acute laminitis are increased digital pulses, difficulty turning, and a short, stilted gait at walk.[86] A typical rocking horse stance is often adopted to shift weight off the front feet. Sensitivity is detected on application of hoof testers over the region of sole underlying the toe of the distal phalanx. Radiographic change can begin within days of onset of clinical signs, while there is still active displacement because of unstable laminae, and persists until alterations to the hoof are made and the inciting cause is resolved.

Diagnosis

The diagnosis of laminitis is currently made via a combination of clinical findings and radiographic evidence of rotation or displacement of the distal phalanx within the hoof capsule. Modeling of the dorsodistal aspect of the distal phalanx develops in chronic cases.

There is no widely accepted set of evidence-based guidelines for the management of laminitis.[89] Continuous digital hypothermia, or cryotherapy, is the sole intervention that has been proven effective in preventing and treating early stages of SIRS-induced laminitis both experimentally and clinically.[99,100] In addition to shoe modifications designed to minimize the biomechanical strain on compromised digital laminae, management strategies for both the treatment and prevention of laminitis should be directed at mitigating the likely inciting cause.

REFERENCES

1. McIlwraith CW. Developmental orthopaedic disease symposium. In: American Quarter Horse Association. Amarillo (TX), April 21–22, 1986.
2. Denoix JM, Jeffcott LB, McIlwraith CW, et al. A review of terminology for equine juvenile osteochondral conditions (JOCC) based on anatomical and functional considerations. Vet J 2013;197(1):29–35.
3. McIlwraith CW. Osteochondrosis. In: Baxter GM, editor. Adams & Stashak's lameness in horses. West Sussex (United Kingdom): Wiley-Blackwell; 2011. p. 1155–64.
4. Hendrix SM, Baxter GM, McIlwraith CW, et al. Concurrent or sequential development of medial meniscal and subchondral cystic lesions within the medial femorotibial joint in horses (1996–2006). Equine Vet J 2010;42(1):5–9.
5. O'Donohue DD, Smith FH, Strickland KL. The incidence of abnormal limb development in the Irish thoroughbred from birth to 18 months. Equine Vet J 1992; 24(4):305–9.

6. Hilla D, Distl O. Prevalence of osteochondral fragments, osteochondrosis dissecans and palmar/plantar osteochondral fragments in Hanoverian warmblood horses. Berl Munch Tierarztl Wochenschr 2013;126(5–6): 236–44.
7. Robert C, Valette JP, Denoix JM. Longitudinal development of equine forelimb conformation from birth to weaning in three different horse breeds. Vet J 2013;198(Suppl 1):e75–80.
8. White KK. Diaphyseal angular deformities in three foals. J Am Vet Med Assoc 1983;182(3):272–9.
9. Ekman S, Carlson CS, van Weeren PR. Workshop report. Third International Workshop on Equine Osteochondrosis, Stockholm, 29–30th May 2008. Equine Vet J 2009;41(5):504–7.
10. Ytrehus B, Carlson CS, Ekman S. Etiology and pathogenesis of osteochondrosis. Vet Pathol 2007;44(4):429–48.
11. Ytrehus B, Carlson CS, Lundeheim N, et al. Vascularisation and osteochondrosis of the epiphyseal growth cartilage of the distal femur in pigs–development with age, growth rate, weight and joint shape. Bone 2004;34(3):454–65.
12. Gee E, Davies M, Firth E, et al. Osteochondrosis and copper: histology of articular cartilage from foals out of copper supplemented and non-supplemented dams. Vet J 2007;173(1):109–17.
13. Olstad K, Ytrehus B, Ekman S, et al. Early lesions of articular osteochondrosis in the distal femur of foals. Vet Pathol 2011;48(6):1165–75.
14. Hyttinen MM, Holopainen J, van Weeren PR, et al. Changes in collagen fibril network organization and proteoglycan distribution in equine articular cartilage during maturation and growth. J Anat 2009;215(5):584–91.
15. Gee EK, Firth EC, Morel PC, et al. Enlargements of the distal third metacarpus and metatarsus in thoroughbred foals at pasture from birth to 160 days of age. N Z Vet J 2005;53(6):438–47.
16. McIlwraith CW. Inferences from referred clinical cases of osteochondritis dissecans. Equine Vet J 1993;25(S16):27–30.
17. Kane AJ, Park RD, McIlwraith CW, et al. Radiographic changes in thoroughbred yearlings. Part 1: prevalence at the time of the yearling sales. Equine Vet J 2003; 35(4):354–65.
18. Butler JA, Colles CM, Dyson SJ, et al. General principles. In: Clinical radiology of the horse. West Sussex (United Kingdom): Wiley-Blackwell; 2008. p. 33–5.
19. McIlwraith CW, Foerner JJ, Davis DM. Osteochondritis dissecans of the tarsocrural joint: results of treatment with arthroscopic surgery. Equine Vet J 1991; 23(3):155–62.
20. McIntosh SC, McIlwraith CW. Natural history of femoropatellar osteochondrosis in three crops of thoroughbreds. Equine Vet J 1993;25(S16):54–61.
21. Dik KJ, Enzerink E, van Weeren PR. Radiographic development of osteochondral abnormalities, in the hock and stifle of Dutch warmblood foals, from age 1 to 11 months. Equine Vet J Suppl 1999;(31):9–15.
22. McIlwraith CW, Nixon AJ, Wright IM. Diagnostic and surgical arthroscopy of the horse. 3rd edition. Edinburgh (United Kingdom): Mosby Elsevier; 2005.
23. McIlwraith CW. Surgical versus conservative management of osteochondrosis. Vet J 2013;197(1):19–28.
24. Fortier LA, Foerner JJ, Nixon AJ. Arthroscopic removal of axial osteochondral fragments of the plantar/palmar proximal aspect of the proximal phalanx in horses: 119 cases (1988–1992). J Am Vet Med Assoc 1995;206(1):71–4.

25. Whitton RC, Kannegieter NJ. Osteochondral fragmentation of the plantar/palmar proximal aspect of the proximal phalanx in racing horses. Aust Vet J 1994; 71(10):318–21.
26. Carmalt JL, Borg H, Näslund H, et al. Racing performance of Swedish standard-bred trotting horses with proximal palmar/plantar first phalangeal (Birkeland) fragments compared to fragment free controls. Vet J 2014;202(1):43–7.
27. Santschi EM, Leibsle SR, Morehead JP, et al. Carpal and fetlock conformation of the juvenile thoroughbred from birth to yearling auction age. Equine Vet J 2006; 38(7):604–9.
28. Stokes IA. Mechanical effects on skeletal growth. J Musculoskelet Neuronal Interact 2002;2(3):277–80.
29. Auer JA, von Rechenberg B. Treatment of angular limb deformities in foals. Clin Tech Equine Pract 2006;5(4):270–81.
30. Witte S, Thorpe PE, Hunt RJ, et al. A lag-screw technique for bridging of the medial aspect of the distal tibial physis in horses. J Am Vet Med Assoc 2004; 225(10):1581–3, 1548.
31. Read EK, Read MR, Townsend HG, et al. Effect of hemi-circumferential periosteal transection and elevation in foals with experimentally induced angular limb deformities. J Am Vet Med Assoc 2002;221(4):536–40.
32. Fretz PB, McIlwraith CW. Wedge osteotomy as a treatment for angular deformity of the fetlock in horses. J Am Vet Med Assoc 1983;182(3):245–50.
33. Anderson TM, McIlwraith CW, Douay P. The role of conformation in musculoskeletal problems in the racing Thoroughbred. Equine Vet J 2004;36(7):571–5.
34. Pinchbeck GL, Clegg PD, Boyde A, et al. Horse-, training- and race-level risk factors for palmar/plantar osteochondral disease in the racing thoroughbred. Equine Vet J 2013;45(5):582–6.
35. Estberg L, Stover SM, Gardner IA, et al. High-speed exercise history and catastrophic racing fracture in thoroughbreds. Am J Vet Res 1996;57(11): 1549–55.
36. Ely ER, Avella CS, Price JS, et al. Descriptive epidemiology of fracture, tendon and suspensory ligament injuries in National Hunt racehorses in training. Equine Vet J 2009;41(4):372–8.
37. Takahashi T, Kasashima Y, Ueno Y. Association between race history and risk of superficial digital flexor tendon injury in thoroughbred racehorses. J Am Vet Med Assoc 2004;225(1):90–3.
38. Valberg SJ, Mickelson JR, Gallant EM, et al. Exertional rhabdomyolysis in quarter horses and thoroughbreds: one syndrome, multiple aetiologies. Equine Vet J Suppl 1999;(30):533–8.
39. Frost HM. Wolff's Law and bone's structural adaptations to mechanical usage: an overview for clinicians. Angle Orthod 1994;64(3):175–88.
40. Kawcak CE, Norrdin RW, Frisbie DD, et al. Effects of osteochondral fragmentation and intra-articular triamcinolone acetonide treatment on subchondral bone in the equine carpus. Equine Vet J 1998;30(1):66–71.
41. Martig S, Chen W, Lee PV, et al. Bone fatigue and its implications for injuries in racehorses. Equine Vet J 2014;46(4):408–15.
42. Whitton RC, Trope GD, Ghasem-Zadeh A, et al. Third metacarpal condylar fatigue fractures in equine athletes occur within previously modelled subchondral bone. Bone 2010;47(4):826–31.
43. Stover SM, Johnson BJ, Daft BM, et al. An association between complete and incomplete stress fractures of the humerus in racehorses. Equine Vet J 1992; 24(4):260–3.

44. Muir P, Peterson AL, Sample SJ, et al. Exercise-induced metacarpophalangeal joint adaptation in the thoroughbred racehorse. J Anat 2008;213(6):706–17.
45. Norrdin RW, Kawcak CE, Capwell BA, et al. Subchondral bone failure in an equine model of overload arthrosis. Bone 1998;22(2):133–9.
46. Tidswell HK, Innes JF, Avery NC, et al. High-intensity exercise induces structural, compositional and metabolic changes in cuboidal bones–findings from an equine athlete model. Bone 2008;43(4):724–33.
47. Carrier TK, Estberg L, Stover SM, et al. Association between long periods without high-speed workouts and risk of complete humeral or pelvic fracture in thoroughbred racehorses: 54 cases (1991–1994). J Am Vet Med Assoc 1998;212(10):1582–7.
48. Frisbie D. Synovial joint biology and pathobiology. Chapter 78. In: Auer JA, Stick JA, editors. Equine surgery. 4th edition. Saint Louis (MO): W.B. Saunders; 2012. p. 1096–114.
49. Berenbaum F. Osteoarthritis as an inflammatory disease (osteoarthritis is not osteoarthrosis!). Osteoarthritis Cartilage 2013;21(1):16–21.
50. McIlwraith CW. Principles of musculoskeletal disease. In: Baxter GM, editor. Adams and Stashak's lameness in horses. West Sussex (United Kingdom): Wiley-Blackwell; 2011. p. 871–89.
51. Scanzello CR, Goldring SR. The role of synovitis in osteoarthritis pathogenesis. Bone 2012;51(2):249–57.
52. Patterson-Kane JC, Firth EC. The pathobiology of exercise-induced superficial digital flexor tendon injury in Thoroughbred racehorses. Vet J 2009;181(2): 79–89.
53. Patterson-Kane JC, Wilson AM, Firth EC, et al. Exercise-related alterations in crimp morphology in the central regions of superficial digital flexor tendons from young thoroughbreds: a controlled study. Equine Vet J 1998;30(1):61–4.
54. Kasashima Y, Smith RK, Birch HL, et al. Exercise-induced tendon hypertrophy: cross-sectional area changes during growth are influenced by exercise. Equine Vet J Suppl 2002;(34):264–8.
55. Macleay J. Acquired myopathies. In: Reed S, Bayly W, Sellon D, editors. Equine internal medicine. St Louis (MO): Saunders; 2010. p. 512–6.
56. Valberg SJ. Muscle injuries and disease. In: Baxter G, editor. Adams and Stashak's lameness in horses. West Sussex (United Kingdom): Blackwell; 2011. p. 939–56.
57. Frisbie DD, Mc Ilwraith CW, Arthur RM, et al. Serum biomarker levels for musculoskeletal disease in two- and three-year-old racing Thoroughbred horses: a prospective study of 130 horses. Equine Vet J 2010;42(7):643–51.
58. McIlwraith CW. Use of synovial fluid and serum biomarkers in equine bone and joint disease: a review. Equine Vet J 2005;37(5):473–82.
59. van Weeren PR, Firth EC. Future tools for early diagnosis and monitoring of musculoskeletal injury: biomarkers and CT. Vet Clin North Am Equine Pract 2008;24(1):153–75.
60. Stockham S, Scott M. Fundamentals of veterinary clinical pathology. 2nd edition. Oxford (United Kingdom): Blackwell; 2008.
61. Tull TM, Bramlage LR. Racing prognosis after cumulative stress-induced injury of the distal portion of the third metacarpal and third metatarsal bones in thoroughbred racehorses: 55 cases (2000–2009). J Am Vet Med Assoc 2011; 238(10):1316–22.
62. Thorpe CT, Clegg PD, Birch HL. A review of tendon injury: why is the equine superficial digital flexor tendon most at risk? Equine Vet J 2010;42(2):174–80.

63. Cohen ND. Causes of and farm management factors associated with disease and death in foals. J Am Vet Med Assoc 1994;204(10):1644–51.
64. Giguere S, Cohen ND, Chaffin MK, et al. *Rhodococcus equi*: clinical manifestations, virulence, and immunity. J Vet Intern Med 2011;25(6):1221–30.
65. Schneider RK, Bramlage LR, Moore RM, et al. A retrospective study of 192 horses affected with septic arthritis/tenosynovitis. Equine Vet J 1992;24(6):436–42.
66. Bertone A. Infectious arthritis and fungal infectious arthritis. In: Ross M, Dyson S, editors. Diagnosis and management of lameness in the horse. St Louis (MO): Elsevier; 2011. p. 677–84.
67. Lew DP, Waldvogel FA. Osteomyelitis. Lancet 2004;364(9431):369–79.
68. Moore RM, Schneider RK, Kowalski J, et al. Antimicrobial susceptibility of bacterial isolates from 233 horses with musculoskeletal infection during 1979–1989. Equine Vet J 1992;24(6):450–6.
69. Vengust M, Arroyo LG, Weese JS, et al. Preliminary evidence for dormant clostridial spores in equine skeletal muscle. Equine Vet J 2003;35(5):514–6.
70. Peek SF, Semrad SD, Perkins GA. Clostridial myonecrosis in horses (37 cases 1985–2000). Equine Vet J 2003;35(1):86–92.
71. Evans AG, White SD. Bacterial diseases. In: Smith BP, editor. Large animal medicine. St Louis (MO): Mosby; 2002. p. 1208–9.
72. Gristina AG, Naylor PT, Myrvik QN. Mechanisms of musculoskeletal sepsis. Orthop Clin North Am 1991;22(3):363–71.
73. Clutterbuck AL, Woods EJ, Knottenbelt DC, et al. Biofilms and their relevance to veterinary medicine. Vet Microbiol 2007;121(1–2):1–17.
74. Wegener WA, Alavi A. Diagnostic imaging of musculoskeletal infection. Roentgenography; gallium, indium-labeled white blood cell, gammaglobulin, bone scintigraphy; and MRI. Orthop Clin North Am 1991;22(3):401–18.
75. Beccati F, Gialletti R, Passamonti F, et al. Ultrasonographic findings in 38 horses with septic arthritis/tenosynovitis. Vet Radiol Ultrasound 2015;56:68–76.
76. Steel CM. Equine synovial fluid analysis. Vet Clin North Am Equine Pract 2008; 24(2):437–54, viii.
77. Dykgraaf S, Dechant JE, Johns JL, et al. Effect of intrathecal amikacin administration and repeated centesis on digital flexor tendon sheath synovial fluid in horses. Vet Surg 2007;36(1):57–63.
78. Jacobsen S, Thomsen MH, Nanni S. Concentrations of serum amyloid A in serum and synovial fluid from healthy horses and horses with joint disease. Am J Vet Res 2006;67(10):1738–42.
79. Belgrave RL, Dickey MM, Arheart KL, et al. Assessment of serum amyloid A testing of horses and its clinical application in a specialized equine practice. J Am Vet Med Assoc 2013;243(1):113–9.
80. Dumoulin M, Pille F, van den Abeele AM, et al. Use of blood culture medium enrichment for synovial fluid culture in horses: a comparison of different culture methods. Equine Vet J 2010;42(6):541–6.
81. Findley JA, Pinchbeck GL, Milner PI, et al. Outcome of horses with synovial structure involvement following solar foot penetrations in four UK veterinary hospitals: 95 cases. Equine Vet J 2014;46(3):352–7.
82. Smith LJ, Mellor DJ, Marr CM, et al. What is the likelihood that a horse treated for septic digital tenosynovitis will return to its previous level of athletic function? Equine Vet J 2006;38(4):337–41.
83. Walmsley EA, Anderson GA, Muurlink MA, et al. Retrospective investigation of prognostic indicators for adult horses with infection of a synovial structure. Aust Vet J 2011;89(6):226–31.

84. Milner PI, Bardell DA, Warner L, et al. Factors associated with survival to hospital discharge following endoscopic treatment for synovial sepsis in 214 horses. Equine Vet J 2014;46(6):701–5.

85. Herdan CL, Acke E, Dicken M, et al. Multi-drug-resistant enterococcus spp. as a cause of non-responsive septic synovitis in three horses. N Z Vet J 2012;60(5): 297–304.

86. Wylie CE, Collins SN, Verheyen KL, et al. A cohort study of equine laminitis in Great Britain 2009–2011: estimation of disease frequency and description of clinical signs in 577 cases. Equine Vet J 2013;45(6):681–7.

87. Parsons CS, Orsini JA, Krafty R, et al. Risk factors for development of acute laminitis in horses during hospitalization: 73 cases (1997–2004). J Am Vet Med Assoc 2007;230(6):885–9.

88. Wylie CE, Newton JR, Bathe AP, et al. Prevalence of supporting limb laminitis in a UK equine practice and referral hospital setting between 2005 and 2013: implications for future epidemiological studies. Vet Rec 2015;176(3):72.

89. Orsini JA. Science-in-brief: equine laminitis research: milestones and goals. Equine Vet J 2014;46(5):529–33.

90. Katz LM, Bailey SR. A review of recent advances and current hypotheses on the pathogenesis of acute laminitis. Equine Vet J 2012;44(6):752–61.

91. Leise BS, Faleiros RR, Watts M, et al. Hindlimb laminar inflammatory response is similar to that present in forelimbs after carbohydrate overload in horses. Equine Vet J 2012;44(6):633–9.

92. de Laat MA, Patterson-Kane JC, Pollitt CC, et al. Histological and morphometric lesions in the pre-clinical, developmental phase of insulin-induced laminitis in Standardbred horses. Vet J 2013;195(3):305–12.

93. Cornelisse CJ, Robinson NE. Glucocorticoid therapy and the risk of equine laminitis. Equine Vet Educ 2013;25(1):39–46.

94. McCluskey MJ, Kavenagh PB. Clinical use of triamcinolone acetonide in the horse (205 cases) and the incidence of glucocorticoid-induced laminitis associated with its use. Equine Vet Educ 2004;16(2):86–9.

95. Bailey SR, Elliott J. The corticosteroid laminitis story: 2. Science of if, when and how. Equine Vet J 2007;39(1):7–11.

96. Medina-Torres CE, Collins SN, Pollitt CC, et al. Examining the contribution of lamellar perfusion and energy failure in supporting limb laminitis. J Equine Vet Sci 2013;33(10):862.

97. Leise BS, Faleiros RR, Burns TA, et al. Inflammation in laminitis: the "itis" in laminitis may not pertain to all. J Equine Vet Sci 2013;33(10):860.

98. Hampson BA, de Laat MA, Beausac C, et al. Histopathological examination of chronic laminitis in Kaimanawa feral horses of New Zealand. N Z Vet J 2012; 60(5):285–9.

99. van Eps AW, Pollitt CC, Underwood C, et al. Continuous digital hypothermia initiated after the onset of lameness prevents lamellar failure in the oligofructose laminitis model. Equine Vet J 2014;46(5):625–30.

100. Kullmann A, Holcombe SJ, Hurcombe SD, et al. Prophylactic digital cryotherapy is associated with decreased incidence of laminitis in horses diagnosed with colitis. Equine Vet J 2014;46(5):554–9.

Ocular Pathology

Bianca S. Bauer, DVM, MSc

KEYWORDS

- Ocular disease • Ocular pathology • Equine ophthalmic disease
- Ocular diagnostic tests

KEY POINTS

- A systematic ophthalmic examination, detailed history, and physical examination combined with ocular diagnostic testing are essential in obtaining an early, accurate diagnosis of equine ocular disorders.
- The eye is a very unforgiving organ and time is usually of the essence when ocular disease is present. The more promptly an ocular condition is diagnosed, the more responsive the condition is to treatment and the better the prognosis in most cases.
- The most common ocular laboratory diagnostic tests include ocular culture and sensitivity, and cytology and/or biopsy for light microscopic examination. When indicated, these diagnostic tests can help the clinician obtain an etiologic diagnosis for the presenting ocular condition which will allow for targeted treatment and in most cases, a better treatment response.
- In unfortunate cases in which ocular disease results in a blind, painful eye necessitating enucleation, submission of the globe for light microscopic evaluation is essential to determine or confirm the cause of the blindness and provide a prognosis for the contralateral eye.

INTRODUCTION

Ocular disease is common in the horse, yet many challenges exist within equine ophthalmology. Horses are more difficult to handle and medicate compared with small animal species and there is a high cost associated with treating a horse. Laboratory diagnostics can aid in obtaining an ophthalmic diagnosis and in determining appropriate therapy. Early diagnosis, treatment, and recovery in turn, will decrease the treatment time and financial burden experienced by many horse owners.

This article is aimed at the equine practitioner and addresses the role of laboratory diagnostics in common equine ophthalmic conditions. Although not the main purpose of this article, the value of performing a complete ophthalmic examination (including Schirmer Tear Test, tonometry, and fluorescein staining) on BOTH eyes should not be underestimated and is essential in the diagnosis of all ocular conditions. This article

Small Animal Clinical Sciences, Western College of Veterinary Medicine, University of Saskatchewan, 52 Campus Drive, Saskatoon, Saskatchewan S7N 5B4, Canada
E-mail address: Bianca.bauer@usask.ca

Vet Clin Equine 31 (2015) 425–448
http://dx.doi.org/10.1016/j.cveq.2015.04.001
0749-0739/15/$ – see front matter © 2015 Elsevier Inc. All rights reserved.

is not intended to be a complete summary of every ophthalmic disease in the horse, but rather to serve as a resource to equine practitioners for when laboratory diagnostics are recommended and beneficial in equine ophthalmic disease. As with any laboratory testing, the clinician should communicate with the laboratory to ensure the method of sample collection, handling, and interpretation of results are correct.

DISEASES OF THE EQUINE ORBIT

The equine orbit completely surrounds and protects the globe; however, the equine orbit is subject to extension of disease from various adjacent structures, including the periorbital sinuses, guttural pouch, ethmoid turbinates, and less commonly from the oral cavity. The large paranasal sinuses are a common location for disease resulting in tissue inflammation that can impinge on the orbital structures and may affect one or both orbits.[1] Typical clinical signs of orbital disease include strabismus, exophthalmos, prolapsed third eyelid, epiphora, and conjunctival hyperemia (**Fig. 1**). Subcutaneous emphysema, altered sinus percussion, bone deformation, and distention of the supraorbital fossa are also possible clinical signs depending on the etiology of the orbital disease.

Orbital Cellulitis

Epidemiology
Common causes of orbital cellulitis include foreign bodies penetrating the orbit, direct trauma, extension of infectious or inflammatory conditions from adjacent sinuses, or seeding of septic emboli. Bacterial (ie, *Actinomyces* spp), parasitic (ie, *Habronema, Strongylus* sp) or fungal (ie, *Cryptococcus*) granulomas have also been reported in the orbit.

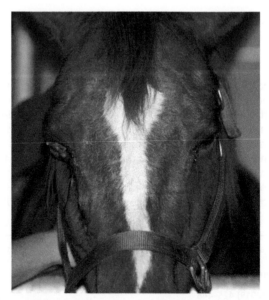

Fig. 1. Exophthalmos, epiphora, and conjunctival hyperemia and chemosis of the right eye secondary to orbital disease.

Diagnosis
Orbital cellulitis may or may not be septic and concurrent systemic illness may be present. Complete blood count is beneficial and may reveal a leukocytosis, hyperfibrinogenemia, and hypergammaglobulinemia. Fine-needle aspiration for cytology and biopsy for histologic examination are helpful in the diagnosis and are recommended to rule out orbital neoplasia, a major differential diagnosis. Microbial culture of the orbital aspirate can rule out a septic cellulitis/abscess and provide targeted antibiotic choices for treatment if indicated. Appropriate diagnostic samples, however, may be difficult to obtain and referral is often indicated in orbital disease. Advanced imaging of the equine orbit and skull should be performed in cases of orbital disease to define the lesion and allow for complete assessment of the patient.

Treatment
Treatment of equine orbital cellulitis includes systemic nonsteroidal anti-inflammatories (NSAIDs) and systemic antimicrobial or antifungal agents based on culture and sensitivity findings, or parasiticides if parasitic orbital disease is diagnosed. The prognosis for cases of equine orbital cellulitis depends on the severity of the disease and response to therapy.

Orbital Neoplasia

Epidemiology
Orbital neoplasia in the horse is uncommon compared with other species. Equine orbital neoplasms may arise primarily from orbital tissues or secondarily from local extension from adjacent tissues or from hematogenous spread. The most common neoplasms of the orbit are neuroendocrine tumors, extra-adrenal paragangliomas, lymphosarcomas (LSA), squamous cell carcinomas (SCCs), and anaplastic sarcomas.

Diagnosis
Advanced imaging of the equine orbit and skull should be performed to define the lesion; however, fine-needle aspirates for cytology and biopsy for histologic examination are necessary to confirm the presence of neoplasia. Fine-needle aspirate of the local lymph nodes is recommended if abnormalities are suspected.

Treatment
Treatment of orbital neoplasia consists of surgical removal with or without adjunctive therapies. Early referral for surgery and imaging is recommended to preserve the globe. Unfortunately most orbital neoplasms are malignant, and prognosis for long-term survival is generally poor.[2]

Orbital Fat Prolapse

Orbital and conjunctival swelling in the horse may be due to fat prolapse through a weakened episcleral fascia or as the result of trauma or nictitans removal. Aspiration or biopsy of the swelling is recommended to confirm the diagnosis. Treatment consists of mass resection and suturing of the overlying conjunctival surface to close the exposed area.

DISEASES OF THE EQUINE EYELID

Eyelid disease is commonly encountered in equine veterinary practice. Although most eyelid conditions are chronic and progressive, some cases of severe, ulcerative blepharitis and some neoplasms may appear as injuries. Therefore, cytology, biopsy, and culture (bacterial ± fungal) are *always* indicated in periocular dermatologic conditions.

Blepharitis

Epidemiology

Blepharitis, in general, appears as inflammation of the eyelid(s) with or without open wounds and can occur with or without conjunctivitis (**Fig. 2**). Infectious forms of blepharitis are not uncommon in the horse and include bacterial, fungal, and parasitic etiologies. Parasitic blepharitis most commonly includes habronemiasis (caused by aberrant migration *Habronema* spp larvae in wounds on or near the eye). This disease is also known as summer sores, granular dermatitis, or swamp cancer.[3] Noninfectious etiologies of blepharitis include trauma, immune-mediated (ie, pemphigus foliaceus), allergic, or actinic blepharitis (**Table 1**).

Diagnosis

Performing cytology, biopsy, and culture will differentiate infectious blepharitis versus noninfectious blepharitis. Treatment of blepharitis should target the specific etiologic agent if known and should include systemic and topical antibiotics based on culture and sensitivity results ± topical or systemic NSAIDs. The prognosis for blepharitis is good with most etiologies, but secondary eyelid defects or ocular damage may occur depending on the severity and chronicity of the blepharitis.

Eyelid Neoplasia

Eyelid neoplasia is relatively common in the horse. Sarcoids and SCC are the most common primary equine eyelid tumors, but papilloma, melanocytoma/melanoma, lymphoma/LSA, neurofibroma, basal cell carcinoma, hemangiosarcoma (HSA), fibroma/fibrosarcoma, mast-cell tumor, and angioma/angiosarcoma are not infrequent.[4,5] Periocular neoplasia should always be confirmed by surgical biopsy and light microscopy. Early diagnosis and aggressive treatment allows for a more successful clinical outcome in most cases of eyelid neoplasia.

Sarcoids

Epidemiology Sarcoids are locally aggressive fibroblastic tumors of the equine skin with proliferative and hyperplastic epithelial components. Sarcoids commonly involve the eyelid either as single or multiple neoplasms, and younger horses (younger than

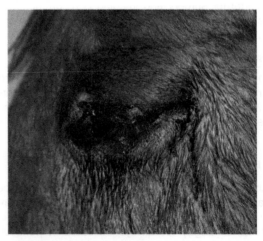

Fig. 2. Blepharitis in an 8-year-old quarter horse.

Table 1
Skin diseases affecting the equine eyelid

Parasitic	Fungal	Bacterial	Other
Habronema spp	*Microsporum* spp	*Moraxella* spp	Trauma
Thelazia lacrymalis	*Trichophyton* spp	*Listeria monocytogenes*	Solar/Actinic
Draschia megastoma	*Histoplasma farciminosum*	*Staphylococcus* spp	Hypersensitivity
Onchocerca cervicalis	*Cryptococcus mirandi*	*Corynebacterium* spp	Immune-mediated
Demodex spp	*Aspergillus* spp	*Dermatophilus congolensis*	Allergic
Flies	*Rhinosporidium seeberi*	*Streptococcus equi*	Neoplasia
Babesia spp	—	—	—

7 years) are more commonly affected. Many breeds develop sarcoids but quarter horses, Arabians, and appaloosas may be at increased risk.[6]

Clinical appearance The clinical appearance of sarcoids varies ranging from small wartlike lesions to large, ulcerated fibrous growths (**Fig. 3**). Sarcoids are classified into 5 types: occult, verrucose, nodular (A and B), fibroblastic, or mixed. Periocular sarcoids are typically nodular, fibroblastic, or mixed.[7]

Diagnosis Sarcoids have been demonstrated to be associated with bovine papilloma virus (BPV).[8] The disease is considered to be a nonproductive infection in which viral DNA exists episomally.[9] The application of BPV DNA as a diagnostic test for sarcoids has, to date, not been fully evaluated or validated. A presumptive diagnosis of sarcoid is based on clinical location and appearance of the lesion with differential diagnoses including exuberant granulation tissue, habronemiasis, melanoma, papilloma, or SCC. A surgical biopsy is always required for definitive diagnosis of a sarcoid. Histologically, periocular sarcoids have proliferation of dermal fibroblasts invading into the subcutis and the deeper muscle structures around the eye with exaggerated epithelial down-growth.

Treatment The treatment of choice for eyelid and periocular sarcoids is surgical debulking and adjunctive therapy (ie, cryotherapy, immunotherapy, chemotherapy,

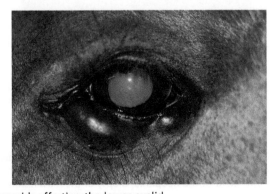

Fig. 3. Nodular sarcoids affecting the lower eyelid.

brachytherapy). Excessive debulking around the eye, however, can be difficult, and in most cases is not possible. Referral to a veterinary ophthalmologist may be necessary to discuss treatment options for many cases of periocular sarcoids. Furthermore, treatment should be done concurrent to the surgical biopsy or shortly after, as the surgical biopsy may stimulate the mass further, resulting in mass proliferation. The prognosis for periocular sarcoids is good to guarded, as failure to induce complete regression will frequently result in aggressive regrowth of the mass.[7]

Squamous cell carcinoma

Epidemiology SCC is the most common neoplasm of the eye and its adnexa in the horse.[4,10] Poorly pigmented horses have a higher prevalence of ocular SCC and animals exposed to higher elevations and increased sunlight have a higher incidence of SCC.[11] The most common eyelid locations for SCC are the third eyelid, medial canthus, and lower eyelid.[10]

Clinical appearance Clinically, lesions vary from a hyperemic erosive plaque to a raised pink, fleshy, cobblestone mass of varying size with variable degrees of inflammation, ulceration, and necrosis[4] (**Fig. 4**).

Differential diagnoses Differential diagnoses for SCC include conjunctivitis (lymphoid hyperplasia and follicular conjunctivitis), inflammatory lesions (foreign body reaction, abscesses, granulation tissue, solar-induced inflammation), parasites (*Habronema, Onchocerca, Thelazia*), and other eyelid tumors (papilloma, melanoma, mast-cell tumor, basal cell carcinoma, schwannoma, hemangioma/HSA, lymphoma/LSA and adenoma/adenocarcinoma). Any chronic infection or irritation causing tissue metaplasia (ie, actinic solar dermatitis) may promote neoplastic change of the epithelium into SCC.

Diagnosis A definitive diagnosis of SCC requires biopsy and histopathology. All abnormal appearing eyelid lesions whether nodular or diffuse (see **Fig. 4**) should be biopsied to determine the extent of neoplastic involvement. Histologically, there are various stages of SCC: dysplastic epithelium, carcinoma in situ, noninvasive SCC, and invasive SCC[12] **Fig. 5**.

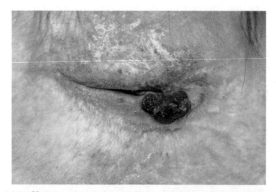

Fig. 4. A nodular SCC affecting the right medial canthus in a poorly pigmented horse. Note the surrounding/upper eyelid alopecia, hyperemia and crusting. To obtain a definitive diagnosis and determine the exent of the neoplasia, biopsy of the mass lesion as well us the upper eyelid are recommended.

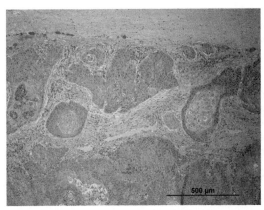

500 μm

Fig. 5. Histologic section (hematoxylin-eosin stain) demonstrating multiple nests of invasive SCC with central keratinization and surrounding inflammation.

Treatment Eyelid SCC requires excision and adjunctive therapy (ie, cryotherapy, intra-lesional chemotherapy, brachytherapy, or photodynamic therapy). Third eyelid/medial canthal SCC generally is treated with excision of the whole third eyelid. All excised tis-sue should be submitted for histologic evaluation to confirm the disease and ensure adequate tissue margins. SCC of the eyelid requires a minimum 2-cm margin on all sides of the mass to be curative. Such margins are almost impossible with eyelid SCC given the nature of the ocular tissue itself and the need to preserve as much func-tioning eyelid margin as possible. Therefore, in many cases of eyelid SCC, referral to a veterinary ophthalmologist for assessment or enucleation or even exenteration may be warranted.

Prognosis The prognosis for eyelid and orbital SCC is worse compared with SCC affecting other sites of the eye.[13] Recurrence of SCC after surgical excision with adjunctive therapy is not uncommon and regular reexaminations, with repeat biopsies of suspicious lesions, are recommended for 3 to 5 years after treatment.[4] Metastasis of ocular SCC is uncommon but when it does occur it is most commonly to the regional (submandibular) lymph nodes, salivary glands, or thorax. Extension into the orbit, sinus, or calvaria also has been reported. Fine-needle aspirate and cytology of the local lymph nodes are recommended if abnormalities are suspected.

Melanocytoma/melanoma
Epidemiology and clinical appearance Gray or white-haired horses, Percherons, and Arabians are at increased risk for developing melanocytic tumors of the eyelid.[14] A slowly progressive, partially alopecic, pigmented cutaneous eyelid mass is most typical of a melanocytic mass; however, such masses need to be differentiated from other eyelid tumors or swellings. Masses may occur as single or multiple eyelid tumors.

Diagnosis Biopsy and histopathology are necessary for definitive diagnosis of mela-nocytoma/melanoma. Equine melanocytic tumors have highly variable histologic and cytologic patterns. Before treatment, careful evaluation of the entire horse is rec-ommended to rule out metastatic disease with biopsy and histopathology of any other lesions evident. Excision of an eyelid melanocytic tumor is the treatment of choice and is usually curative.

Lymphosarcoma

Epidemiology Compared with other species, LSA is relatively uncommon in the horse. Unilateral or bilateral neoplastic infiltration of the eyelids and conjunctiva is the most common ocular manifestation of equine LSA.

Diagnosis Biopsy and histopathology are required to differentiate LSA from other masses, such as habronemiasis, sarcoids, papilloma, melanoma, and SCC. In most cases, LSA is considered to represent a systemic disease and nonspecific systemic signs, including fever, weight loss, respiratory ailments, peripheral lymphadenopathy, and anemia, may accompany the ophthalmic signs. A complete systemic workup (ie, blood work, lymph node aspiration or biopsy, and visceral imaging) is indicated to stage the disease. The long-term prognosis for survival is guarded to poor for most horses with LSA.[15] Horses diagnosed with the nodular form of extraocular lymphoma that undergo complete excision appear to have the best prognosis.[16]

DISEASES OF THE EQUINE CONJUNCTIVA

Conjunctivitis is common in the equine, yet the conjunctiva is more often secondarily affected and inflamed as a result of another ocular condition (ie, nonulcerative or ulcerative keratitis, uveitis) versus a primary conjunctival disease. Differentiating primary conjunctivitis from the more severe secondary causes of conjunctivitis is essential and a complete and thorough ophthalmic examination is imperative first and foremost to rule out ocular disease resulting in a secondary conjunctivitis.

Primary Conjunctivitis

Clinical appearance

Many causes of primary conjunctivitis also cause systemic disease. See **Table 2** and **Table 6** for causes of primary conjunctivitis in the horse. The typical clinical signs of conjunctivitis include conjunctival hyperemia and chemosis but mucopurulent discharge and lymphoid follicle formation also can be present.

Diagnosis

A conjunctival bacterial culture and sensitivity with cytologic examination of conjunctival scrapings should be done on all eyes with chronic conjunctivitis and ocular discharge. The normal equine ocular surface (corneal and conjunctival) microflora consists mainly of gram-positive bacteria and fungi. Many of these normal microflora may act as opportunistic ocular pathogens. For interpretation of results it is essential that the clinician have a thorough understanding of the normal equine conjunctival cytology and bacterial and fungal flora (**Table 3**). If infectious etiologies are suspected,

Table 2
Causes of primary conjunctivitis in the equine

Parasitic	Fungal	Bacterial	Viral	Other
Habronema spp	*Aspergillus* spp	*Moraxella* spp	EHV 1 & 2	Trauma
Thelazia lacrymalis	Histoplasmosis	Chlamydophila	EVA	Solar/Actinic
Onchocerca	Blastomycosis	spp	Adenovirus	Hypersensitivity
cervicalis	*Rhinosporidium*	*Mycoplasma* spp		Immune-
Trypanosoma	*seeberi*	*Streptococcus*		mediated
evansi		*equi*		Allergic
Babesia spp				Neoplasia

Abbreviations: EHV, equine herpes virus; EVA, equine viral arteritis.

Table 3
Microbial isolates from conjunctival/corneal collections in healthy horses

Gram Positive	Gram Negative	Fungal
Actinomyces	Acinetobacter[a]	Alternaria
Bacillus[a]	Actinobacillus	Aspergillus[a]
Corynebacterium[a]	Alcaligenes	Cladosporium[a]
Dermatophilus	Citrobacter	Fusarium
Diphtheroid	Enterobacter[a]	Penicillium
Enterococcus	Escherichia[a]	Scopulariopsis
Lactobacillus	Klebsiella	
Micrococcus	Moraxella[a]	
Rhodococcus	Neisseria	
Staphylococcus[a]	Pasteurella	
Streptococcus[a]	Proteus	
Streptomyces[a]	Pseudomonas[a]	
	Sphingomonas	
	Stenotrophomonas	

[a] Most common isolates.

then viral or fungal isolation, culture, or polymerase chain reaction (PCR) should be performed by the veterinary practitioner. In many cases of conjunctivitis, however, conjunctival biopsy and histology may be necessary to obtain a definitive diagnosis and rule out other conjunctival disease processes.

Treatment
Treatment of conjunctivitis is based on culture and sensitivity, cytology, and histopathology results. Antibiotic, antiviral, antifungal, or parasiticide therapy may be required pending the cause of the conjunctivitis.

Nodular Lymphocytic Conjunctivitis

Nodular lymphocytic conjunctivitis appears clinically as unilateral or bilateral, smooth or nodular, pink conjunctival masses.[17] To differentiate this type of conjunctivitis from other masses, biopsy and histopathology are required. On light microscopic evaluation, characteristic lymphoid follicles with lymphocytes, plasma cells, and histiocytes are evident.[17] Treatment consists of excision of the lesion with topical administration of anti-inflammatory agents.

Conjunctival Neoplasia

Similar to the equine eyelid, the conjunctiva can be affected with neoplasia, including SCC, melanoma, LSA, papilloma, mastocytoma, basal cell carcinoma, schwannoma, hemangioma/HSA, adenoma/adenocarcinoma, and angioma/angiosarcoma. Many conjunctival masses also may affect the cornea; see Corneal Neoplasia for more information. Biopsy and histopathology are required to obtain a definitive diagnosis.

DISEASES OF THE NASOLACRIMAL SYSTEM

Nasolacrimal duct (NLD) obstruction is a very common problem in horses, with causes of obstruction including congenital atresia, obstruction from inflammation (dacryocystitis), strictures, foreign bodies, and trauma. Clinical signs of NLD obstruction include epiphora, conjunctivitis, and mucopurulent discharge (**Fig. 6**). Diagnostic methods in horses with nasolacrimal obstruction or suspected dacryocystitis should include

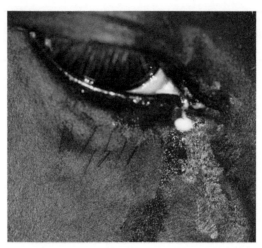

Fig. 6. Nasolacrimal duct obstruction resulting in mucopurulent ocular discharge.

bacterial culture and sensitivity and cytology of the discharge. After these tests are performed, a retrograde nasolacrimal flushing under sedation should be attempted. If the NLD cannot be flushed, then referral for a dacryocystorhinogram and/or computed tomography is recommended to examine the NLD and surrounding bone to determine the exact location of the obstruction. Treatment for the NLD obstruction depends on the etiology and consists of treating any infection present with oral and topical antibiotics and surgery for the creation of a new NLD opening in cases of atresia. The prognosis for most NLD obstruction and dacryocystitis cases is good.

DISEASES OF THE EQUINE CORNEA

Diseases of the equine cornea are very common and a frequent cause of presentation of horses to veterinarians.

Ulcerative Keratitis

Clinical appearance
A presumptive diagnosis of corneal ulceration is based on clinical signs, including epiphora, blepharospasm, conjunctival hyperemia, and corneal opacification with or without varying degrees of anterior uveitis. Collagenolysis (ie, keratomalacia or corneal melting) may or may not be present, but if present, typically appears as a gelatinous, yellow to white corneal stromal opacity (**Fig. 7**).

Pathogenesis and diagnosis
The corneal epithelium normally prevents infection of normal resident ocular microflora. When the epithelium is damaged, normally nonpathogenic and pathogenic bacteria can adhere to and invade the exposed stroma, establishing infection and prompting inflammatory cell influx. The diagnosis of a corneal ulcer is confirmed by positive fluorescein staining of the corneal defect. Differential diagnoses for ulcerative keratitis include other ulcerative corneal diseases, such as equine herpes virus (EHV) keratitis, foreign body, immune-mediated keratitis or eosinophilic keratitis, or nonulcerative conditions, such as stromal abscess, nonulcerative keratouveitis, corneal degeneration, or corneal neoplasia.

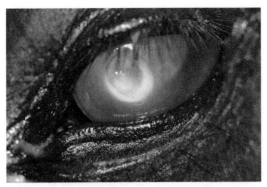

Fig. 7. Gelatinous, yellow to white corneal stromal opacification consistent with collagenolysis in a complex corneal ulcer.

There are 3 categories of ulcerative keratitis: simple, indolent, or complex. Simple ulcers are acute, superficial, and noninfected. Indolent ulcers are also superficial and noninfected but are chronic in nature. Simple and indolent ulcers typically do not require diagnostic testing other than a complete ophthalmic examination to rule out any underlying ocular disease resulting in the ulcer. However, before surgical treatment of an indolent ulcer (ie, grid keratotomy), it is reasonable to ensure that the ulcer is not infected by performing aerobic and anaerobic culture and sensitivity testing for bacteria and fungi. Complex corneal ulcers include any deep, melting/infected, or perforating corneal ulcers. These types of ulcers are the most severe type of corneal ulcers and they may be acute or chronic. When a clinician suspects a complex ulcer, diagnostic tests should include cytologic examination of a corneal scraping with Gram staining and aerobic and anaerobic culture and sensitivity for bacteria and fungi (**Figs. 8** and **9**). These tests are extremely important in *ALL* cases of complex ulceration to ascertain whether or not infection is present so appropriate therapy can be instituted as soon as possible. Not all melting ulcers are infected, as an influx of inflammatory leukocytes may also release proteolytic enzymes that can readily induce

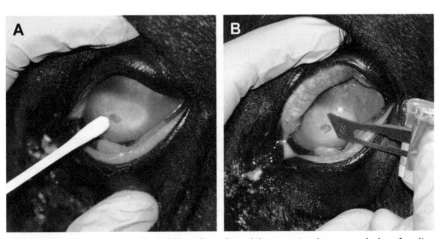

Fig. 8. Performing corneal culture (*A*) and cytology (*B*) on a complex corneal ulcer for diagnostic purposes.

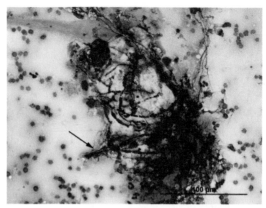

Fig. 9. Corneal cytology from an ulcerative keratitis demonstrating multiple fungal hyphae (*arrow*) (Wright-Giemsa).

collagenolysis. If, however, infection with either bacterial or fungal organisms is present, these invading organisms will contribute to corneal collagenolysis. Therefore, infection should be assumed with the presence of keratomalacia until proven otherwise. Ideally, cultures should be performed before application of any topical medications, as the common preservative benzalkonium chloride, which exists in topical medications, such as proparacaine, may inhibit microbial growth.[18]

Microbiology
In equine ulcerative keratitis, the most frequently isolated bacterial pathogens include gram-negative organisms, such as *Pseudomonas* spp, *Klebsiella* spp, and *Enterobacter* spp, but gram-positive bacteria, such as *Staphylococcus* spp, *Streptococcus* spp, and *Clostridium* spp are also commonly cultured.[19] Common fungal pathogens cultured in infected corneal ulcers include *Aspergillus* spp and *Fusarium* spp.[19] Although cytology and culture are effective means of diagnosing fungal keratitis, keratectomy by a veterinary ophthalmologist with tissue submission for histopathologic examination is the most effective.[20]

Treatment
For complex ulcers, once the complete ophthalmic examination and initial diagnostic tests (ie, cytology and culture/sensitivity) have been performed, referral to a veterinary ophthalmologist for assessment for surgical treatment is recommended, as any complex ulcer can result in the loss of an eye within 24 to 48 hours. Before referral, however, initiation of topical and systemic medications is warranted. Therapy should include placement of a subpalpebral lavage system and aggressive treatment (ie, every 1–2 hours) with broad-spectrum topical antibiotics based on cytology and culture/sensitivity to treat any underlying infection as well an anticollagenolytic agent, such as autologous serum, to prevent further collagenolysis (ie, every 1–2 hours). In the presence of increasing antibiotic resistance patterns, the importance of performing culture and sensitivity cannot be overemphasized. A topical mydriatic, such as atropine sulfate 1% given every 6 to 12 hours, is essential for its mydriatic, cycloplegic, and blood-aqueous barrier–stabilizing effects. Given the extent of secondary uveitis that is present with complex corneal ulceration in the horse, the author also recommends the use of systemic nonsteroidal anti-inflammatories as well as topical NSAIDs minimally every 8 hours. In human ophthalmology, corneal collagenolysis has been

reported with the use of topical NSAIDs and, therefore, the use of topical NSAIDs in the face of corneal ulceration is controversial among veterinary ophthalmologists. A definite link between topical NSAID use and human corneal collagenolysis remains tenuous, and in the author's experience, application of topical NSAIDs in equine corneal ulcers with proper monitoring appears safe. In most cases of complex corneal ulceration, referral surgical treatment consists of corneal debridement and a grafting procedure using conjunctiva, cornea, or natural (ie, amnion) or biosynthetic/synthetic (ie, BioSIS (R), A-cell) tissues. The prognosis for complex corneal ulcers without referral surgery is guarded but with surgery is good.

Corneal Stromal Abscess

Clinical appearance

An equine corneal abscess appears clinically as a yellow to white corneal stromal opacity with varying degrees of secondary uveitis (**Fig. 10**). Clinical signs accompanying the abscess include epiphora, blepharospasm, enophthalmos, variable corneal vascularization, and corneal edema. Most stromal abscesses are fluorescein negative due to an intact overlying corneal epithelium.

Differential diagnoses

Differential diagnoses for a stromal abscess with associated anterior uveitis include a corneal foreign body, a nonulcerative keratouveitis, eosinophilic keratoconjunctivitis, parasitic infection (ie, *Onchocerca*), granulation tissue, neoplasia, calcific band keratopathy, corneal degeneration, and an ulcerative keratitis.

Pathogenesis, diagnosis, and treatment

The cause of a corneal stromal abscess in the horse is suspected to be due to a corneal puncture where opportunistic organisms (bacteria and/or fungi) and/or foreign material are trapped within corneal stroma underneath corneal epithelium that has since sealed.[21] Cytology and culture of the fluorescein-negative lesion often do not identify any infectious agents due to the healed corneal epithelium. Diagnosis of a corneal stromal abscess is mainly based on clinical signs. Corneal stromal abscesses may respond poorly to medical therapy due to inadequate penetration of the medication to the stromal abscess, the presence of resistant organisms, or the presence of a corneal stromal foreign body. Referral surgery is, therefore, the recommended treatment of choice with a keratectomy and either a conjunctival or corneal graft or keratoplasty depending on the location/depth of the abscess. Definitive diagnosis typically

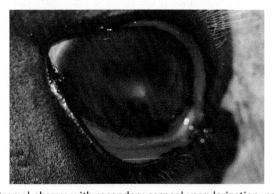

Fig. 10. Equine stromal abscess with secondary corneal vascularization, edema and uveitis.

occurs after referral surgery, biopsy, and histopathology. With surgery, the prognosis for a corneal stromal abscess is good.

Eosinophilic Keratoconjunctivitis

Clinical appearance

Eosinophilic keratoconjunctivitis is a relatively uncommon condition of the equine cornea, typically characterized by corneal ulcers covered by raised, white to gray necrotic plaques. Accompanying clinical signs often include blepharospasm, conjunctival hyperemia, and caseous mucoid discharge.[22]

Pathogenesis, diagnosis, and treatment

The etiology of eosinophilic keratitis is unknown, although an allergic, immune-mediated condition or inflammatory response from chronic ivermectin administration against parasitic microfilaria have all been speculated.[22] Differential diagnoses include parasitic keratitis (ie, onchocerciasis, habronemiasis); bacterial, fungal, or viral keratitis; foreign body; neoplasia; and calcium or lipid degeneration. Definitive diagnosis is based on clinical signs and corneal cytology demonstrating abundant eosinophils and occasional mast cells, neutrophils, lymphocytes, plasma cells, and macrophages.[23] Although there is an ulcerative component to this condition and corticosteroid treatment is contraindicated in ulcerative keratitis, treatment is directed at the inflammatory response and includes prolonged use of topical corticosteroids. Although treatment is often prolonged, the prognosis for resolution of eosinophilic keratitis with treatment is good.

Equine Herpes Virus

Epidemiology and clinical appearance

Although systemic infection with EHV-2 is common, EHV-2 keratitis or keratoconjunctivitis is relatively uncommon in horses.[24] Systemic infection with EHV-1 is less common than EHV-2 and can cause other ocular signs such as chorioretinitis as well as, strabismus, ptosis, keratoconjunctivitis sicca, lagophthalmos, optic neuritis, and blindness due to neurologic dysfunction.[25] Horses or foals affected with EHV-2 keratitis present with multiple, white, punctate, or linear corneal opacities with or without fluorescein uptake. Epiphora, blepharospasm, conjunctivitis, corneal edema, superficial vascularization, and miosis can be also associated with EHV-2 keratoconjunctivitis.

Pathogenesis

EHV keratitis is caused by replication of the epitheliotropic gammaherpesvirus[26] within the cornea. Once a horse is infected with the virus, infection is lifelong due to the virus establishing latency and, as such, clinical signs and disease may recur when the immune system is stressed or compromised.

Diagnosis

The primary differential diagnosis is early ulcerative keratitis secondary to fungi, although foreign bodies and equine recurrent uveitis are also differentials. A complete ophthalmic examination and corneal cytology and bacterial and fungal culture should be performed to rule out these differentials. Definitive diagnosis is obtained by identification of the virus from an affected cornea via PCR or virus isolation.

Treatment

Treatment includes aggressive antiviral therapy, and symptomatic treatment of any corneal ulcers or uveitis is recommended with broad-spectrum antibiotics to prevent a secondary bacterial infection and topical NSAIDs. EHV-2 keratitis is a challenging disease to treat, as recurrence is common.

Corneal Neoplasia

Similar to the equine eyelid and conjunctiva, the equine cornea can be affected with neoplasia with the corneoscleral limbus being predisposed. The most common types of corneal neoplasia include SCC, hemangioma/HSA, angioma/angiosarcoma, melanoma, papilloma, LSA, and mast-cell tumor. Of these tumors, SCC is the most common.

Corneal squamous cell carcinoma

Clinical appearance As with SCC affecting the eyelid, poorly pigmented horses such as appaloosas, pintos, and paints are at increased risk for the development of corneal SCC.[11] Draft horses, including Belgians and Clydesdales also have a high prevalence of SCC despite having pigmented periocular skin and eyelid margins.[11] Corneal SCC most often appears at the limbus, although any corneal location is possible. Typically, lesions appear as a pink, raised, fleshy mass, although nonraised infiltrative lesions also are possible (**Fig. 11**).

Diagnosis Differential diagnoses include other corneal neoplasms, eosinophilic keratitis, corneal granulation tissue, and nonulcerative keratouveitis. Biopsy and histopathology are required to obtain a definitive diagnosis.

Treatment Referral surgery under general anesthesia to perform a lamellar keratectomy/keratoconjunctivectomy with adjunctive therapy (such as photodynamic therapy, beta radiation, cryosurgery) is the treatment of choice for corneal/limbal SCC. With resection, the prognosis for corneal/limbal SCC is good.

DISEASES OF THE EQUINE UVEA
Acute Uveitis

Clinical appearance

Uveitis can involve the anterior portion of the uvea (iris and ciliary body), posterior portion (choroid), or both. The clinical signs associated with acute uveitis are due to damage of the uveal tract, subsequent compromise of the blood-aqueous barrier, and release of inflammatory mediators (**Fig. 12**). **Table 4** summarizes the most common clinical signs associated with acute uveitis.

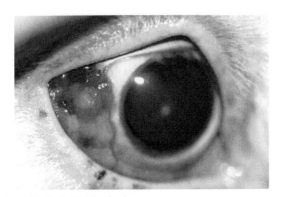

Fig. 11. Corneoscleral (limbal) SCC in the horse.

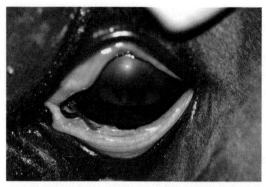

Fig. 12. Enophthalmos, conjunctival hyperemia, corneal edema, and miosis consistent with anterior uveitis.

Diagnosis

The definitive diagnosis of uveitis is based on the presence of clinical signs consistent with uveitis and a low intraocular pressure. The etiologies of uveitis are abundant (**Table 5**) and, in general, any infectious or parasitic agent that is hematogenously disseminated is capable of causing uveitis. Therefore, in addition to a complete ophthalmic examination, a physical examination and laboratory diagnostics are recommended in all cases of uveitis with the hopes of obtaining an etiologic diagnosis. Typical laboratory tests recommended in cases of uveitis include complete blood count, serum biochemistry profile, and serologic tests for specific infectious causes (**Table 6**).

Treatment

If an etiologic agent is detected, specific therapy against the agent should be initiated, otherwise medical therapy for acute uveitis is symptomatic and aimed at controlling the intraocular inflammation by using systemic and topical NSAIDs, topical steroids,

---

Table 4
Clinical manifestations of acute uveitis

Blepharospasm
Enophthalmos
Epiphora
Conjunctival hyperemia
Corneal edema
Corneal vascularization
Keratic precipitates
Fibrin in anterior chamber
Aqueous flare
Hyphema
Hypopyon
Miosis
+/− Haziness to vitreous[a]
+/− Chorioretinal edema, hemorrhage[a]
+/− Retinal detachment[a]

[a] If the posterior uvea is involved.

Table 5			
Etiologies of acute uveitis			
Parasitic	**Bacterial**	**Viral**	**Other**
Halicephalobus gingivalis	*Anaplasma phagocytophilum*	Adenovirus	Corneal ulceration
Onchocerca spp	*Borrelia burgdorferi*	EHV-1	Trauma
Strongylus spp	*Brucella* spp	EIA	Neoplasia
Toxoplasma gondii	*Escherichia coli*	Equine influenza	Lens-induced
Setaria spp	*Leptospira* spp	EVA	Tooth root abscess
	Rhodococcus equi	Parainfluenza Type 3	Hoof abscess
	Streptococcus spp	West Nile	Idiopathic
	Salmonella spp		
	Generalized septicemia		

Abbreviations: EHV, equine herpes virus; EIA, equine infectious anemia; EVA, equine viral arteritis.

and topical atropine. Most horses with acute uveitis respond well to symptomatic treatment; however, patients should be monitored closely for recurrence (see the next section, Equine Recurrent Uveitis). Long-term sequelae of uveitis include corneal scarring, cataract formation, retinal degeneration, glaucoma, and blindness.

Equine Recurrent Uveitis

Equine recurrent uveitis (ERU) is the most common cause of equine blindness with a reported prevalence of up to 25% in horses in the United States.[27] Appaloosas, warmbloods, and draft horses appear to be at increased risk for the development of ERU.[28] This syndrome is characterized classically by recurrent episodes of uveitis, followed, in many horses, by periods of quiescence of variable length. Some cases of ERU, however, are insidious such that a low-grade uveitis persists chronically with no documentation of quiescence.

Clinical appearance

The clinical signs of ERU are variable and include any of the signs in **Table 4**. In the chronic stages of ERU, iris hyperpigmentation, corpora nigra atrophy, posterior synechia, cataract, or lens luxation can be evident (**Fig. 13**).

Pathogenesis

ERU typically develops after an initial bout of primary uveitis,[29] but it is important to note that not every case of equine uveitis will develop into ERU (see the earlier section, Acute Uveitis). Horses experiencing an initial episode of uveitis of any etiology are at risk for development of this syndrome but are not classified as ERU until 2 or more episodes of inflammation have been observed.[28] The pathophysiology of ERU is very complex with the cause of the primary uveitis, environmental factors, and genetic makeup of the horse all playing a role in the development of ERU. Research studies suggest that the pathogenesis of ERU involves a dysregulated immune response to infectious agents, with *Leptospira interrogans* serotypes Pomona or Grippotyphosa being most often incriminated.[29–31] Other bacterial (ie, *Escherichia coli, Rhodococcus equi*, borreliosis, actinobacillus, brucellosis, salmonellosis, *Streptococcus* spp), viral (equine viral arteritis [EVA], equine influenza virus, EHV-1, equine infectious anemia [EIA]), protozoan (toxoplasmosis), and parasitic (onchocerciasis, intestinal strongylus), as well as noninfectious etiologies, have also, however, been associated with the syndrome.[32]

Table 6
Laboratory testing for systemic diseases with ocular manifestations

Disease	Ocular Manifestation(s)	Diagnostic Test(s)
Developmental		
IgM Deficiency	Uveitis	Serum IgM concentrations: will be reduced or absent
Acquired		
Neonatal isoerythrolysis	Conjunctival pallor, jaundice, hemorrhages or hyphema	Hemolytic cross-match between dam's serum or colostrum with foal's RBCs
Equine motor neuron disease	Honeycomb pattern of yellow/brown pigment (ceroid/lipofuscin) within the tapetal fundus	Vitamin E blood levels: typically reduced
Bacterial		
Lyme disease (*Borrelia burgdorferi*)	Uveitis	Serology (IFA, ELISA, or Western blot) or PCR on skin/synovia/connective tissue samples
Leptospirosis	Anterior uveitis and chorioretinitis	ELISA or microscopic agglutination test to identify the presence of circulating anti-*Leptospira* antibodies; dark-field microscopy of urine to identify organisms
Rhodococcus equi	Uveitis, panophthalmitis, or keratouveitis	Culture fluid obtained from transtracheal wash or bronchoalveolar lavage
Salmonellosis	Uveitis	Fecal, blood, or tissue culture
Streptococcus equi (also known as strangles)	Serous followed by mucopurulent ocular discharge, panophthalmitis, chorioretinitis, or blindness due to brain abscess	Culture abscesses
Septicemia	Uveitis, keratitis, chorioretinitis, optic neuritis	Bacterial culture and sensitivity of blood and/or bodily fluids (ie, transtracheal wash samples from lungs, joint fluid)

Mycotic		
Cryptococcosis	Orbital disease	Culture, cytology or histopathology of infected tissue
Dermatophytosis	Blepharitis	Culture and/or histopathology of skin biopsy
Histoplasmosis	Blepharitis +/− keratitis	Culture or cytology or fluorescent antibody/ELISA
Parasitic		
Demodicosis	Blepharitis	Skin scrapings
Sarcoptic mange	Blepharitis	Skin scrapings
Habronemiasis	Raised, irregular, ulcerative, granulomatous masses at mucocutaneous junction, third eyelid, or palpebral conjunctiva	Histopathology of skin biopsy identifying nematode
Halicephalobus deletrix	Anterior uveitis, chorioretinitis, optic neuritis, blindness	Biopsy of affected tissue with histopathology identifying nematode
Onchocerciasis	Anterior uveitis, chorioretinitis, keratoconjunctivitis, lateral conjunctival vitiligo	Histopathology of skin/conjunctival biopsy identifying nematode
Babesiosis	Blepharitis, icterus of conjunctiva, or ecchymotic hemorrhages over conjunctiva	Blood smear identifying organism within erythrocytes, blood culture, ELISA, Western blot, IFA, PCR
Equine protozoal myeloencephalitis	Blindness	CSF anti-*Sarcocystis neurona* antibody titers; PCR or immunohistochemical detection of parasites in CNS
Toxoplasmosis	Anterior uveitis, chorioretinitis	*Toxoplasma gondii* serum antibody titers; PCR
Anaplasma phagocytophila	Conjunctival petechiation, uveitis	PCR; circulating anti-*Anaplasma* antibodies, identification of organism within granulocytes

(continued on next page)

Table 6
(continued)

Disease	Ocular Manifestation(s)	Diagnostic Test(s)
Viral		
Adenovirus	Conjunctivitis, uveitis	Intranuclear viral inclusion bodies in exfoliated epithelial cells; virus isolation, serum antibody tires
African horse sickness	Conjunctivitis/petechial hemorrhages, swelling of eyelids and supraorbital fossa	Virus isolation, RT-PCR
Borna disease	Altered PLRs and central blindness	Serum and CSF antibody titers
EHV-1	Chorioretinitis	Virus isolation; PCR
EHV-2	Keratoconjunctivitis	Virus isolation; PCR
EIA	Conjunctival and intraocular hemorrhages	Agar-gel immunodiffusion test (ie, Coggins test); ELISA
EVA	Conjunctivitis, uveitis	Serum antibody titers, virus isolation, RT-PCR
Equine viral encephalomyelitis	Blindness	Serum antibody titers; virus isolation from CSF; RT-PCR
Rabies	Nystagmus, strabismus, blindness	Virus detection via RT-PCR
West Nile virus	Blindness	IgM concentrations in serum and/or CSF; PCR or virus isolation
Nutritional		
Thiamine deficiency	Blindness	Demonstration of low serum thiamine levels
Equine Leukoencephalomalacia	Blindness	Culture of *Fusarium moniliforme* and isolation of fumonisin toxins from feed source

Abbreviations: CNS, central nervous system; CSF, cerebral spinal fluid; EHV, equine herpes virus; EIA, equine infectious anemia; ELISA, enzyme-linked immunosorbent assay; EVA, Equine viral arteritis; IFA, Immunofluorescence assay; Ig, immunoglobulin; PCR, polymerase chain reaction; PLR, pupillary light reflexes; RBCs, red blood cells; RT-PCR, reverse-transcriptase PCR.

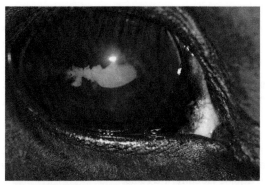

Fig. 13. Corneal edema, iridal hyperpigmentation, corpora nigra atrophy, posterior syne-chia, and cataract secondary to chronic uveitis.

Diagnosis

The diagnosis of ERU is based on clinical signs and a history of recurrent or insidious uveitis. A thorough ophthalmic examination of BOTH eyes is imperative to rule out other differential diagnoses or causes of uveitis. Diagnostic workup of ERU includes a full physical examination, complete blood count, and serum biochemical profile to assess for systemic infection and serologic testing for leptospirosis, brucellosis, and toxoplasmosis. Blood may also be submitted to test for exposure to EVA and/or Lyme disease. Equine leukocyte antigen (ELA) typing also may be helpful in determining the animal's genetic susceptibility.[33] Fecal parasite analysis is also recommended to rule out intestinal parasites. Referral to a board-certified veterinary ophthalmologist may be necessary in many cases of suspected ERU to help the clinician differentiate between acute/primary uveitis and ERU. The veterinary ophthalmologist also may elect to perform aqueous or vitreal titers to compare to serologic titers.

Differential diagnoses for ERU include other causes of non-ERU uveitis (ie, acute uveitis due to trauma, ulcerative keratitis, septicemia, neoplasia) and other causes of recurrent or persistent ocular inflammation, such as stromal abscessation, immune-mediated keratitis, and EHV keratitis. Unfortunately, in most cases of ERU, confirmation of an exact etiology is uncommon and, therefore, most cases of ERU are classified as idiopathic, immune-mediated disease based on negative serology and cultures.

Treatment

If an etiologic agent is detected, specific therapy against the agent should be initiated, otherwise, aggressive medical therapy for ERU is symptomatic and aimed at controlling the intraocular inflammation by using systemic and topical NSAIDs, topical steroids, and topical atropine. Recent surgical therapies for ERU have focused on the use of a suprachoroidal cyclosporine sustained release implant, and with use of this device, decreased recurrence rates and improved long-term control were noted.[34] Despite aggressive medical and surgical therapies, however, the long-term visual prognosis for ERU remains poor. Many horses with ERU eventually develop glaucoma or phthisis bulbi secondary to the chronic inflammation necessitating enucleation for palliative reasons. In such cases when enucleation is performed, histopathology is *essential* to rule out other ocular or systemic disease processes potentially causing the recurring uveitis. Histopathology demonstrating predominately a lymphocytic, plasmacytic uveal inflammatory infiltrate; the presence of a thick, noncellular hyaline membrane overlying the nonpigmented ciliary epithelium (NPE); and eosinophilic linear inclusions within the cytoplasm of the NPE is highly suggestive of the presence of ERU.[35]

Uveal Neoplasia

Uveal neoplasia is relatively rare in the horse with uveal melanocytic tumors and LSA being most commonly reported.

DISEASES OF THE EQUINE LENS

The most common disorders of the lens are cataract and lens luxation or subluxation. In the horse, these conditions are typically associated with chronic uveitis or ERU. See the earlier section, Equine Recurrent Uveitis.

OCULAR MANIFESTATIONS OF SYSTEMIC DISEASE

Performing a complete ophthalmic examination is essential in horses with systemic disease, as numerous systemic diseases can cause ocular changes. In particular, diseases affecting the vascular and nervous systems are more prone to ocular manifestations. In most cases of systemic disease with ocular manifestations, blood work for serology, virus isolation, enzyme-linked immunosorbent assay, or PCR testing is often necessary to determine a definitive diagnosis. See **Table 6** for recommended diagnostic testing for systemic diseases with ocular manifestations.

SUMMARY

Although not comprehensive of all ocular conditions in the equine species, this article concentrates on various ophthalmic conditions observed in the horse where laboratory diagnostics are recommended. The importance of laboratory diagnostic testing cannot be underestimated with equine ophthalmic disease. In many cases, laboratory diagnostics can aid in obtaining an early diagnosis and determining appropriate therapy, which in turn, can provide a better prognosis. In unfortunate cases in which ocular disease results in a blind, painful eye necessitating enucleation, light microscopic evaluation of the affected globe is *imperative* to determine or confirm the cause of the blindness and provide a prognosis for the contralateral eye.

REFERENCES

1. van Maanen C, Klein WR, Dik KJ, et al. Three cases of carcinoid in the equine nasal cavity and maxillary sinuses: histologic and immunohistochemical features. Vet Pathol 1996;33(1):92–5.
2. Baptiste KE, Grahn BH. Equine orbital neoplasia: a review of 10 cases (1983-1998). Can Vet J 2000;41(4):291–5.
3. Rebhun WC, Mirro EJ, Georgi ME, et al. Habronemic blepharoconjunctivitis in horses. J Am Vet Med Assoc 1981;179(5):469–72.
4. Giuliano E. Equine ocular adnexal and nasolacrimal disease. In: Gilger BC, editor. Equine ophthalmology. 2nd edition; 2011. p. 133–80.
5. Gilger BC. Equine Ophthalmology. In: K.N.G., Gilger BC, Kern TJ, editors. Vet ophthalmol. 2. 5th edition. Ames (IA): John Wiley & Sons, Inc; 2013. p. 1560–609.
6. Mohammed HO, Rebhun WC, Antczak DF. Factors associated with the risk of developing sarcoid tumours in horses. Equine Vet J 1992;24(3):165–8.
7. Knottenbelt DC, Kelly DF. The diagnosis and treatment of periorbital sarcoid in the horse: 445 cases from 1974 to 1999. Vet Ophthalmol 2000;3(2–3):169–91.

8. Martens A, De Moor A, Ducatelle R. PCR detection of bovine papilloma virus DNA in superficial swabs and scrapings from equine sarcoids. Vet J 2001;161(3): 280–6.

9. Lancaster WD. Apparent lack of integration of bovine papillomavirus DNA in virus-induced equine and bovine tumor cells and virus-transformed mouse cells. Virology 1981;108(2):251–5.

10. Lavach JD, Severin GA. Neoplasia of the equine eye, adnexa, and orbit: a review of 68 cases. J Am Vet Med Assoc 1977;170(2):202–3.

11. Dugan SJ, Curtis CR, Roberts SM, et al. Epidemiologic study of ocular/adnexal squamous cell carcinoma in horses. J Am Vet Med Assoc 1991;198(2):251–6.

12. Dubielzig RR, Ketring KL, McLellan GJ, et al. Veterinary ocular pathology - a comparative review. 1st edition. Edinburgh (UK): Sauders Elsevier; 2010.

13. Dugan SJ, Roberts SM, Curtis CR, et al. Prognostic factors and survival of horses with ocular/adnexal squamous cell carcinoma: 147 cases (1978-1988). J Am Vet Med Assoc 1991;198(2):298–303.

14. Hamor RE, Ramsey DT, Wiedmeyer CE, et al. Melanoma of the conjunctiva and cornea in a horse. Veterinary and Comparative Ophthalmology 1997;7(1):52–5.

15. Lavach JD. Large animal ophthalmology. St Louis (MO): Mosby Co.; 1990.

16. Schnoke AT, Brooks DE, Wilkie DA, et al. Extraocular lymphoma in the horse. Vet Ophthalmol 2013;16(1):35–42.

17. Stoppini R, Gilger BC, Malarkey DE, et al. Bilateral nodular lymphocytic conjunctivitis in a horse. Vet Ophthalmol 2005;8(2):129–34.

18. Kleinfeld J, Ellis PP. Inhibition of microorganisms by topical anesthetics. Appl Microbiol 1967;15(6):1296–8.

19. Clode AB. Diseases and surgery of the cornea. In: Gilger BC, editor. Equine ophthalmology. Maryland Heights (MO): Elsevier; 2011. p. 181–266.

20. Andrew SE, Brooks DE, Smith PJ, et al. Equine ulcerative keratomycosis: visual outcome and ocular survival in 39 cases (1987-1996). Equine Vet J 1998;30(2): 109–16.

21. Hendrix DVH, Brooks DE, Smith PJ, et al. Corneal stromal abscesses in the horse: a review of 24 cases. Equine Vet J 1995;27(6):440–7.

22. Yamagata M, Wilkie DA, Gilger BC. Eosinophilic keratoconjunctivitis in seven horses. J Am Vet Med Assoc 1996;209(7):1283–6.

23. Ramsey DT, Whiteley HE, Gerding PA Jr, et al. Eosinophilic keratoconjunctivitis in a horse. J Am Vet Med Assoc 1994;205(9):1308–11.

24. Kershaw O, von Oppen T, Glitz F, et al. Detection of equine herpesvirus type 2 (EHV-2) in horses with keratoconjunctivitis. Virus Res 2001;80(1–2):93–9.

25. Cullen CL, Webb AA. Ocular manifestations of systemic disease part 3: the horse. In: Gelatt KN, editor. Veterinary ophthalmology. Ames (IA): John-Wiley & Sons, Inc; 2013. p. 2037–70.

26. Telford EA, Studdert MJ, Agius CT, et al. Equine herpesviruses 2 and 5 are gamma-herpesviruses. Virology 1993;195(2):492–9.

27. Barnett KC. Equine periodic ophthalmia: a continuing aetiological riddle. Equine Vet J 1987;19(2):90–1.

28. Gilger BC. Equine ophthalmology. 2nd edition. Maryland Heights (MO): Elsevier Saunders; 2011.

29. Dwyer AE, Crockett RS, Kalsow CM. Association of leptospiral seroreactivity and breed with uveitis and blindness in horses: 372 cases (1986-1993). J Am Vet Med Assoc 1995;207(10):1327–31.

30. Romeike A, Brugmann M, Drommer W. Immunohistochemical studies in equine recurrent uveitis (ERU). Vet Pathol 1998;35(6):515–26.

31. Deeg CA. Ocular immunology in equine recurrent uveitis. Vet Ophthalmol 2008; 11(Suppl 1):61–5.
32. Gilger BC, Salmon JH, Yi NY, et al. Role of bacteria in the pathogenesis of recurrent uveitis in horses from the southeastern United States. Am J Vet Res 2008; 69(10):1329–35.
33. Deeg CA, Marti E, Gaillard C, et al. Equine recurrent uveitis is strongly associated with the MHC class I haplotype ELA-A9. Equine Vet J 2004;36:73–5.
34. Gilger BC, Wilkie DA, Clode AB, et al. Long-term outcome after implantation of a suprachoroidal cyclosporine drug delivery device in horses with recurrent uveitis. Vet Ophthalmol 2010;13(5):294–300.
35. Dubielzig RR, Render JA, Morreale RJ. Distinctive morphologic features of the ciliary body in equine recurrent uveitis. Veterinary and Comparative Ophthalmology 1997;7(3):163–7.

Index

Note: Page numbers of article titles are in **boldface** type.

A

Abortion
    reproductive disorders in female related to, 390–392
Abscess(es)
    corneal stromal, 437–438
Accessory sex glands
    pathology of
        reproductive disorders of male related to, 399–400
Acetate tape impressions
    in skin disease diagnosis, 359–360
Acute uveitis, 439–441
Alopecia areata, 368
Alopecic dermatoses, 367–369
Anagen/telogen effluvium, 368–369
Angular limb deformities
    prognosis of, 412
    treatment of, 411
Arboviral encephalomyelitides, 291–292
Atopy, 367–368

B

Bacterial agents
    reproductive disorders of female related to, 391
Bacterial disease(s)
    enteritis and colitis related to, 343–350
BAL. *See* Bronchoalveolar lavage (BAL)
Basophil responses
    in hematology assessment, 252
Biliary system
    toxins affecting, 271–272
Biochemical changes
    in clinical pathology, 253–264
        enteric diseases, 255–258
        liver disease, 258–261
        metabolic diseases, 263–264
        musculoskeletal disease, 261
        neurologic disease, 262
        respiratory disease, 262–263
        urinary system disease, 261–262
Biopsy
    in skin disease diagnosis, 360

Vet Clin Equine 31 (2015) 449–461
http://dx.doi.org/10.1016/S0749-0739(15)00044-9
0749-0739/15/$ – see front matter © 2015 Elsevier Inc. All rights reserved.

Moving?

Make sure your subscription moves with you!

To notify us of your new address, find your **Clinics Account Number** (located on your mailing label above your name), and contact customer service at:

Email: journalscustomerservice-usa@elsevier.com

800-654-2452 (subscribers in the U.S. & Canada)
314-447-8871 (subscribers outside of the U.S. & Canada)

Fax number: 314-447-8029

Elsevier Health Sciences Division
Subscription Customer Service
3251 Riverport Lane
Maryland Heights, MO 63043

*To ensure uninterrupted delivery of your subscription, please notify us at least 4 weeks in advance of move.